Bentham Briefs in Biomedicine and Pharmacotherapy

(Volume 2)

Botanicals and Natural Bioactives: Prevention and Treatment of Diseases

Edited by

Pardeep Kaur
Post Graduate Department of Botany
Khalsa College, Amritsar
Punjab, India

Tewin Tencomnao
Natural Products for Neuroprotection
and Anti-Ageing Research Unit &
Department of Clinical Chemistry
Faculty of Allied Health Sciences
Chulalongkorn University
Bangkok, Thailand

Robin

Agilent Technologies India Pvt. Ltd;
Regional Water Testing Laboratory- Amritsar
Department of Water Supply and
Sanitation, Punjab
India

&

Rajendra G. Mehta

Cancer Biology Division
IIT Research Institute and
Department of Biological Sciences
Illinois Institute of Technology
Chicago, Illinois
U.S.A.

Bentham Briefs in Biomedicine and Pharmacotherapy

(Volume 2)

Botanicals and Natural Bioactives: Prevention and Treatment of Diseases

Editors: Pardeep Kaur, Tewin Tencomnao, Robin & Rajendra G. Mehta

ISSN (Online): 2810-997X

ISSN (Print): 2810-9988

ISBN (Online): 978-981-5238-27-3

ISBN (Print): 978-981-5238-28-0

ISBN (Paperback): 978-981-5238-29-7

First published in 2024.

need for a court order if at any point you breach any terms of this License Agreement. In no event will any delay or failure by Bentham Science Publishers in enforcing your compliance with this License Agreement constitute a waiver of any of its rights.

3. You acknowledge that you have read this License Agreement, and agree to be bound by its terms and conditions. To the extent that any other terms and conditions presented on any website of Bentham Science Publishers conflict with, or are inconsistent with, the terms and conditions set out in this License Agreement, you acknowledge that the terms and conditions set out in this License Agreement shall prevail.

Bentham Science Publishers Pte. Ltd.
80 Robinson Road #02-00
Singapore 068898
Singapore
Email: subscriptions@benthamscience.net

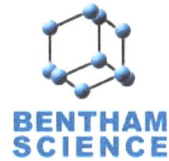

BENTHAM SCIENCE

CONTENTS

FOREWORD

I am pleased to write this foreword for the e-book '*Botanicals and Natural Bioactives: Prevention and Treatment of Diseases*'. This outstanding endeavour by the editors represents a multi-disciplinary coverage of research in preventing and treating many diseases. This book embodies a compelling compilation of chapters on therapeutic aspects of natural bioactives against various physiological disorders. The authors deserve credit for their time and efforts to contribute excellent chapters relevant to their expertise. These chapters include timely discussions on ageing, infectious diseases, neurodegenerative diseases, osteoporosis, coronary heart diseases, and autoimmune disorders. I am confident this book will be a valuable addition to the bookshelves of teaching faculty, recognized investigators, and young graduate students. I wish you all the success for the launch of this book.

Rajeshwari R. Mehta
Cancer Biology Division
IIT Research Institute
Chicago, Illinois
U.S.A.

PREFACE

Scientific research in the diverse domains of biomedicine and pharmacotherapy has contributed much to the recent advancements in enhancing global health. Researchers have shown a great interest in exploring and enhancing the therapeutic assistance for a variety of diseases *via* vital understanding in areas of molecular diagnostics, immunobiology, regenerative medicine, drug development and discovery, cancer biology, functional genomics, pharmaceutics, chemical biology, human biology, and primary or scientific research. Following these, the book series *Bentham Briefs in Biomedicine and Pharmacotherapy* seeks to cover recent developments in various domains *via* various volumes.

The second volume *"Botanicals and Natural Bioactives: Prevention and Treatment of Diseases"* offers immense knowledge of the current research in the prevention and treatment of many diseases. This book volume provides recent and future trends in therapeutic aspects of natural bioactives against various physiological disorders. The pathogenic intervention of chronic ailments like cardiovascular diseases, neurodegenerative diseases, infectious diseases, age-associated diseases, and many cancers involves oxidative damage. The intensified pro-oxidant factors cause structural and functional defects at enzymatic and DNA levels. This leads to mutations and aberrations at the genetic level. The book chapters will captivate interest in the researchers for investigation and augmentation of the use of botanicals and natural bioactives in the remedial assistance against various ailments.

Pardeep Kaur
Post Graduate Department of Botany
Khalsa College, Amritsar
Punjab, India

Tewin Tencomnao
Natural Products for Neuroprotection
and Anti-Ageing Research Unit &
Department of Clinical Chemistry
Faculty of Allied Health Sciences
Chulalongkorn University
Bangkok, Thailand

Robin
Agilent Technologies India Pvt. Ltd;
Regional Water Testing Laboratory- Amritsar
Department of Water Supply and
Sanitation, Punjab
India

&

Rajendra G. Mehta
Cancer Biology Division
IIT Research Institute and
Department of Biological Sciences
Illinois Institute of Technology
Chicago, Illinois
U.S.A.

List of Contributors

Ami P. Thakkar	Shobhaben Pratapbhai Patel School of Pharmacy and Technology Management, Shri Vile Parle Kelavani Mandal's Narsee Monjee Institute of Management Studies, Mumbai, India
Amisha Vora	Shobhaben Pratapbhai Patel School of Pharmacy and Technology Management, Shri Vile Parle Kelavani Mandal's Narsee Monjee Institute of Management Studies, Mumbai, India
Douglas W. Wilson	Formerly, School of Medicine Pharmacy and Health, Durham University, Thornaby, Durham, UK
Dicson Sheeja Malar	Natural Products for Neuroprotection and Anti-ageing Research Unit, Chulalongkorn University, Bangkok-10330, Thailand Department of Clinical Chemistry, Faculty of Allied Health Sciences, Chulalongkorn University, Bangkok-10330, Thailand
Fabien De Meester	TsimTsoum Institute, Krakow, Poland
Ginpreet Kaur	Shobhaben Pratapbhai Patel School of Pharmacy and Technology Management, Shri Vile Parle Kelavani Mandal's Narsee Monjee Institute of Management Studies, Mumbai, India
Harpal S. Buttar	Department of Pathology & Laboratory Medicine, Faculty of Medicine, University of Ottawa, Ottawa, ON, K1H 8M5, Canada
Istvan G. Telessy	Department of Pharmaceutics, Faculty of Pharmacy, University of Pécs, Hungary, and MedBioFit Lpc. Fácán sor 25. Gödöllö, Hungary
Maushmi S. Kumar	Somaiya Institute for Research and Consultancy, Somaiya Vidyavihar University, Vidyavihar (East), Mumbai-400077, India
Mani Iyer Prasanth	Natural Products for Neuroprotection and Anti-ageing Research Unit, Chulalongkorn University, Bangkok-10330, Thailand Department of Clinical Chemistry, Faculty of Allied Health Sciences, Chulalongkorn University, Bangkok-10330, Thailand
Paweena Pradniwat	Department of Clinical Microscopy, Faculty of Allied Health Sciences, Chulalongkorn University, Bangkok, Thailand Immunomodulation of Natural Products Research Unit, Chulalongkorn University, Bangkok, Thailand
Palak Parekh	Shobhaben Pratapbhai Patel School of Pharmacy and Technology Management, SVKM's NMIMS, V. L. Mehta Road, Vile Parle (West), Mumbai-400056, India
Prabhnain Kaur	Department of Pharmacology, Delhi Pharmaceutical Sciences and Research University, Pushp Vihar, New Delhi, India
Ram B. Singh	Halberg Hospital and Research Institute, Civil Lines, Moradabad (UP 244001), India
Riya Patel	Shobhaben Pratapbhai Patel School of Pharmacy and Technology Management, SVKM's NMIMS, V. L. Mehta Road, Vile Parle West, Mumbai-400056, India
Ritu Dahiya	Department of Pharmacology, Delhi Pharmaceutical Sciences and Research University, Pushp Vihar, New Delhi, India

Sharika Rajasekharan Pillai Immunomodulation of Natural Products Research Unit, Faculty of Allied Health Sciences, Chulalongkorn University, Bangkok-10330, Thailand

Siriporn Chuchawankul Immunomodulation of Natural Products Research Group & Department of Transfusion Medicine and Clinical Microbiology, Faculty of Allied Health Sciences, Chulalongkorn University, Bangkok 10330, Thailand

Shravya Shanbhag Shobhaben Pratapbhai Patel School of Pharmacy and Technology Management, SVKM's NMIMS, V. L. Mehta Road, Vile Parle (West), Mumbai-400056, India

Toru Takahashi Department of Nutrition, Faculty of Nutrition, Kanazawa Gakuin University, 10 Sue, Kanazawa City, Ishikawa Prefecture, 920-1392, Japan

Tushar Oak Shobhaben Pratapbhai Patel School of Pharmacy and Technology Management, SVKM's NMIMS, V. L. Mehta Road, Vile Parle West, Mumbai-400056, India

Tewin Tencomnao Natural Products for Neuroprotection and Anti-ageing Research Unit, Chulalongkorn University, Bangkok-10330, Thailand
Department of Clinical Chemistry, Faculty of Allied Health Sciences, Chulalongkorn University, Bangkok-10330, Thailand

CHAPTER 1

Food Color, Taste, Smell, Culinary Plate, Flavor, Locale, and their Impact on Nutrition: Present and Future Multisensory Food Augmentation and Non-communicable Disease Prevention: An Overview

Douglas W. Wilson[1], Fabien De Meester[2], Toru Takahashi[3], Ram B. Singh[4] and Harpal S. Buttar[5,*]

[1] *Formerly, School of Medicine Pharmacy and Health, Durham University, Thornaby, Durham, UK*

[2] *TsimTsoum Institute, Krakow, Poland*

[3] *Department of Nutrition, Faculty of Nutrition, Kanazawa Gakuin University, 10 Sue, Kanazawa City, Ishikawa Prefecture, 920-1392, Japan*

[4] *Halberg Hospital and Research Institute, Civil Lines, Moradabad (UP 244001), India*

[5] *Department of Pathology & Laboratory Medicine, Faculty of Medicine, University of Ottawa, Ottawa, ON, K1H 8M5, Canada*

Abstract: Cognizant that 'the world is one family', this overview describes chemosensory characteristics of food and related issues that may enable global inequalities in healthy food consumption to be improved with a reduction in non-communicable diseases (NCDs), preventatively. Past and modern aspects of food tradition are briefly described followed by titular chemosensory characteristics and their potential application to improving health in nutrition in the sense intended, including the culinary plate. Human-computer interface and food augmentation reality and commensal dining, in association with chemosensory properties, including sound concerning oral food processing, are described. Future research on arresting trends in the prevalence of NCD is suggested based on the literature. Visual cues for in-store food choice are discussed that potentially allow the consumer, through psychological processes and behavior outcomes, to be more discerning. Advertisements and store architecture *per se* are not discussed. The relatively high prevalence of anosmia caused by COVID-19 infection relative to non-infected subjects may alter taste and flavor perception and lead to changed dietary habits and metabolism. Most global consumers can practice the 'how' and 'when' to beneficially eat but food insecurity poses a global problem.

---

* **Corresponding author Harpal S. Buttar:** Department of Pathology & Laboratory Medicine, Faculty of Medicine, University of Ottawa, Ottawa, ON, K1H 8M5, Canada; E-mail: hsbuttar@bell.net

Keywords: Commensal dining, Food augmentation, Global NCDs, Hidden hunger, Marketing, Robotics, Visual cues.

INTRODUCTION

The subject matter of this overview topic is vast and only relevant scientific snippets and definitions have been embodied into a general framework of life on this planet. From a human perspective [1], sociological [2, 3], accessibility [4], environmental [5], locale [3], historiography [1], scientific [6 - 8], economic [9], feeding habits [10] and cultural [11] are among key factors/terms for food security [3, 12 - 14] and sustainability [5]; and even longevity [11]. From a philosophical/ religious point of view, food has a place in the concept that 'the world is one family' ('Vashudayo Kutumbakam' which comes from ancient Sanskrit वसुधैव कुटुम्बकम in the Maha Upanishad (VI,71-73) [15]), a motivation for the authors to write this overview in this world of inequality [16, 17]; *e.g.* low-income countries'-CVD deaths [18]. The layout of this article concerning the reduction in global NCDs using food chemosensory properties is shown in Fig. (**1**).

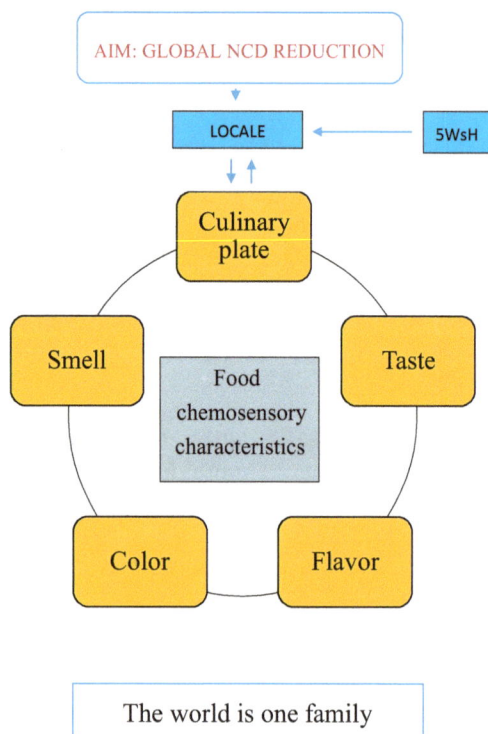

Fig. (1). Schema for reducing global NCDs using food chemosensory characteristics: health inequalities implicitly incorporate the '5WsH' circumstances which refer to the who, what, where, when, why and 'how' of food consumption.

Food

This is a source of chemical energy [19]. The human body requires food, and just as the entire universe has been reportedly made up of the five elements *Viz.* earth, water, fire, air, and space, which according to Hinduism [20] ((assumed to be traced back to the Veda) are Prithvi/Bhudevi (Sanskrit: पृथ्वी Earth), Apas/Varuna/Jal (Sanskrit: अप: Water), Agni (Sanskrit: अग्नि Fire), Vayu (Sanskrit: वायु Air), and Akasha/Dyaus (Sanskrit: आकाश Space/Atmosphere/Ether)) whereas a similar system of cosmic rather than natural substances, arose in East Asia [21]. In Ancient Mediterranean tradition, food utility could be construed to involve the four classical Greek elements [22] *Viz.* fire (energy), earth (chemicals), air (oxygen/carbon dioxide), and water (*q.v.* Empedocles (c450 BCE) ([23], pp 62,75)), later aether (space) (*q.v.* Aristotle [22, 19], 350 BCE). It has been said, "No animal can live without food….(which) is about the most important influence in determining the organization of the brain and the behavior that the brain organization dictates." [24]. From birth, humans have different taste propensities [25], and presumably, this has developed throughout evolution [26, 27] and migration [28]: hence the subsection herein on 'locale'. Today researchers think of food as being necessary for sustaining metabolic processes essential for life [29] including reproduction and fertility [30] in terms of thermodynamic properties associated with evolved anaerobic and aerobic pathways involving the metabolism of fats [31], carbohydrates, proteins, *etc.*, and other essential ingredients. Descriptions of sensory and related characteristics are as follows.

Color

This does not exist in the external world but luminance along with wavelength (color) is extremely important in natural selection and behavior. Color, which arose in common ancestors in Cambrian times in the Metazoa, arises from the visual perception by the brain of the light-spectrum (390-700nm) in humans and other animals [32 - 34] emanating from absorption, emission, and reflection from objects interacting with different retinal cells [35]. In humans "Color is the general name for all sensations arising from the activity of the retina of the eye and its attached nervous mechanisms, this activity being, in nearly every case in the normal individual, a specific response to radiant energy of certain wavelengths and intensities [36]". As a sensory property, this sense can affect food choice [37, 38]. Though in animals 'one cap does not fit all' there is an interplay between luminance and wavelength processing [32] *e.g.*, identifying brown [39], which drives behavior. Luminance and wavelength color/contrast are important in the co-evolution in plants and animals [40, 41]. Also, visual pictures of high-calorific food with contrasts were shown to women with binge-eating disorder or bulimia nervosa (with controls) and differential brain activation was found using functional magnetic imaging [42]. Of practical value in marketing (FDM), is the CIELAB 3-dimensional color space tool [43] which represents the gamut of human photopic vision that allows the detection of small numerical differences in color and has utility in the wine [44] and food [45, 46] industries. It has been reported, for example, that blue light reduces the hedonic impression of food appearance but not the willingness to eat: men consumed less breakfast (omelets and mini-pancakes) than women under conditions of blue light unlike yellow or white light [47]. Taste and smell may affect our visual choice of food [48] which are now described.

Taste

In humans/primates taste [49] (disambiguate sentiment and judgment in society [50, 51]), which comprises sensory afferents from intra- and extra-taste buds (epiglottis, soft palate, and esophagus) from food in the mouth and tongue [52, 53] arising from texture [54, 55] (and temperature and mechanical stress/ pain in the trigeminal system [56] in the taste cortex (anterior insula) [49], and inputs from the neurons of the orbitofrontal cortex (taste and smell of food) and amygdala. In humans, there is a learning curve in infants for taste and food preferences [57] and a genetic sensitivity to taste [58]. In the evolution of animals, particularly in herbivory, it is necessary for mutual survival to recognize categories of taste (*e.g.*, sweet, sour, salty bitter, pungent, astringent [59], and smell). Singh *et al.* [60] have devised a 10-point hedonic scale for the perception of taste among Asians with some possible reservations for adjustment/expansion for a locale, vide infra *e.g.*, Middle East and South Asia. Before the advent of bioelectronic tongues [61], understanding mechanisms of neuronal action that are satiety-specific *e.g.*, fats, and calcium that may lead to designer foods [54, 62] to aid nutrition and combat eating disorders, it is preferable that taste, akin to other senses remains a 'window onto the world' with its evolutionary focus on specificity and sensitivity. It seems that taste can influence GLP-1 (Glucagon-like peptide) levels [63], which is important for insulin secretion and sensitivity, therefore in the prevention of metabolic syndrome which is an NCD. Methods have been developed to simulate human taste, but these are in their infancy and may be used to monitor food adulteration [64].

Smell

The olfactory system in human pregnant mothers develops in utero, possibly from conception (certainly in the first trimester) when the olfactory bulb differentiates from the forebrain [65 - 67]: and odor learning begins before birth in response to maternal consumption of volatile foods and may be important in 'latching on' as breast milk from natural mother or wet nurse has a characteristic odor (Jocelyn

Baber-midwife-personal communication). Associative learning in odor perception of infants, based on food volatiles consumed by the mother [68] may be important for next-generation food consumption and nutrition, preconditioning in maternal diet through perspiration and lactation. In some animals, smell is more sensitive than humans due to anatomy and inhalation *e.g.*, canines [69], and detailed descriptions of animal food-searching and nutrition are beyond the remit of this overview. Smell and food have relevance in the marketing of perfume [65]. Perhaps supermarkets may prime customers with fragrances, in a non-attentive way that influences food choice [70] and consequently nutrition. In a subtle/insidious way, perfumes could be used to promote food products *e.g.*, 'eau de stilton' for Stilton cheese or 'flame' for red meat [65] marketed by the Stilton Cheese Company and Burger King, respectively. Odors also have 'colors' as adjudged by tasters of white wine adulterated with odorless dye assessed to be red; thus, olfactory information was probably ignored at the verbalization phase of this perceptual illusion [71].

'Smell' in insects is complex and mediated through receptor genes for chemical cues acting as signals for a range of non-social to eusocial cuticular hydrocarbons important in the evolution of communication in social insects, particularly concerning foraging and fertility [72]. Therefore, smell has evolved and is used in conjunction with other senses, as an important agent in safe food consumption in planetary life. The development of odor measurements can provide 'fingerprint' patterns of chemical species revealed from gas chromatographic/mass spectrographic [73] or specific devices *e.g* [74]. measurements obtained from odor-sample space analysis under control conditions. Given the role of vision, taste, and smell in food choice, and the appearance [75] and content of food on the plate [76], these being important factors in food consumption are now described as follows.

Culinary Plate

The factors that influence the safety (*e.g.* microfluidic technologies [77]) and nature of food consumption on the plate include hygiene standards [78], farming/fishery/aquaculture practices [79 - 81], food processing [82, 83], storage technologies (potential improvements [84]) and transport to point-of-sale (*e.g.* refrigeration [85] (functional food could reduce food waste, and added antioxidant dietary fiber, *e.g.* by-products of plant processing, can bring added health value [86]), psychological cognitive-affective aspects of food choice [87], plate size and food amount/spacing/calorific value [88 - 91], communal and shared eating [92], printing [6, 93, 94], labeling information/in color/size [95], gustatory competence in animal evolution [96], *etc.*). Cooking and cooking skills of chosen foods also relate to cultural, environmental, and socioeconomic factors leading to health inequalities [97] which are beyond the remit of this paper.

Flavor

Flavor may be described as a perception drawn from multisensory inputs which can be core intrinsic (smell, some elements of touch, taste) or extrinsic (shape, color, sound,) [98, 99]. Cowart [100] has divided flavor into two parts: sensitivity to chemical stimuli (threshold, sensitivity, adaption, *etc.*); hedonism (preferences, pleasantness, *etc.*); and the chemoaesthetic sensations described by Lawless and Heyman [101]. A review of flavor preferences of children and adults found that children had preferences for sweet and salty flavors cf. to adults [102] and possibly *Vice versa* for children and adolescents for sour and bitter flavor preferences, which may have a bearing on NCD risk depending on their flavor preference and dietary consumption in childhood and adolescence and later.

Locale

As men and women have developed differentially in anatomy, physiology, and morphology, over evolutionary time, in different parts of the world with multifarious food preparations that have been developed, they have evolved different dietary and nutritional needs. In isolation, cautious causal interpretation of sensory data is the watchword because ethnicity, gender, age, diet, alcohol consumption, social class, occupation, exercise (inactivity), shift work, smoking, environment, *etc.*, and sensory measurement may influence erroneous conclusions about causation, but correlations indicate the strength and direction of association *e.g.*, factors associated with non-communicable diseases such as cardiovascular disease. The experiment design and analysis are paramount for national studies *e.g.*, cross-section design with sufficient participants for prescribed statistically significant differences. Singh *et al.* [60] cite the work of the University of Nottingham's Sensory Science Centre which studied 223 volunteers who were pheno- (PTS (6-n-propylthiouracil (PROP) Taster Status [103]; SLS (Sweet Liking Status); TTS (Thermal Taster Status)) and genotyped for TAS2R38 –rs713598 (encoding a bitter taste receptor) and the salivary trophic factor Gustin –rs2274333; single nucleotide polymorphism is indicated. The taste phenotypes were found to be independent, but differences between Asians and Caucasians existed, the former being more likely to be PROP supertasters, as well as more likely to be thermal tasters or Low Sweet Likers, than the latter. Gender was also significantly associated with SLS, where males were more likely to be High Sweet Likers. For perceived taste intensity, traditional ANOVA analysis proved to be challenging. The alternative approach, using regression trees, was shown to be an effective tool to provide a visualized framework to demonstrate the multiple interactions in this dataset. For example, ethnicity was the most influencing factor for perceived sour and metallic taste intensity, where Asians had a heightened response compared to Caucasians. The regression tree analysis also highlighted that the PTS effect was dependent on ethnicity for sour taste, and PTS and TTS effects were dependent on ethnicity for metallic taste. The quest now is to determine if all these food-choice sensory and related factors are possibly associated with nutritional outcomes and the future prevalence of NCDs.

Impact on Nutrition and Non-communicable Disease Prevention

Non-communicable diseases included herein are cancer, cardiovascular disease (CVD), diabetes, and obesity [104] (these also include dementias, bone and joint diseases, liver and GI diseases, *etc.*) and evidence-based counter-high-risk dietary constituents include nuts, fruit, vegetable oils, non-starchy vegetables, legumes, and fish whereas increased risk is associated with red meat, trans fat, sugar, refined grains, starch, *etc.* and a recent notable reviewed 51-chapter publication by Singh and colleagues is relevant [3, 105 - 113] which includes a chapter on Ancient Chinese medicine [109]. It would seem logical to assume that when chemo-senses are impaired the choice of dietary constituents is changed, possibly increasing adverse factors for NCDs [114]. Liu *et al.* [115], as part of the National Health and Nutrition Examination Survey of the USA for self-reporting adults ≥40y, building on a previous study of smell and taste dysfunction by Hoffman *et al.* [116], found that ethnicity (non-Hispanic Blacks), a CVD history, and high alcohol consumption was associated with a higher prevalence of taste impairment. The prevalence of smell impairment was independently associated with cancer, age, gender ethnicity, family income and educational attainment. The scale of the smell and taste impairment was estimated overall to be approximately 21 (14%) and 26(17%) million Americans for smell and taste, respectively; there were also significant differences, in univariate analysis, for diabetes as per hypertension and cancer for smell impairment [115]. It follows that prospective and objective measures of smell and taste are needed to progress towards more definitive outcomes of association of non-communicable disease and chemo-senses.

However, it is a Herculean task to design studies, using multisensory human-food information, to prevent non-communicable diseases: but we invoke Elpis, the spirit of hope [117], to make progress: by suggesting one alters people's behavior on food choices through marketing (FDM) [118, 119], based on functional foods (in a predictable way) without causing adverse health effects, using human-computer interactive flavor augmentation (HCIFA) (enhancing, boosting, modifying flavor: perceived/imagined [99]) technologies/methodologies [99, 120]. The human visual experience of food (shape, color) in the UK, and elsewhere, may influence choice through logical semantics, concerned with presupposition and implication, *e.g.*, round rosy red apples, 'wonky'/misshapen grubby vegetables/mushrooms but on a global basis, orthonasal olfaction is beyond the remit of this overview *e.g.* odor is not discernible in some packaged products, particularly in supermarkets. However, Velasco *et al.* [121] demonstrated a Stroop [122] like effect when searching for the product packaging which exhibited rapid searching by participants when congruent characteristics, *e.g.*, color/flavor label, were present cf. non-congruent (*e.g.* red/tomato *Vs.* yellow/tomato) [121].

Elpis, the Spirit of Hope, will traverse the gap between HCIFA in a limited setting to one of the large-scale designs involving psychologists, computer experts, statisticians, social and behavioral scientists, regulatory and monitoring bodies, operating through expert practitioners, which will lead consumers/diners (food and beverages) towards a healthier lifestyle; including a reduction in non-communicable diseases [123] (NCD). Beginning with VATMA (Visual, Auditory, Tactic, Multisense, Augmentation) [99], visual perception in appetite science can be enhanced by pairing the main dish, comprising putative low-risk NCD constituents, with a garnish [124], or including the same with herbs and spices which may have cultural outcomes [125] or trends towards vegetarianism [126]. One can change the luminance of food on a plate to convey the mental imagery of freshness [127] or by the neatness of the plating of food [128]. All such augmentations may involve factors, vide supra, *e.g.*, color, shape, and more, *e.g.*, sound [129] (auditory flavor augmentation [130]; necklace device [131]; commensal dining robotics [132]; *etc.*).

The use of extended reality (XR) technology, comprises augmented reality (AR), mixed reality, and virtual reality and the former has used a pro-cam AR system to modify the shape and appearance of food on a plate (sponge-cake & chips) such that increased food chroma can increase the taste-sweetness of sponge-cake. Experiments have been conducted on the hedonics of taste and flavor wherein tableware (EducaTableware) has been introduced which emits sounds/music according to the electrical resistance of the food through fork (EaTheremin) or TeaTheremin (which is a cup-type device used for drinking) [133, 134] which can be linked to mealtime and used as possibly one tool for increasing cardiometabolic health [135], including NCDs, particularly if children are initiated through acoustic media *e.g.* nursery rhymes [136]. From a tactile perspective, the flavor may be influenced by the weight, and size of cutlery [137, 138]; prevention of NCD using the 'gravitamine spice' system [139] may potentially encourage people to eat less (of the correct food). Although future augmentation reality processes may be combined, they are not sufficiently developed to enhance any NCD prevention strategies and are not discussed further. However, experiment design will be critical and expensive as one progresses from a laboratory-style setting through to a pilot field experiment and thence to large-scale trials.

DISCUSSION

Global NCD: Future Research

An important question asked of food research for reducing global NCDs, especially in low- and middle-income countries [140] (where the burden of NCDs is the highest and rapidly growing [141]), is 'its effectiveness' given (the oft conflicting) research/activities undertaken by public health bodies and the food and beverage industry [142], and NGOs (Singh *et al e.g* [143].) and individual practices. Effectiveness is a questionable measurement for a variety of reasons including food insecurity [144, 145] and economic constraints (women) [146, 147]. Aware (authors) of the Katha Upanishad idiom (c5 century BCE) [148] on so-called personal ignorance, it is important to set the work in this overview from the perspective of health priorities on global 'hidden hunger' [149, 150], NCDs and the sustainability of feeding the world's population [151]. According to FAO data [152] an acceleration of the 'present' reduction of hunger and malnutrition is needed (see Fig. (**2**) for future food research by global networks of centers of excellence). It has been reported that 800 million are chronically underfed from an energy perspective, 2 billion have micronutrient deficiency and 1.9 billion are overweight or obese [153, 154]. Importantly, 4.7 million premature deaths are linked to obesity, 13% of the adult population (39% overweight) and 1 in 5 children/adolescents are obese or overweight, respectively [155]. Reference [155] has an important interactive feature for providing information on children, women, men, and adult obesity over several recent decades.

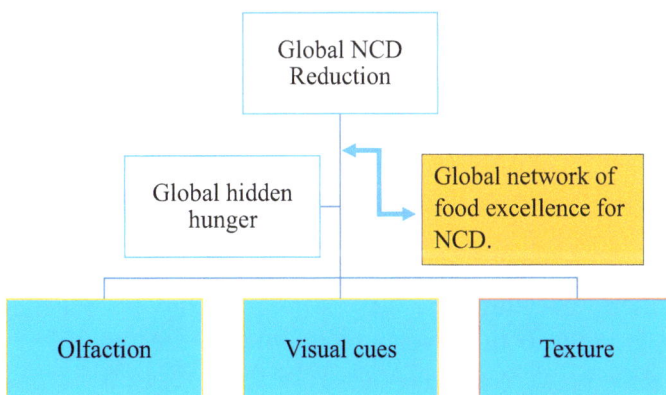

Fig. (2). Avenues of future food research by global networks of centers of excellence.

It is reasonable, amid the multifarious global risk factors for NCDs, that the salient feature of this overview enables future niche activities to reduce NCDs through the creation of centers or networks of excellence which translate properly statistically 'significant and powered' findings through paired or networked public health bodies within or between countries akin to those reported [141] and so enhancing global research platforms rather than being largely forgotten [156].

Visual Cues

In a global context, it is important to consider the visual design cues for food choice [157] affecting behavioral outcome or psychological processes [119, 158, 159]. A consumer's interpretation of health claims on the packaging labels of functional food products [160] will motivate them to purchase or otherwise (*q.v.* health star rating rather than nutrition information [161]). More of the product, particularly if they have a perceived need, poses higher risks, *e.g.* an elevated NCD risk. There are 74 categories of future research items (*e.g.*, FR 73 is a long-term choice needed for making unappealing products appealing) [157]: this is a complex situation to be unraveled in NCD reduction research programs because not all are related to in-store food marketing *per se*. Price and inflationary socioeconomic pressure may force consumers to choose cheaper and possibly foods that are less healthy [162]. Populations in nations that were formerly very adherent to the Mediterranean Diet (MD) are choosing not to do so, which may indicate less reduced CVD (*e.g.*, among children or adolescents) [163 - 165]. Media information about food can be a target for public health policies such as NCD reduction, particularly from food corporations adjudged to be sometimes cautious in providing food-health information or who have alternative views or promotions that are often directed towards unhealthy food [166 - 168]. Advertisements [169] are not discussed further in this overview.

Olfaction

It remains to be seen how COVID-19 [170] in low-, medium- and high-income countries may change the prevalence of NCDs due to its high prevalence (though not exclusive and variable [171, 172] of anosmia (short term (or longer) effect [173]) compared to non-infected tested subjects (3:1 [174]) which alters taste and flavor perception [175], through possibly differential mechanisms [176] potentially leading to malnutrition, weight loss, fatigue, poorer mental health, *etc* [175]. Importantly, an infection may affect comorbidities including NCDs such as diabetes progression [177] which is not part of this overview.

Texture

Food texture may affect oral processing and if dietary management advice increases the number of masticatory cycles before bolus, this may reduce dietary intake, and increase satiety [178], and consequently 'how to eat' and 'when to eat [179]' may, given the appropriate low-ultra-processed food, reduce NCDs [180].

CONCLUSION

Cognizant that 'the world is one family', this overview describes chemosensory characteristics of food and related issues that may enable global inequalities in healthy food consumption to be improved with a reduction in non-communicable diseases (NCDs). Food color, taste, smell, culinary plate, flavor, locale, and the disposition of food on the culinary plate all have the potential to have a favorable impact on nutrition and non-communicable disease, particularly in concert with researchers around the world. Human-computer interface and food augmentation reality and commensal dining in association with chemosensory properties, including sound concerning oral food processing are described. Future research on arresting trends in the prevalence of NCD is suggested based on the literature. Visual cues for in-store food choice are discussed that potentially allow the consumer, through psychological processes and behavior outcomes, to be more discerning. The relatively high prevalence of anosmia caused by COVID-19 infection relative to non-infected subjects may alter taste and flavor perception and lead to changed dietary habits and metabolism. Food insecurity poses a global problem and the authors recognize the global plight of 800 million or so who are chronically underfed, the 2 billion who have micronutrient deficiency and 1.9 billion who are overweight or obese, and the 4.7 million premature deaths that are linked to obesity. For many, life is difficult, but alternative crops may yield promise subject to healthy nutrition [*e.g.*, 181, 182] (Non-vivere bonum est, sed bene vivere [183] (To live is not a blessing, but to live well)); and Elpis with the relevant author-citations herein (and others in the past, present and future) will substantially overcome this scourge on humanity.

AUTHORSHIP ATTRIBUTION

DW mainly wrote the paper; FDM provided marketing advice; RBS was the expert on NCDs and nutrition; TT provided information on dietary fiber; and HSB reviewed the structure and edited content.

ABBREVIATIONS

ANOVA	Analysis of Variance
AR	Augmented Reality

BCE	Before the Common Era
CIELAB	The CIE 1976 L*a*b* color space
COVID-19	Coronavirus Disease 2019
CVD	Cardiovascular Disease
FAO	Food and Agriculture Organization
FDM	Fabien De Meester
FR	Future Research
GI	Gastrointestinal
GLP-1	Glucagon-like Peptide-1
HCIFA	Human-computer Interactive Flavor Augmentation
i.a.	Inter Alia
NCD	Non-Communicable Disease
NGO	Non-Governmental Organization
Nm	Nanometer
PROP	6-n-propylthiouracil
PTS	PROP Taster Status
q.v.	Quod Vide
SLS	Sweet Liking Status
TTS	Thermal Taster Status
VATMA	Visual, Auditory, Tactic, Multi-sense, Augmentation
XR	Extended Reality

REFERENCES

[1]   Wikipedia. Food history. Available from: Http://en.wikipedia.org/wiki/food_history

[2]   Ward P, Coveney J, Henderson J. Editorial: A sociology of food and eating. J Sociol 2010; 46(4): 347-51.
[http://dx.doi.org/10.1177/1440783310384448]

[3]   Wilson DW, Nash P, Singh RB, De Meester F, Takahashi T, Buttar H. Functional foods and nutraceuticals in metabolic and non-communicable diseases. In: Singh RB, Watanabe S, Isaza AA, Eds. International food security directed toward older adults: an overview. London: Academic Press 2020; pp. 619-40.
[http://dx.doi.org/10.1016/B978-0-12-819815-5.00010]

[4]   Caspi CE, Sorensen G, Subramanian SV, Kawachi I. The local food environment and diet: A systematic review. Health Place 2012; 18(5): 1172-87.
[http://dx.doi.org/10.1016/j.healthplace.2012.05.006]

[5]   Alsaffar AA. Sustainable diets: The interaction between food industry, nutrition, health and the environment. Food Sci Technol Int 2016; 22(2): 102-11.
[http://dx.doi.org/10.1177/1082013215572029]

[6]   He C, Zhang M, Fang Z. 3D printing of food: Pretreatment and post-treatment of materials. Crit Rev Food Sci Nutr 2020; 60(14): 2379-92.

[http://dx.doi.org/10.1080/10408398.2019.1641065]

[7]   Kingsbury N. The history and science of plant breeding. Chicago: The University of Chicago Press 2009.
        [http://dx.doi.org/10.7208/chicago/9780226437057.001.0001]

[8]   Mantihal S, Kobun R, Lee BB. 3D food printing of as the new way of preparing food: A review. Int J Gastron Food Sci 2020; 22: 100260.
        [http://dx.doi.org/10.1016/j.ijgfs.2020.100260]

[9]   Lo YT, Chang YH, Lee MS, Wahlqvist ML. Health and nutrition economics: Diet costs are associated with diet quality. Asia Pac J Clin Nutr 2009; 18(4): 598-604.

[10]   Wilson D, Nash P, Buttar H, *et al.* The role of food antioxidants, benefits of functional foods, and influence of feeding habits on the health of the older person: An overview. Antioxidants 2017; 6(4): 81.
        [http://dx.doi.org/10.3390/antiox6040081]

[11]   Wahlqvist ML, Darmadi-Blackberry I, Kouris-Blazos A, *et al.* Does diet matter for survival in long-lived cultures? Asia Pac J Clin Nutr 2005; 14(1): 2-6.

[12]   Godfray HCJ, Beddington JR, Crute IR, *et al.* Food security: The challenge of feeding 9 billion people. Science 2010; 327(5967): 812-8.
        [http://dx.doi.org/10.1126/science.1185383]

[13]   Singh RB, Watson RR, Takahashi T. The role of functional food security in global health. Edinburgh: Academic Press Elsevier Inc 2019.
        [http://dx.doi.org/10.1016/C2016-0-04169-4]

[14]   USDA ERS - Measurement. Available from: https://www.ers.usda.gov/topics/food-nutrition-assistance/food-security-in-the-us/measurement/

[15]   Seelan R. Deconstructing global citizenship. Routledge: Lexington Books 2015; 143

[16]   Fanzo J, Davis C. Can diets be healthy, sustainable, and equitable? Curr Obes Rep 2019; 8(4): 495-503.
        [http://dx.doi.org/10.1007/s13679-019-00362-0]

[17]   OECD. Income Distribution Database: by country. Available from: https://stats.oecd.org/index.aspx?queryid=66670

[18]   Schutte AE, Srinivasapura Venkateshmurthy N, Mohan S, Prabhakaran D. Hypertension in low and middle income countries. Circ Res 2021; 128(7): 808-26.
        [http://dx.doi.org/10.1161/CIRCRESAHA.120.318729]

[19]   Wikipedia. Food energy. Available from: https://en.wikipedia.org/wiki/Food_energy#:~: text= Food%20energy%20is%20chemical%20energy%20that%20animals%20%28including,with%20oxygen%20from%20air%20or%20dissolved%20in%20water

[20]   Wikipedia. Pancha. Available from: https://en.wikipedia.org/wiki/Pancha_Bhoota#:~:text= These %20elements%20are%3A%20Prithvi%2FBhudevi,Space%2FAtmosphere%2FEther

[21]   Deng Y, Zhu S, Xu P, Deng H. Characteristics and a New English Translation of Wu Xing and Yin-Yang. Chin J Integr Med 2000; 20(12): 937.

[22]   Wikipedia. Aristotle, On the Heavens, translated by J.L. Stocks, III.3.302a17-19. Available from: https://en.wikipedia.org/wiki/Aristotle

[23]   Russell B. History of Western philosophy. London: Routledge 1995.

[24]   Young JZ. Influence of the mouth on the evolution of the brain. In: Person P Eds. Biology of the mouth: A symposium presented at the Washington meeting of the American Association for the Advancement of Science. New York: American Association for the Advancement of Science. 1968; pp.21-35.

[25]   Spence C. Multisensory flavor perception. Cell 2015; 161(1): 24-35.
[http://dx.doi.org/10.1016/j.cell.2015.03.007]

[26]   Breslin PAS. An evolutionary perspective on food and human taste. Curr Biol 2013; 23(9): R409-18.
[http://dx.doi.org/10.1016/j.cub.2013.04.010]

[27]   Krebs JR. The gourmet ape: Evolution and human food preferences. Am J Clin Nutr 2009; 90(3): 707S-11S.
[http://dx.doi.org/10.3945/ajcn.2009.27462B]

[28]   Creanza N, Feldman MW. Worldwide genetic and cultural change in human evolution. Curr Opin Genet Dev 2016; 41: 85-92.
[http://dx.doi.org/10.1016/j.gde.2016.08.006]

[29]   Jeffrey SF. Regulating energy balance: The substrate strikes back. Science 2006; 312(5775): 861-4.

[30]   Garruti G, Depalo R, De Angelis M. Weighing the impact of diet and lifestyle on female reproductive function. Curr Med Chem 2019; 26(19): 3584-92.
[http://dx.doi.org/10.2174/0929867324666170518101008]

[31]   Crawford MA. The early development and evolution of the human brain. Ups J Med Sci Suppl 1990; 48: 43-78.

[32]   Kelber A, Osorio D. From spectral information to animal colour vision: Experiments and concepts. Proc Biol Sci 2010; 277(1688): 1617-25.
[http://dx.doi.org/10.1098/rspb.2009.2118]

[33]   Mollon JD. John Elliot MD (1747–1787). Nature 1987; 329(6134): 19-20.
[http://dx.doi.org/10.1038/329019a0]

[34]   Stoerig P. Wavelength information processing versus color perception: evidence from blindsight and color-blind sight. In: Backhaus WGK, Kliegl R, Werner JS, Eds. Color vision: perspectives from different disciplines. Berlin: DeGruyter 1998; pp. 131-47.
[http://dx.doi.org/10.1515/9783110806984.131]

[35]   Longden KD. Central brain circuitry for color-vision-modulated behaviors. Curr Biol 2016; 26(20): R981-8.
[http://dx.doi.org/10.1016/j.cub.2016.07.071]

[36]   Troland LT. Report of Committee on Colorimetry for 1920–21. J Opt Soc Am 1922; 6(6): 527-96.
[http://dx.doi.org/10.1364/JOSA.6.000527]

[37]   Oxford Academic Literature and Taste. 1700–1800 : Oxford Handbooks. Available from: https://www.oxfordhandbooks.com/view/10.1093/oxfordhb/9780199935338.001.0001/oxfordhb-9780199935338-e-108

[38]   Leigh Gibson E. Emotional influences on food choice: Sensory, physiological and psychological pathways. Physiol Behav 2006; 89(1): 53-61.
[http://dx.doi.org/10.1016/j.physbeh.2006.01.024]

[39]   DeLawyer T, Morimoto T, Buck SL. Dichoptic perception of brown. J Opt Soc Am A Opt Image Sci Vis 2016; 33(3): A123-8.
[http://dx.doi.org/10.1364/JOSAA.33.00A123]

[40]   Miller R, Owens SJ, Rørslett B. Plants and colour: Flowers and pollination. Opt Laser Technol 2011; 43(2): 282-94.
[http://dx.doi.org/10.1016/j.optlastec.2008.12.018]

[41]   Nevo O, Valenta K, Razafimandimby D, Melin AD, Ayasse M, Chapman CA. Frugivores and the evolution of fruit colour. Biol Lett 2018; 14(9): 20180377.
[http://dx.doi.org/10.1098/rsbl.2018.0377]

[42]   Schienle A, Schäfer A, Hermann A, Vaitl D. Binge-eating disorder: Reward sensitivity and brain

activation to images of food. Biol Psychiatry 2009; 65(8): 654-61.
[http://dx.doi.org/10.1016/j.biopsych.2008.09.028]

[43]   e-ILV CIE Homepage on the internet. 1976 L*a*b* colour space http:/eilv.cie.co.at/term/157

[44]   Aleixandre-Tudo JL, Buica A, Nieuwoudt H, Aleixandre JL, du Toit W. Spectrophotometric analysis of phenolic compounds in grapes and wines. J Agric Food Chem 2017; 65(20): 4009-26.
[http://dx.doi.org/10.1021/acs.jafc.7b01724]

[45]   Macdougall DB. Colour measurement of food: Principles and practice. In: Gulrajani ML, Ed. Woodhead Publishing Series in Textiles Colour measurement. Oxford: Woodhead Publishing 2010; pp. 312-42.
[http://dx.doi.org/10.1533/9780857090195.2.312]

[46]   Hernández Salueña B, Sáenz Gamasa C, Diñeiro Rubial JM, Alberdi Odriozola C. CIELAB color paths during meat shelf life. Meat Sci 2019; 157: 107889.
[http://dx.doi.org/10.1016/j.meatsci.2019.107889]

[47]   Cho S, Han A, Taylor MH, *et al.* Blue lighting decreases the amount of food consumed in men, but not in women. Appetite 2015; 85: 111-7.
[http://dx.doi.org/10.1016/j.appet.2014.11.020]

[48]   Barnes S, Prasain J, Kim H. In: Nutrition, can we "see" what is good for us? Adv Nutr 2013; 4(3): 327S-34S.
[http://dx.doi.org/10.3945/an.112.003558]

[49]   Rolls ET. Taste and smell processing in the brain. Handb Clin Neurol 2019; 164: 97-118.
[http://dx.doi.org/10.1016/B978-0-444-63855-7.00007-1]

[50]   Hume D. Of the standard of taste. In: Eliott CW, Ed. English essays from Sir Philip Sidney to Macaulay. New York: P F Collier & Son 1910; pp. 215-36.

[51]   Hume D. Four dissertations. 1st. London: A. Millar in the Strand 1757.

[52]   Breslin PAS. An evolutionary perspective on food and human taste. Curr Biol 2013; 23(9): R409-18.
[http://dx.doi.org/10.1016/j.cub.2013.04.010]

[53]   Breslin PA, Huang L. Human taste: Peripheral anatomy, taste transduction, and coding. Adv Otorhinolaryngol 2006; 63: 152-90.
[http://dx.doi.org/10.1159/000093760]

[54]   Rolls ET. The texture and taste of food in the brain. J Texture Stud 2020; 51(1): 23-44.
[http://dx.doi.org/10.1111/jtxs.12488]

[55]   Rolls E. Taste, olfactory, and food texture processing in the brain, and the control of food intake. Physiol Behav 2005; 85(1): 45-56.
[http://dx.doi.org/10.1016/j.physbeh.2005.04.012]

[56]   Gutierrez R, Simon SA. Physiology of taste processing in the tongue, gut, and brain. Compr Physiol 2021; 11(4): 2489-523.
[http://dx.doi.org/10.1002/cphy.c210002]

[57]   Mennella JA, Jagnow CP, Beauchamp GK. Prenatal and postnatal flavor learning by human infants. Pediatrics 2001; 107(6): e88.
[http://dx.doi.org/10.1542/peds.107.6.e88]

[58]   Mennella JA, Pepino MY, Reed DR. Genetic and environmental determinants of bitter perception and sweet preferences. Pediatrics 2005; 115(2): e216-22.
[http://dx.doi.org/10.1542/peds.2004-1582]

[59]   The six tastes in Ayurveda | Banyan Botanicals. Available from: https://www.banyanbotanicals.com/info/ayurvedic-living/living-ayurveda/diet/six-tastes/

[60]   Singh RB, Onsaard E, Tripathi AK, Chauhan AK, Horuichi R. The modified ten point hedonic scale

for perception of taste in Asians. Int J Clin Nutrition 2007; 7: 6-10.

[61]   Wasilewski T, Kamysz W, Gębicki J. Bioelectronic tongue: Current status and perspectives. Biosens Bioelectron 2020; 150: 111923.
[http://dx.doi.org/10.1016/j.bios.2019.111923]

[62]   Tordoff MG, Alarcón LK, Valmeki S, Jiang P. T1R3: A human calcium taste receptor. Sci Rep 2012; 2(1): 496.
[http://dx.doi.org/10.1038/srep00496]

[63]   Jang HJ, Kokrashvili Z, Theodorakis MJ, *et al.* Gut-expressed gustducin and taste receptors regulate secretion of glucagon-like peptide-1. Proc Natl Acad Sci 2007; 104(38): 15069-74.
[http://dx.doi.org/10.1073/pnas.0706890104]

[64]   Makkliang F, Kanatharana P, Thavarungkul P, Thammakhet C. Development of magnetic micro-solid phase extraction for analysis of phthalate esters in packaged food. Food Chem 2015; 166: 275-82.
[http://dx.doi.org/10.1016/j.foodchem.2014.06.036]

[65]   Herz RS. Perfume. In: Gottfried JA, Ed. Neurobiology of sensation and reward. Boca Raton: CRC Press/Taylor & Francis 2011.

[66]   Winberg J, Porter RH. Olfaction and human neonatal behaviour: Clinical implications. Acta Paediatr 1998; 87(1): 6-10.
[http://dx.doi.org/10.1111/j.1651-2227.1998.tb01376.x]

[67]   Ventura AK, Worobey J. Early influences on the development of food preferences. Curr Biol 2013; 23(9): R401-8.
[http://dx.doi.org/10.1016/j.cub.2013.02.037]

[68]   Mennella JA, Johnson A, Beauchamp GK. Garlic ingestion by pregnant women alters the odor of amniotic fluid. Chem Senses 1995; 20(2): 207-9.
[http://dx.doi.org/10.1093/chemse/20.2.207]

[69]   Kokocińska-Kusiak A, Woszczyło M, Zybala M, Maciocha J, Barłowska K, Dzięcioł M. Canine olfaction: Physiology, behavior, and possibilities for practical applications. Animals 2021; 11(8): 2463.
[http://dx.doi.org/10.3390/ani11082463]

[70]   Gaillet-Torrent M, Sulmont-Rossé C, Issanchou S, Chabanet C, Chambaron S. Impact of a non-attentively perceived odour on subsequent food choices. Appetite 2014; 76: 17-22.
[http://dx.doi.org/10.1016/j.appet.2014.01.009]

[71]   Morrot G, Brochet F, Dubourdieu D. The color of odors. Brain Lang 2001; 79(2): 309-20.
[http://dx.doi.org/10.1006/brln.2001.2493]

[72]   Leonhardt SD, Menzel F, Nehring V, Schmitt T. Ecology and evolution of communication in social insects. Cell 2016; 164(6): 1277-87.
[http://dx.doi.org/10.1016/j.cell.2016.01.035]

[73]   Schwieterman ML, Colquhoun TA, Jaworski EA, *et al.* Strawberry flavor: Diverse chemical compositions, a seasonal influence, and effects on sensory perception. PLoS One 2014; 9(2): e88446.
[http://dx.doi.org/10.1371/journal.pone.0088446]

[74]   Olfactometers, VOC emission test chambers & odour measurement devices | Olfasense. Available from: https://www.olfasense.com/odour-measurement-equipment/

[75]   Wansink B. From mindless eating to mindlessly eating better. Physiol Behav 2010; 100(5): 454-63.
[http://dx.doi.org/10.1016/j.physbeh.2010.05.003]

[76]   Slavin JL, Lloyd B. Health benefits of fruits and vegetables. Adv Nutr 2012; 3(4): 506-16.
[http://dx.doi.org/10.3945/an.112.002154]

[77]   Zhao X, Li M, Liu Y. Microfluidic-based approaches for foodborne pathogen detection. Microorganisms 2019; 7(10): 381.

[http://dx.doi.org/10.3390/microorganisms7100381]

[78] Food standard agency. Food hygiene rating scheme. Available from: https://www.food.gov.uk/safety-hygiene/food-hygiene-rating-scheme [cited: 12th Aug 2002].

[79] A plus topper. What is agriculture and what are agricultural practices. Available from: https://www.aplustopper.com/agriculture-and-agricultural-practices/#:~:text=Agricultural%20Prac-tices%201%20Soil%20Preparation.%20Soil%20is%20the,before%20they%20are%20made%20availa ble%20for%20consumption.%20

[80] Chen H, Kinchla AJ, Richard N, Shaw A, Feng Y. Produce growers' on-farm food safety education: A review. J Food Prot 2021; 84(4): 704-16.
[http://dx.doi.org/10.4315/JFP-20-320]

[81] Sabo-Attwood T, Apul OG, Bisesi JH Jr, Kane AS, Saleh NB. Nano-scale applications in aquaculture: Opportunities for improved production and disease control. J Fish Dis 2021; 44(4): 359-70.
[http://dx.doi.org/10.1111/jfd.13332]

[82] Kontominas MG, Badeka AV, Kosma IS, Nathanailides CI. Innovative seafood preservation technologies: recent developments. Animals 2021; 11(1): 92.
[http://dx.doi.org/10.3390/ani11010092]

[83] Kontominas MG, Badeka AV, Kosma IS, Nathanailides CI. Recent developments in seafood packaging technologies. Foods 2021; 10(5): 940.
[http://dx.doi.org/10.3390/foods10050940]

[84] Oliveira M, Tiwari BK, Duffy G. Emerging technologies for aerial decontamination of food storage environments to eliminate microbial cross-contamination. Foods 2020; 9(12): 1779.
[http://dx.doi.org/10.3390/foods9121779]

[85] UN Economic Commission for Europe – Inland Transport Committee. 2003. Available from: http://www.unece.org/trans/main/wp11/atp.html

[86] Eskicioglu V, Kamiloglu S, Nilufer-Erdil D. Antioxidant dietary fibres: Potential functional food ingredients from plant processing by-products. Czech J Food Sci 2015; 33(6): 487-99.
[http://dx.doi.org/10.17221/42/2015-CJFS]

[87] Leng G, Adan RAH, Belot M, *et al.* The determinants of food choice. Proc Nutr Soc 2017; 76(3): 316-27.
[http://dx.doi.org/10.1017/S002966511600286X]

[88] Jia W, Wu Z, Ren Y, Cao S, Mao ZH, Sun M. Estimating dining plate size from an egocentric image sequence without a fiducial marker. Front Nutr 2021; 7: 519444.
[http://dx.doi.org/10.3389/fnut.2020.519444]

[89] Jia SS, Liu Q, Allman-Farinelli M, *et al.* The use of portion control plates to promote healthy eating and diet-related outcomes: A scoping review. Nutrients 2022; 14(4): 892.
[http://dx.doi.org/10.3390/nu14040892]

[90] Hetherington MM, Blundell-Birtill P, Caton SJ, *et al.* Understanding the science of portion control and the art of downsizing. Proc Nutr Soc 2018; 77(3): 347-55.
[http://dx.doi.org/10.1017/S0029665118000435]

[91] Almiron-Roig E, Forde CG, Hollands GJ, Vargas MÁ, Brunstrom JM. A review of evidence supporting current strategies, challenges, and opportunities to reduce portion sizes. Nutr Rev 2020; 78(2): 91-114.
[http://dx.doi.org/10.1093/nutrit/nuz047]

[92] Burrows T, Collins C, Adam M, Duncanson K, Rollo M. Dietary assessment of shared plate eating: A missing link. Nutrients 2019; 11(4): 789.
[http://dx.doi.org/10.3390/nu11040789]

[93] Varvara RA, Szabo K, Vodnar DC. 3D Food printing: Principles of obtaining digitally designed

nourishment. Nutrients 2021; 13(10): 3617.
[http://dx.doi.org/10.3390/nu13103617]

[94]   Pereira T, Barroso S, Gil MM. Food texture design by 3D printing: A review. Foods 2021; 10(2): 320.
        [http://dx.doi.org/10.3390/foods10020320]

[95]   Reyes M, Garmendia ML, Olivares S, Aqueveque C, Zacarías I, Corvalán C. Development of the
        chilean front of package food warning label. BMC Public Health 2019; 19(1): 906.
        [http://dx.doi.org/10.1186/s12889-019-7118-1]

[96]   Thoma V, Kobayashi K, Tanimoto H. The role of the gustatory system in the coordination of feeding.
        eNeuro 2017; 4(6).
        [http://dx.doi.org/10.1523/ENEURO.0324-17.2017]

[97]   Engler-Stringer R. Food, cooking skills, and health: A literature review. Can J Diet Pract Res 2010;
        71(3): 141-5.
        [http://dx.doi.org/10.3148/71.3.2010.141]

[98]   Prescott J. Multisensory processes in flavour perception and their influence on food choice. Curr Opin
        Food Sci 2015; 3: 47-52.
        [http://dx.doi.org/10.1016/j.cofs.2015.02.007]

[99]   Velasco C, Obrist M, Petit O, Spence C. Multisensory technology for flavor augmentation: A mini
        review. Front Psychol 2018; 9: 26.
        [http://dx.doi.org/10.3389/fpsyg.2018.00026]

[100]   Cowart B, Beauchamp G, Mennella J. Development of taste and smell in the neonate. In: Polin R, Fox
        W, Abman S, Eds. Fetal and neonatal physiology. Philadelphia: Saunders Elsevier 2011; pp. 1899-
        907.
        [http://dx.doi.org/10.1016/B978-1-4160-3479-7.10172-7]

[101]   Lawless H, Heyman H. Sensory evaluation of food. NY: Springer Science & Business Media 2010.
        [http://dx.doi.org/10.1007/978-1-4419-6488-5]

[102]   Hoffman AC, Salgado RV, Dresler C, Faller RW, Bartlett C. Flavour preferences in youth versus
        adults: A review. Tob Control 2016; 25 (2): ii32-9.
        [http://dx.doi.org/10.1136/tobaccocontrol-2016-053192]

[103]   Prescott J, Tepper BJ. Genetic variation in taste sensitivity. New York: Marcel Dekker, Inc. 2004.
        [http://dx.doi.org/10.1201/9780203023433]

[104]   Mozaffarian D. Dietary and policy priorities for cardiovascular disease, diabetes, and obesity: a
        comprehensive review. Circulation 2016; 133(2): 187-225.
        [http://dx.doi.org/10.1161/CIRCULATIONAHA.115.018585]

[105]   Singh RB, Watanabe S, Isaza AA. Functional foods and nutraceuticals in metabolic and non-
        communicable diseases. London: Academic Press 2022; pp. 799-821.
        [http://dx.doi.org/10.1016/B978-0-12-819815-5.00060-4]

[106]   Fedacko J, Takahashi T, Singh RB, *et al.* Western diets and risk of non-communicable diseases. In:
        Singh RB, Watanabe S, Isaza AA, Eds. Functional foods and nutraceuticals in metabolic and non-
        communicable diseases. London: Academic Press 2022; pp. 3-21.
        [http://dx.doi.org/10.1016/B978-0-12-819815-5.00042-2]

[107]   Mishra R, Tripathi AD, Singh RB, Tomar RS, Wilson DW, Smail MMA. Estimates of functional food
        and nutraceutical availability in the world, with reference to food peroxidation and food safety. In:
        Singh RB, Watanabe S, Isaza AA, Eds. Functional foods and nutraceuticals in metabolic and non-
        communicable diseases. London: Academic Press 2022; pp. 23-42.
        [http://dx.doi.org/10.1016/B978-0-12-819815-5.00025-2]

[108]   Singh RB, Wilson DW, Chibisov S, Kharlitskaya E, Abromova M, Smail MMA. Effects of guava fruit
        intake on cardiometabolic diseases. In: Singh RB, Watanabe S, Isaza AA, Eds. Functional foods and
        nutraceuticals in metabolic and non-communicable diseases. London: Academic Press 2022; pp. 79-

85.
[http://dx.doi.org/10.1016/B978-0-12-819815-5.00051-3]

[109] Shahrajabian MH, Sun W, Cheng Q, Khoshkharam M. Exploring the quality of foods from ancient China based on traditional Chinese medicine. In: Singh RB, Watanabe S, Isaza AA, Eds. Functional foods and nutraceuticals in metabolic and non-communicable diseases. London: Academic Press 2022; pp. 87-105.
[http://dx.doi.org/10.1016/B978-0-12-819815-5.00048-3]

[110] Singh RB, Watanabe S, Li D, *et al.* Effects of polyunsaturated fatty acid–rich diets and risk of non-communicable diseases. In: Singh RB, Watanabe S, Isaza AA, Eds. Functional foods and nutraceuticals in metabolic and non-communicable diseases. London: Academic Press 2022; pp. 165-85.
[http://dx.doi.org/10.1016/B978-0-12-819815-5.00011-2]

[111] Singh R, Singh RB, Mojto V, *et al.* Cocoa and chocolate consumption and prevention of cardiovascular diseases and other chronic diseases. In: Singh RB, Watanabe S, Isaza AA, Eds. Functional foods and nutraceuticals in metabolic and non-communicable diseases. 279-99.
[http://dx.doi.org/10.1016/B978-0-12-819815-5.00012-4]

[112] Jaglan P, Buttar HS, Al-bawareed OA, Chibisov S. Potential health benefits of selected fruits: Apples, blueberries, grapes, guavas, mangos. pomegranates, and tomatoes. In: Singh RB, Watanabe S, Isaza AA, Eds. Functional foods and nutraceuticals in metabolic and non-communicable diseases. 359-70.
[http://dx.doi.org/10.1016/B978-0-12-819815-5.00026-4]

[113] Jain E, Tripathi AD, Agarwal A, *et al.* Anticancerous compounds in fruits, their extraction, and relevance to food. In: Singh RB, Watanabe S, Isaza AA, Eds. Functional foods and nutraceuticals in metabolic and non-communicable diseases. 517-32.
[http://dx.doi.org/10.1016/B978-0-12-819815-5.00022-7]

[114] WHO. Available from: https://www.euro.who.int/en/health-topics/noncommunicable-diseases/n-d-background-information/what-are-noncommunicable-diseases#:~:text=Noncommunicable%20di-seases%20%E2%80%93%20a%20group%20of%20conditions%20that,the%20disease%20burden%20 in%20the%20WHO%20European%20Region

[115] Liu G, Zong G, Doty RL, Sun Q. Prevalence and risk factors of taste and smell impairment in a nationwide representative sample of the US population: A cross-sectional study. BMJ Open 2016; 6(11): e013246.
[http://dx.doi.org/10.1136/bmjopen-2016-013246]

[116] Hoffman HJ, Cruickshanks KJ, Davis B. Perspectives on population-based epidemiological studies of olfactory and taste impairment. Ann N Y Acad Sci 2009; 1170(1): 514-30.
[http://dx.doi.org/10.1111/j.1749-6632.2009.04597.x]

[117] Hesiod. Montanari F, Rengakos A, Tsagalis C. (Eds) Brill's Companion to Hesiod. pp. xii + 430. Leiden and Boston: Brill 2009.

[118] Petit O, Cheok A, Spence C, Velasco C, Karunanayaka KT. Sensory marketing in light of new technologies. Proceedings of the 12th International Conference on Advances in Computer Entertainment Technology (ACE '15). New York, NY: ACM 2015.
[http://dx.doi.org/10.1145/2832932.2837006]

[119] Labrecque LI, Patrick VM, Milne GR. The marketers' prismatic palette: A review of colour research and future directions. Psychol Mark 2013; 30(2): 187-202.
[http://dx.doi.org/10.1002/mar.20597]

[120] Obrist M, Velasco C, Vi C, *et al.* Sensing the future of HCI. Interactions 2016; 23(5): 40-9.
[http://dx.doi.org/10.1145/2973568]

[121] Velasco C, Wan X, Knoeferle K, Zhou X, Salgado-Montejo A, Spence C. Searching for flavor labels in food products: The influence of color-flavor congruence and association strength. Front Psychol 2015; 6: 301.

[http://dx.doi.org/10.3389/fpsyg.2015.00301]

[122]   Stroop JR. Studies of interference in serial verbal reactions. J Exp Psychol 1935; 18(6): 643-62.
[http://dx.doi.org/10.1037/h0054651]

[123]   Velasco C, Carvalho FR, Petit O, Nijholt A. A multisensory approach for the design of food and drink enhancing sonic systems. Proceedings of the 1st Workshop on multi-sensorial approaches to human-food interaction (MHFI '16). New York: ACM 2016.
[http://dx.doi.org/10.1145/3007577.3007578]

[124]   Kokaji N, Nakatani M. With a hint of sudachi: Food plating can facilitate the fondness of food. Front Psychol 2021; 12: 699218.
[http://dx.doi.org/10.3389/fpsyg.2021.699218]

[125]   Carney EM, Stein WM, Reigh NA, *et al.* Increasing flavor variety with herbs and spices improves relative vegetable intake in children who are propylthiouracil (PROP) tasters relative to nontasters. Physiol Behav 2018; 188: 48-57.
[http://dx.doi.org/10.1016/j.physbeh.2018.01.021]

[126]   Spencer M, Guinard JX. The Flexitarian Flip™: Testing the modalities of flavor as sensory strategies to accomplish the shift from meat-centered to vegetable-forward mixed dishes. J Food Sci 2018; 83(1): 175-87.
[http://dx.doi.org/10.1111/1750-3841.13991]

[127]   Arce-Lopera C, Masuda T, Kimura A, Wada Y, Okajima K. Luminance distribution modifies the perceived freshness of strawberries. Perception 2012; 3(5): 338-55.
[http://dx.doi.org/10.1068/i0471]

[128]   Zellner DA, Loss CR, Zearfoss J, Remolina S. It tastes as good as it looks! The effect of food presentation on liking for the flavor of food. Appetite 2014; 77: 31-5.
[http://dx.doi.org/10.1016/j.appet.2014.02.009]

[129]   Wang Y, Li Z, Jarvis R, Khot RA, Mueller FF. The singing carrot: Designing playful experiences with food sounds Proceedings of the 2018 Annual Symposium on Computer-Human Interaction in Play Companion Extended abstracts, CHI PLAY '18 Extended Abstracts. New York: ACM;2018, pp. 669–676.
[http://dx.doi.org/10.1145/3270316.3271512]

[130]   Niewiadomski R, Ceccaldi E, Huisman G, Volpe G, Mancini M. Computational commensality: From theories to computational models for social food preparation and consumption in HCI. Front Robotics AI 2019; 6: 119.
[http://dx.doi.org/10.3389/frobt.2019.00119]

[131]   Bi Y, Xu W, Guan N, Wei Y, Yi W. Pervasive eating habits monitoring and recognition through a wearable acoustic sensor. Proceedings of the 8th International Conference on Pervasive Computing Technologies for Healthcare Pervasive Health '14. 174-7.
[http://dx.doi.org/10.4108/icst.pervasivehealth.2014.255423]

[132]   Khot RA, Arza ES, Kurra H, Wang Y. FoBo: Towards designing a robotic companion for solo dining. Extended abstracts of the 2019 CHI conference on human factors in computing systems, CHIEA '19. New York: ACM 2019; pp. 1-6.
[http://dx.doi.org/10.1145/3290607.3313069]

[133]   Kadomura A, Nakamori R, Tsukada K, Siio I. EaTheremin Proceedings of the SIGGRAPH Asia 2011 Emerging Technologies (SA '11). New York, NY: ACM 2011; p. 1.
[http://dx.doi.org/10.1145/2073370.2073376]

[134]   Kadomura A, Tsukada K, Siio I. EducaTableware: Computer augmented tableware to enhance the eating experiences. Proceedings of the CHI '13 extended abstracts on human factors in computing systems (CHIEA '13). New York: ACM 2013; pp. 3071-4.
[http://dx.doi.org/10.1145/2468356.2479613]

[135] St-Onge MP, Ard J, Baskin ML, *et al.* Meal timing and frequency: Implications for cardiovascular disease prevention: A scientific statement from the american heart association. Circulation 2017; 135(9): e96-e121.
[http://dx.doi.org/10.1161/CIR.0000000000000476]

[136] Wikipedia. Old MacDonald had a farm. Available from: https://en.wikipedia.org/wiki/Old_MacDonald_Had_a_Farm#:~:text=%22%20Old%20MacDonald%20Had%20a%20Farm%20%22%20%28sometimes,%22moo%22%20would%20be%20used%20as%20the%20animal%27s%20sound

[137] Slocombe BG, Carmichael DA, Simner J. Cross-modal tactile–taste interactions in food evaluations. Neuropsychologia 2016; 88: 58-64.
[http://dx.doi.org/10.1016/j.neuropsychologia.2015.07.011]

[138] Van Rompay TJL, Finger F, Saakes D, Fenko A. "See me, feel me": Effects of 3D-printed surface patterns on beverage evaluation. Food Qual Prefer 2017; 62: 332-9.
[http://dx.doi.org/10.1016/j.foodqual.2016.12.002]

[139] Hirose M, Iwazaki K, Nojiri K, Takeda M, Sugiura Y, Inami M. Gravitamine spice: a system that changes the perception of eating through virtual weight sensation. Proceedings of the 6th Augmented Human International Conference (AH '15). New York, NY: ACM 2015; pp. 33-40.
[http://dx.doi.org/10.1145/2735711.2735795]

[140] Worldbank.org. WDI : The world by income and region. Available from: https://datatopics.worldbank.org/world-development-indicators/the-world-by-income-and-region.html

[141] Engelgau MM, Sampson UK, Rabadan-Diehl C, *et al.* Tackling NCD in LMIC: Achievements and lessons learned from the nhlbi—unitedhealth global health centers of excellence program. Glob Heart 2016; 11(1): 5-15.
[http://dx.doi.org/10.1016/j.gheart.2015.12.016]

[142] Mercer JG, Johnstone AM, Halford JCG. Approaches to influencing food choice across the age groups: From children to the elderly. Proc Nutr Soc 2015; 74(2): 149-57.
[http://dx.doi.org/10.1017/S0029665114001712]

[143] Singh RB, Rastogi SS, Rao PV, *et al.* Diet and lifestyle guidelines and desirable levels of risk factors for the prevention of diabetes and its vascular complications in Indians: A scientific statement of The International College of Nutrition. J Cardiovasc Risk 1997; 4(3): 201-8.
[http://dx.doi.org/10.1097/00043798-199706000-00007]

[144] USDA ERS . Measurement. Available from: https://www.ers.usda.gov/topics/food-nutrition-assistance/food-security-in-the-us/measurement/

[145] Te Vazquez J, Feng SN, Orr CJ, Berkowitz SA. Food insecurity and cardiometabolic conditions: A review of recent research. Curr Nutr Rep 2021; 10(4): 243-54.
[http://dx.doi.org/10.1007/s13668-021-00364-2]

[146] Wikipedia. Ellen Swallow Richards. Available from: https://en.wikipedia.org/wiki/Ellen_Swallow_Richards

[147] Mclaughlin C, Tarasuk V, Kreiger N. An examination of at-home food preparation activity among low-income, food-insecure women. J Am Diet Assoc 2003; 103(11): 1506-12.
[http://dx.doi.org/10.1016/j.jada.2003.08.022]

[148] Juan Mascaró. (tr) The Upanishads. London: Penguin Classics 1965; p. 58.

[149] Muthayya S, Rah JH, Sugimoto JD, Roos FF, Kraemer K, Black RE. The global hidden hunger indices and maps: an advocacy tool for action. PLoS One 2013; 8(6): e67860.
[http://dx.doi.org/10.1371/journal.pone.0067860]

[150] Eggersdorfer M, Akobundu U, Bailey R, *et al.* Hidden hunger: Solutions for America's aging populations. Nutrients 2018; 10(9): 1210.
[http://dx.doi.org/10.3390/nu10091210]

[151] Fróna D, Szenderák J, Harangi-Rákos M. The challenge of feeding the world. Sustainability 2019; 11(20): 5816.
[http://dx.doi.org/10.3390/su11205816]

[152] McGuire S. WHO, World Food Programme, and International Fund for Agricultural Development. 2012. The State of Food Insecurity in the World 2012. Economic growth is necessary but not sufficient to accelerate reduction of hunger and malnutrition. Rome, FAO. Adv Nutr 2013; 4(1): 126-7.
[http://dx.doi.org/10.3945/an.112.003343]

[153] McGuire S. FAO, IFAD, and WFP. The state of food insecurity in the world 2015: Meeting the 2015 international hunger targets: Taking stock of uneven progress. Rome: FAO, 2015. Adv Nutr 2015; 6(5): 623-4.
[http://dx.doi.org/10.3945/an.115.009936]

[154] Haddad L, Achadi E, Bendech MA, *et al.* The global nutrition report 2014: Actions and accountability to accelerate the world's progress on nutrition. J Nutr 2015; 145(4): 663-71.
[http://dx.doi.org/10.3945/jn.114.206078]

[155] Ritchie H, Roser M. Obesity. Available from: https://ourworldindata.org/obesity

[156] Singh RB, Reddy KK, Fedacko J, De Meester F, Wilczynska A, Wilson DW. Ancient concepts of nutrition and the diet in hunter-gatherers. Open Nutraceuticals J 2011; 4(1): 130-5.
[http://dx.doi.org/10.2174/1876396001104010130]

[157] Vermeir I, Roose G. Visual design cues impacting food choice: A review and future research agenda. Foods 2020; 9(10): 1495.
[http://dx.doi.org/10.3390/foods9101495]

[158] Sample KL, Hagtvedt H, Brasel SA. Components of visual perception in marketing contexts: A conceptual framework and review. J Acad Mark Sci 2020; 48(3): 405-21.
[http://dx.doi.org/10.1007/s11747-019-00684-4]

[159] Adaval R, Saluja G, Jiang Y. Seeing and thinking in pictures: A review of visual information processing. Consum Psychol Rev 2018; 2(1): 50-69.
[http://dx.doi.org/10.1002/arcp.1049]

[160] Van Buul VJ, Brouns FJ. Nutrition and health claims as marketing tools. Crit Rev Food Sci Nutr 2015; 55(11): 1552-60.
[http://dx.doi.org/10.1080/10408398.2012.754738]

[161] Talati Z, Norman R, Kelly B, *et al.* A randomized trial assessing the effects of health claims on choice of foods in the presence of front-of-pack labels. Am J Clin Nutr 2018; 108(6): 1275-82.
[http://dx.doi.org/10.1093/ajcn/nqy248]

[162] Backholer K, Sacks G, Cameron AJ. Food and beverage price promotions: An untapped policy target for improving population diets and health. Curr Nutr Rep 2019; 8(3): 250-5.
[http://dx.doi.org/10.1007/s13668-019-00287-z]

[163] Martínez-González MA, Gea A, Ruiz-Canela M. The Mediterranean Diet and cardiovascular health. Circ Res 2019; 124(5): 779-98.
[http://dx.doi.org/10.1161/CIRCRESAHA.118.313348]

[164] Castronuovo L, Guarnieri L, Tiscornia MV, Allemandi L. Food marketing and gender among children and adolescents: A scoping review. Nutr J 2021; 20(1): 52.
[http://dx.doi.org/10.1186/s12937-021-00706-4]

[165] Bonaccio M, Bes-Rastrollo M, de Gaetano G, Iacoviello L. Challenges to the mediterranean diet at a time of economic crisis. Nutr Metab Cardiovasc Dis 2016; 26(12): 1057-63.
[http://dx.doi.org/10.1016/j.numecd.2016.07.005]

[166] Weishaar H, Dorfman L, Freudenberg N, *et al.* Why media representations of corporations matter for public health policy: A scoping review. BMC Public Health 2016; 16(1): 899.

[http://dx.doi.org/10.1186/s12889-016-3594-8]

[167] BBC Kellogg's in court battle over new rules for high-sugar cereals : BBC News. Available from: https://www.bbc.co.uk/news/business-61238630

[168] Kaur A, Lewis T, Lipkova V, *et al.* A systematic review, and meta-analysis, examining the prevalence of price promotions on foods and whether they are more likely to be found on less-healthy foods. Public Health Nutr 2020; 23(8): 1281-96.
[http://dx.doi.org/10.1017/S1368980019004129]

[169] Sadeghirad B, Duhaney T, Motaghipisheh S, Campbell NRC, Johnston BC. Influence of unhealthy food and beverage marketing on children's dietary intake and preference: A systematic review and meta-analysis of randomized trials. Obes Rev 2016; 17(10): 945-59.
[http://dx.doi.org/10.1111/obr.12445]

[170] Asselah T, Durantel D, Pasmant E, Lau G, Schinazi RF. COVID-19: Discovery, diagnostics and drug development. J Hepatol 2021; 74(1): 168-84.
[http://dx.doi.org/10.1016/j.jhep.2020.09.031]

[171] Meng X, Deng Y, Dai Z, Meng Z. COVID-19 and anosmia: A review based on up-to-date knowledge. Am J Otolaryngol 2020; 41(5): 102581.
[http://dx.doi.org/10.1016/j.amjoto.2020.102581]

[172] Parma V, Ohla K, Veldhuizen MG, *et al.* More than smell : COVID-19 is associated with severe impairment of smell, taste, and chemesthesis. Chem Senses 2020; 45(7): 609-22.
[http://dx.doi.org/10.1093/chemse/bjaa041]

[173] Hopkins C, Surda P, Whitehead E, Kumar BN. Early recovery following new onset anosmia during the COVID-19 pandemic : An observational cohort study. J Otolaryngol Head Neck Surg 2020; 49(1): 26.
[http://dx.doi.org/10.1186/s40463-020-00423-8]

[174] Menni C, Valdes AM, Freidin MB, *et al.* Real-time tracking of self-reported symptoms to predict potential COVID-19. Nat Med 2020; 26(7): 1037-40.
[http://dx.doi.org/10.1038/s41591-020-0916-2]

[175] Glezer I, Bruni-Cardoso A, Schechtman D, Malnic B. Viral infection and smell loss: The case of COVID-19. J Neurochem 2021; 157(4): 930-43.
[http://dx.doi.org/10.1111/jnc.15197]

[176] Boesveldt S, de Graaf K. The differential role of smell and taste for eating behavior. Perception 2017; 46(3-4): 307-19.
[http://dx.doi.org/10.1177/0301006616685576]

[177] Kaur R, Singh S, Singh TG, Sood P, Robert J. Covid-19: Pharmacotherapeutic insights on various curative approaches in terms of vulnerability, comorbidities, and vaccination. Inflammopharmacology 2022; 30(1): 1-21.
[http://dx.doi.org/10.1007/s10787-021-00904-w]

[178] Hollis JH. The effect of mastication on food intake, satiety and body weight. Physiol Behav 2018; 193: 242-5.
[http://dx.doi.org/10.1016/j.physbeh.2018.04.027]

[179] Halberg F. Some aspects of the chronobiology of nutrition: More work is needed on 'when to eat'. J Nutr 1989; 119(3): 333-43.
[http://dx.doi.org/10.1093/jn/119.3.333]

[180] Elizabeth L, Machado P, Zinöcker M, Baker P, Lawrence M. Ultra-Processed foods and health outcomes: A narrative review. Nutrients 2020; 12(7): 1955.
[http://dx.doi.org/10.3390/nu12071955]

[181] Brandt SA, Spring A, Hiesch C, McCabe ST, Endale T, *et al.* The Tree against Hunger Enset-Based Agricultural Systems in Ethiopia American Association for the Advancement of Science, with Awassa

Agricultural Research Center, Kyota University Center for Africa Area Studies and University of Flora. Washington, DC: American Association for the Advancement of Science 1997.

[182] Borrell JS, Biswas MK, Goodwin M, *et al.* Enset in Ethiopia: A poorly characterized but resilient starch staple. Ann Bot 2019; 123(5): 747-66.
[http://dx.doi.org/10.1093/aob/mcy214]

[183] The Epistles of Seneca: Epistle LXX. Loeb Classical Library. Available from: https://www.loebclassics.com/view/seneca_younger-epistles/1917/pb_LCL076.59.xml?readMode=reader

CHAPTER 2

Oxidative Stress and Protein Misfolding in Skin Aging

Tushar Oak[1], **Riya Patel**[1] and **Maushmi S. Kumar**[2,*]

[1] *Shobhaben Pratapbhai Patel School of Pharmacy and Technology Management, SVKM's NMIMS, V. L. Mehta Road, Vile Parle West, Mumbai-400056, India*

[2] *Somaiya Institute for Research and Consultancy, Somaiya Vidyavihar University, Vidyavihar (East), Mumbai-400077, India*

Abstract: Aging is a visible indicator of malfunctioning or toxic proteins that sensitize other proteins to oxidative damage which is most prominently observed on the skin. Protein misfolding is caused by the protein following an incorrect folding pathway which may lead to spontaneous misfolding while oxidative stress refers to the disruption of the balance between antioxidant defenses and reactive oxygen species production. Oxidation may alter noncovalent interactions within proteins, peptide chain fragmentation, and protein cross-linking, which causes protein misfolding and further skin aging. A feedback loop is observed in all three processes. A proper understanding of these events is significant in the formulation of anti-aging preparations and further understanding of the mechanism of aging. In this Chapter, we will be discussing some natural antioxidants available to combat oxidative stress which facilitate healthy aging and normal functioning of the body. We will be elaborating on the body's natural defense mechanism against these problems such as the role of Chaperones. We will be looking at the detailed mechanism of oxidative stress, protein misfolding, and their correlation with skin aging along with factors influencing it. The biomarkers for oxidative stress will be enlisted. A brief correlation between these processes in a test worm and how it correlates to humans and its importance will be explained in this chapter.

Keywords: Antioxidants, Biomarkers, Chaperones, *Caenorhabditis elegans*, Oxidative stress, Protein misfolding, Reactive oxygen species, Skin aging.

INTRODUCTION

The term "oxidative stress" refers to an imbalance favoring oxidants over-reactive oxygen species in an antioxidant defense system [1]. Protein misfolding is caused by the protein following an incorrect folding pathway which may lead to spontaneous misfolding. Aging is a visible indicator of the accumulation of mal-

---
* **Corresponding author Maushmi S. Kumar:** Somaiya Institute for Research and Consultancy, Somaiya Vidyavihar University, Vidyavihar (East), Mumbai-400077, India; E-mail: maushmiskumar@gmail.com

Pardeep Kaur, Tewin Tencomnao, Robin and Rajendra G. Mehta (Eds.)

functioning or toxic proteins that sensitize other proteins to oxidative damage which is most prominently observed on the skin [2].

Oxidative Stress – The Underlying Mechanism

The term "oxidative stress" refers to an imbalance favoring oxidants over the antioxidant defense system, which disrupts redox signaling and may be accompanied by molecular damage [1]. Reactive oxygen species (ROS) that are commonly involved include hydroxyl radicals (OH), superoxide radicals (O_2), singlet oxygen, and hydrogen peroxide (H_2O_2), which are metabolic by-products of biological systems [3, 4]. Apoptosis, immunity, differentiation, and phosphory-lation of proteins are a few processes depending upon correct ROS production and occurrence within cells and both should be maintained at a low level [2]. As ROS production increases, crucial cellular components like proteins, nucleic acids, and lipids are negatively impacted [5]. The fundamental premise is that there is a maintenance of a constant balance of redox in an open metabolic system at a specific setpoint, providing the redox tone a base. Any change from the constant redox balance is considered stress, triggering a stress response. According to the definition of oxidative stress, there are two types of aberrations: physiological deviations, known as "oxidative eustress", and supraphysiological deviations, known as "oxidative distress". Redox regulation and physiological redox signaling depend on oxidative eustress. This idea and the redox equilibrium being the "golden mean" are related [1, 6, 7]. Oxidant signaling is specific to a target while higher exposure of oxidants beyond the normal causes damage due to reaching unspecified targets. Fig. (1) exhibits the oxidative stress mechanisms and its therapy.

Biomarkers Involved in Oxidative Stress

Biomarkers are biomolecules altered upon interaction with antioxidant system molecules or ROS' in the microenvironment and those that change in response to increased redox stress are two categories of biomarkers of oxidative stress. Molecules like proteins, carbohydrates, lipids (including phospholipids), and DNA are some of those that can be altered *in vivo* owing to too many ROS'. A crucial factor involved in the determination of the validity of the marker is the causal effect or the functional importance of oxidative alteration on the functioning of the cells, organs, and the system. The availability of a suitable biological specimen, the biomarker's stability when subjected to various storage conditions and during preparation of the specimen process, and the specificity, sensitivity, and repeatability of the assay used to measure the modification are additional factors that affect a ROS biomarker's clinical applicability [8]. Table **1** enlists the various biomarkers of oxidative stress along with their advantages, and problems encountered along with some remarks regarding the same.

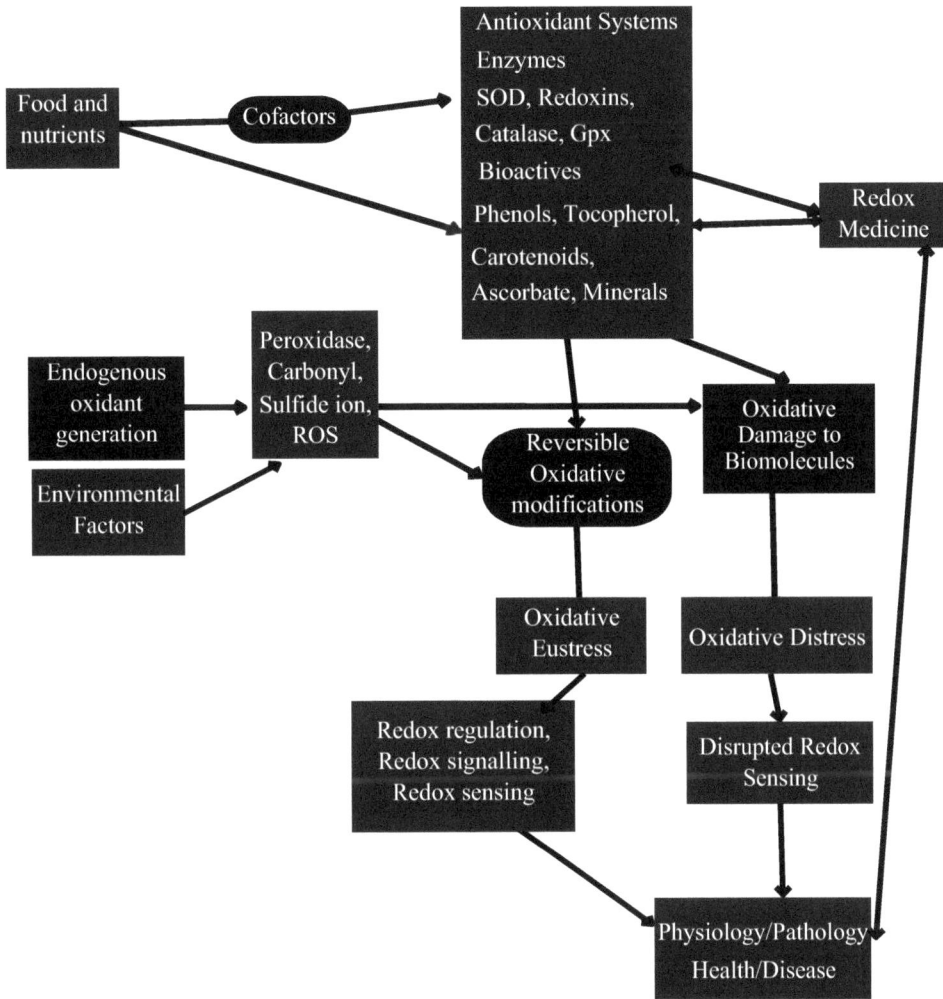

Fig. (1). Oxidative stress mechanism and therapy.

Table 1. Biomarkers, their advantages, and disadvantages.

Biomarker	Advantages	Problems	Remarks	References
IsoPs	Detectable in various samples (urine, serum) easily.	Current quantification techniques are not suitable, and modifications are required.	Lack of evidence linking biomarkers to their clinical outcomes.	[9 - 11]

(Table 1) cont.....

Biomarker	Advantages	Problems	Remarks	References
OxLDL	An elevated OxLDL is linked to increased clinical seriousness. It is indicative of future complications in healthy people. It is easy to reproduce from frozen samples.	A decrease in OxLDL is not linked with an improvement in clinical conditions.	ELISAs for OxLDL detection are easily available.	[12 - 15]
S-glutathionylation	S-glutathionylation of SERCA, eNOS, and Na^+–K^+ pump are biomarkers and have pathological functions as well.	Detection of S-glutathionylation is not generally an accurate representation. Access to the clinical source is an obstacle.	Modified Hb is currently being investigated as a biomarker.	[16 - 19]
MDA	ELISA kits can easily detect MDA with good performance, and TRABS assay is easy to perform.	TBARS assay sample preparation can affect the results and is non-specific.	Serves as a promising clinical biomarker.	[20 - 22]
ROS-mediated gene levels and expression alterations	The expression of genes can be analyzed by microarray.	Microarray technology needs computational and manual expertise.	It is ambiguous whether the expression profile of cells in biological samples reflects that in cardiovascular tissues.	[23]

Antioxidants prevent the spread of free radicals or prevent their synthesis through a variety of processes, which inhibit autoxidation. These substances aid in quenching $\cdot O_2$, quenching the chain reaction of auto-oxidation, scavenging species that cause the peroxidation, and inhibiting the production of peroxides [24]. Antioxidants with the capacity to thwart the free radical chain reaction are the most potent. These antioxidants can contribute H$\cdot$ to the free radicals produced in the course of oxidative reactions because of the phenolic or aromatic rings that they contain. The resonance delocalizes electrons within the aromatic ring and then stabilizes the radical intermediate [25]. By eliminating the free radical intermediates, antioxidants play a crucial part in stopping oxidative chain reactions [26]. Numerous studies show that mitochondrial activity and ROS-mediated signaling depend critically on the cellular redox condition [27]. The mitochondrial ROS production is considerably increased, and the mitochondrial membrane becomes depolarized when intracellular glutathione (GSH) levels are low [28]. The action of antioxidative defense enzymes along with intracellular GSH modification as a stress response depends critically on the Nrf2/ARE pathway being stimulated [29]. Tocopherol (vitamin E) and Ascorbic acid (vitamin C) are both low molecular weight antioxidants that a human body cannot synthesize [30, 31].

Glutathione

Glutathione shields cells from the harm caused by ROS, such as peroxides, lipid peroxides, heavy metals, and heavy metals [32]. Through enzymatic and non-enzymatic processes, glutathione can remove ROS [33]. Glutathione has a free thiol group contributing to the non-enzymatic antioxidant action. Detoxification of oxidants and electrophiles is also done by glutathione *via* enzymatic processes involving peroxidase, glutathione reductase, and glutathione-S transferase [34]. Glutathione facilitates thiol-disulfide exchange concurrently with protein disulfide isomerases and glutaredoxin which modulates the correct tertiary protein structure and in turn, regulates the redox status of the cell. For humans, glutathione is regarded as non-essential because the body can make it from amino acids like glycine, L-cysteine, and L-glutamic acid [35].

Polyphenols

Plants produce polyphenols as secondary metabolites, which are frequently found in fruits and vegetables [29]. The group of polyphenols that have been studied the most are called flavonoids. Flavonoids have a diphenyl propane skeleton as their fundamental structure of a closed pyran ring formed by two benzene (A and B) rings joined by 3 carbon chains [36]. Flavonoids have antioxidant properties that include scavenging ROS [37], preventing ROS production by enzyme inhibition [38], trace element chelation, and enhancing antioxidant defenses [39]. Due to their low redox potential, flavonoids can be used to donate protons to reduce highly oxidized free radicals such as peroxyl, hydroxyl, and alkoxyl radicals [40]. Superoxide anion is synthesized enzymatically including protein kinase C and xanthine oxidase which are inhibited *via* flavonoids [38]. Other ROS-producing enzymes, such as COX, lipoxygenase, mitochondrial succinoxidase, microsomal monooxygenase, and NADH oxidase, have also been reported to be inhibited by flavonoids [41]. Coumarin derivatives also show good free radical scavenging properties [42].

Carotenoids

Organic pigments produced in plastids of many bacteria, fungi, plants, and algae are Carotenoids. Carotenoids (*Acyrthosiphon pisum*) are only generated by the spider mite (*Tetranychus urticae*) and the red pea aphid [43]. More than 600 different carotenoids have currently been found to serve a variety of purposes [44]. Based on their chemistry, carotenes, and xanthophylls are the two types of carotenoids [45]. In addition to their antioxidant effects, carotenoids also influence the cell cycle, apoptosis, and differentiation of cells [46], boost the immune response and system, control cell signaling pathways [47], and increase growth factors [48] and adhesion molecules [49]. Highly lipophilic carotenoids live inside the cells to protect the membrane from oxidative damage [50].

Dietary Minerals

These are elements with fixed chemical formulae and universal structures occurring naturally. All living things need certain chemical compounds, which are found in dietary minerals. For physical health to be maintained, each dietary mineral must be consumed in sufficient amounts.

Macrominerals and trace minerals are the two major categories into which dietary minerals are divided. The macrominerals that the body needs in greater proportions are phosphorus, calcium, potassium, sodium, magnesium, and chloride. Contrarily, trace elements are dietary minerals including copper, selenium, zinc, iodine, fluoride, and iron that are needed in very small levels for normal cellular activity [51]. Minerals with antioxidant characteristics include magnesium, zinc, selenium, and copper. Zinc regulates the metabolism of glutathione, inhibits the enzyme nicotinamide adenine dinucleotide phosphate-oxidase (NADPH-oxidase) [52], and is a cofactor for the superoxide dismutase enzyme to function as an antioxidant in the body [53]. Non-enzymatic antioxidants used as the first line of defense are considered preventative antioxidants. These antioxidants interact with the transition metal ions to block new reactive species' emergence [54]. Non-enzymatic antioxidants play a vital role in both the first and second lines of defense against ROS, which are represented by molecules having the capacity to neutralize oxidants and radicals [54].

Ascorbic Acid

Ascorbic acid is a hydrosoluble antioxidant, also known as vitamin C. In numerous enzyme-catalyzed activities, Ascorbic acid acts as a cofactor including preserving the integrity of connective and vascular tissue and strengthening collagen [55]. Decreasing ascorbate levels in tissues and the aging process have been linked, according to data from both animal and population-based research. Age-related ascorbate decline is caused by several complex mechanisms, including increasing use, decreased cellular uptake, decreased absorption/ reabsorption, and accelerated turnover of cells. When used in combination, ascorbic acid is a valuable nutritional supplement for the prevention of secondary diseases associated with aging. Ascorbic acid has a myriad of functions. It scavenges the free radicals and acts as a reducing agent along with quenching singlet oxygen.

Vitamin E

Vitamin E is made up of eight structurally related lipophilic chromanol congeners. Vitamin E is made up of phytyl tails of eight tocopherols and eight tocotrienols which are typically found in food containing three double bonds and four saturated bonds, respectively. Vitamin E is mainly found in the diet as tocopherol which has strong antioxidant properties [46]. It is the isoform of vitamin E that is mostly found in mammalian tissue. Overall, tocotrienols and tocopherols may be effective agents for reducing oxidative stress and avoiding illnesses associated with aging. Comparative randomized clinical trials need to be performed for further examination of the possible effects of tocopherols and tocotrienols on age-related illnesses.

Ubiquinone

Coenzyme Q10, commonly known as ubiquinone (UQ), is created by the body's cells, or can alternatively be consumed through food [56]. The best sources of dietary UQ are meat and fish [51]. Additionally, liver, soy oil, sardines' kidney, beef, heart, and peanuts all contain UQ. A redox-active benzoquinone head group with a poly-isoprenoid side chain of species-specific length attachment creates UQ, a naturally occurring vitamin-like molecule. UQ levels, on the other hand, decline as we age and eventually lead to several aging-related ailments. A prominent contributing cause to the onset of chronic diseases may be the decline in UQ levels with age. Ubiquinone is a very effective antioxidant to neutralize ROS. To protect mitochondrial oxidative damage, many antioxidants targeting mitochondrial oxidative damage have been developed of which MitoQ is a great option [51].

Organosulfur Compounds

Vegetable species are mostly found in the Brassicaceae family and the *Allium* genus contains organosulfur compounds. Allium sulfur compounds are essential for defense [16]. For the action of enzymes, sulfur is a molecule made up of several amino acids along with Fe-S clusters. For biogenesis, clusters of Fe-S are crucial, especially for acetyl-CoA, RNA, and DNA [57]. Phase II and glutathione enzymes are modulated by organosulfur compounds, which also suppress inflammatory mediators. However, the medicinal potential of these antioxidants is constrained by their weak water solubility and low stability [58].

PROTEIN MISFOLDING AND ITS MECHANISM

It is an improper folding caused by the synthesis of proteins with a conformation not analogous to its native folding. Several factors can cause proteins to misfold, including:

i. Gene sequence undergoes somatic mutations resulting in the production of a protein incapable of adopting its native folding.

ii. Errors in transcription or translation result in modified protein production incapable of correct folding.

iii. Failure of the chaperone as folding machinery.

iv. Errors on the post-translational modifications (PTM).

v. Structural modifications resulting from environmental changes.

vi. Seeding and cross-seeding mechanism induced misfolding [59].

Misfolding of proteins often leads to self-aggregation because of the improper exposure of solvent to protein fragments that causes a high level of stickiness. The β-sheet, which can hold virtually interminable numbers of polypeptide chains, provides the most beneficial arrangement for these intermolecular aggregates [60]. Misfolded proteins thus are found in a broad and heterogeneous continuum of polymeric sizes, often categorized in poorly defined and nonspecific categories like oligomers, fibrils, and protofibrils. The most toxic species in the folding and aggregation pathway might be the Oligomers [61 - 63]. Protein misfolding and aggregation are explained by the so-called "seeding-nucleation" paradigm [63]. A fast elongation stage is followed by a sluggish and thermodynamically unfavorable nucleation phase throughout the process. Stable seed creation or protein-polymerized nucleus is the rate-determining step in the nucleation phase. Incorporating monomeric protein into the polymer allows the seeds to develop quickly after they are formed. Large polymers may fragment *in vivo* by an unknown method to produce additional seeds for the reaction. The ability of prepared seeds to significantly speed up the process of aggregation *via* the attraction of normal soluble protein into the expanding aggregate is a characteristic aspect of the seeding-nucleation paradigm [63]. From a biophysical perspective, the protein aggregation and misfolding processes entail reorganizing the structure of protein into numerous strands that are negatively charged. Hydrogen bonds along with hydrophobic interactions help in the stabilization of these strands. They then reveal "sticky" ends that draw in molecules of folded or partially unfolded proteins, causing their misfolding to fit into the cross-polymeric structure. Although the main structure of the wrongly folded aggregates resembles, individual molecules can adopt different arrangements. Fig. (**2**) depicts the mechanism at a glance.

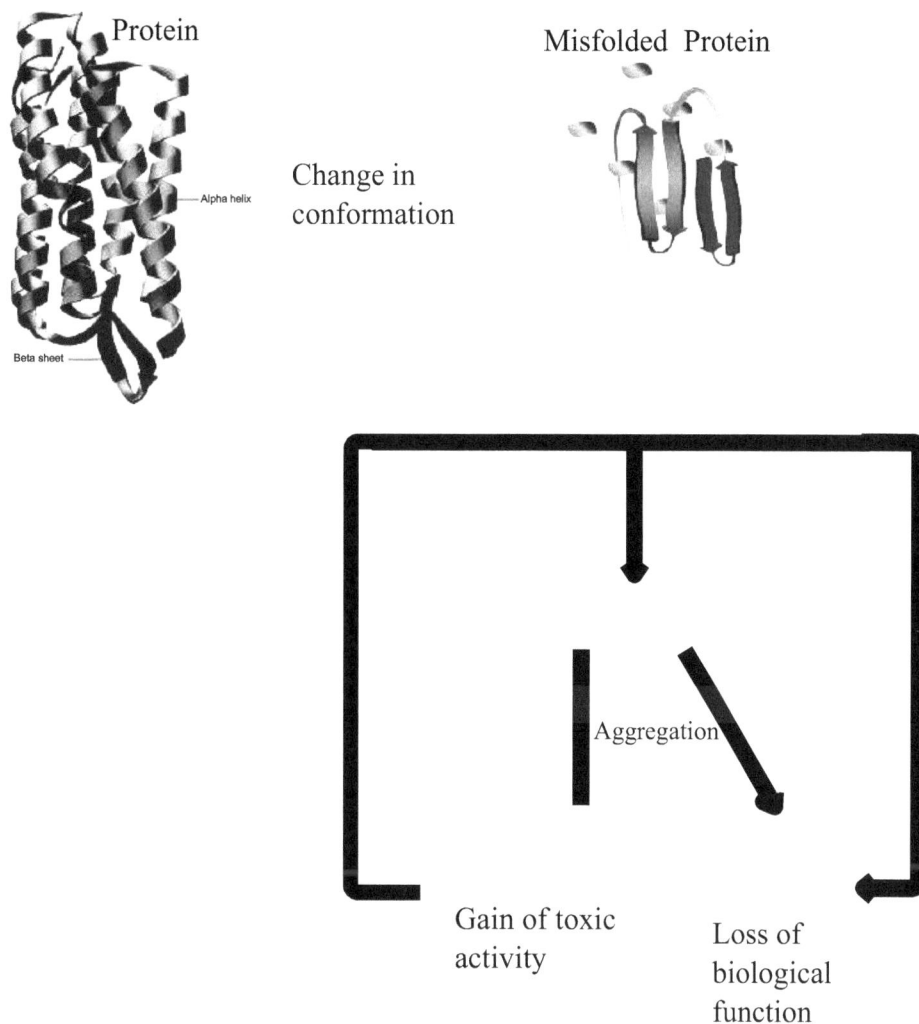

Fig. (2). Protein misfolding mechanism.

Chaperones

The numerous families of multidomain proteins known as molecular chaperones have evolved to help developing proteins attain their natural fold, inhibit protein aggregation, shield subunits from heat shock during complex assembly, or mediate selective unfolding and disassembly. Cell health and an organism's longevity are drastically influenced by their enhanced expression in responding to stress. Proteostasis, another name for protein quality control, is the control of protein production, folding, unfolding, and turnover.

Chaperone and protease systems, as well as cellular elimination processes including autophagy and lysosomal degradation, mediate it. These quality control mechanisms are crucial to the survival of cells because they guarantee the correct folding of proteins and perform their functions at the appropriate time and location. They are essential for reducing the harmful effects of protein aggregation and misfolding.

Controlling protein quality and recovering from stressful situations are important functions of molecular chaperones. They aid in folding, unfolding, and stopping or reversal in the aggregation of various substrates, however, as people age, their functions become less effective, resulting in disorders with late-onset misfolding. The main cellular chaperone systems, heat shock protein 60 (HSP60), heat shock protein 70 (HSP70), heat shock protein 90 (HSP90), and heat shock protein 100 (HSP100), function by stabilizing non-native proteins, unfolding misfolded proteins or folded proteins that are intended for proteolysis, and promoting favorable folding conditions. With several uncovered binding sites for co-chaperones that control their activities in various biological pathways, HSP70 and HSP90 are highly interacting, open structures. HSP60 and HSP100, in contrast, have internalized active sites, few collaborating partners, and are self-contained. Chaperones are dynamic, highly adaptable machines. Their domains rotate up to 100° and are displaced up to 50 or more to function on their substrates.

The availability and kinetics of binding sites for non-native proteins are affected by ATP binding and hydrolysis. For instance, when HSP70 interacts with the ATPase domain, the lid subdomain of the substrate-binding domain fully opens, whereas an open ring is transformed into an enclosed container for protein folding by HSP60 [64].

Skin Aging

Aging is a visible indicator of the accumulation of malfunctioning or toxic proteins that sensitize other proteins to oxidative damage which is most prominently observed on the skin [65]. Skin aging is determined by characteristics like elasticity loss, wrinkles, an appearance of rough texture, and laxity. The aging process is followed by phenotypic alterations in cells of skin along with functional and structural changes in extracellular matrix elements like elastin and collagen [66]. The following paragraphs describe the role of various elements responsible for their role in skin aging.

Collagen

The primary modifications seen in aging skin are structural and quantitative in collagen fibers [67]. Collagen fibrils in the skin that has aged are fractured and unevenly dispersed, contrary to those in youthful skin, which are plentiful, compactly stuffed, and arranged whole collagen fibrils [67, 68]. Clinical modifications brought on by this process include loss of suppleness and skin wrinkling, which are seen in the two photoaged and naturally aging skin. ECM proteins include collagen, fibronectin, and elastin which are crucial for maintaining the integrity of the skin. The following three factors influence ECM by different mechanisms which directly affect skin aging.

Increase in Matrix Metalloproteinase Levels (MMPs)

MMPs are a group of ubiquitous endopeptidases that can break down ECM proteins [69]. MMPs can be divided into five main subgroups, namely: (1) matrilysins (MMP-7 and MMP-26); (2) gelatinases (MMP-2 and MMP-9); (3) membrane-type (MT) MMPs (MMP-14, MMP-15, and MMP-16) (4) Collagenases (MMP-1, MMP-8, and MMP-13); and (5) stromelysins (MMP-3, MMP-10, and MMP-11) [70]. Collagen fibers, primarily types I and III in human skin, are fragmented by the main protease known as MMP-1. Collagen can be further broken down by MMP-3 and MMP-9 after being first cleaved by MMP-1. MMPs can be made by endothelial cells and immunocytes, however dermal fibroblasts and epidermal keratinocytes are the main sources of MMPs in the skin. The specific endogenous tissue inhibitors of metalloproteinases (TIMPs), a group of four protease inhibitors made up of TIMP-1, TIMP-2, TIMP-3, and TIMP-4, control MMPs physiologically [71]. MMP-1, MMP-2, MMP-3, MMP-9, MMP-10, MMP-11, MMP-13, MMP-17, MMP-26, and MMP-27 levels have been observed to be higher in old human skin in some research [72 - 75]. MMPs and TIMPs are frequently controlled together to reduce excessive MMP activity. However, the levels of endogenous MMP inhibitors do not rise in parallel with the elevation of MMP in old skin [72, 73]. Even less TIMP-1 may be present in the skin that has undergone photoaging and intrinsic aging. This imbalance hastens the dermal collagen fragmentation process, which hastens skin aging [76]. An important factor driving the rise in MMP levels in aging skin is reactive oxygen species (ROS) [67, 77]. UV rays and metabolically produced pro-oxidants are two external and intrinsic sources of ROS that are produced in the skin. C-Jun NH2-terminal kinase and Extracellular signal-regulated kinase (ERK), p38, are family of the mitogen-activated protein kinase (MAPK) family that are triggered by ROS (JNK). This activation activates the activator protein 1 (AP-1) transcription factor, which is crucial for controlling the transcription of MMP-1, MMP-3, MMP-9, and MMP-12. Another transcription factor that is activated by ROS is nuclear factor-B (NF-B) [78]. Importantly, NF-B mediates the reactions to UV exposure and photoaging. The elevation of MMPs like MMP-1 and MMP-3 in dermal fibroblasts is brought on by NF-kB activation [70, 79, 80]. In general, photoaged skin exhibits higher oxidative damage, which may account for more noticeable accompanying aging characteristics such as deep wrinkles. MMPs are mostly produced by dermal fibroblasts in intrinsic aging, although epidermal keratinocytes also create MMPs in photoaging [70, 73].

Impaired Transforming Growth Factor-β Signalling During Aging

A key regulator of ECM production is the transforming growth factor (TGF) [81]. Through the Smad route, TGF- regulates collagen synthesis and breakdown in human dermal fibroblasts, which in turn controls collagen homeostasis. TGF- first attaches to a TGF- type II receptor (TRII), causing it to phosphorylate and draw in a TGF- type I receptor (TRI). The transcription factors Smad2 and Smad3 are triggered because of this phosphorylation of TRI. Heteromeric Smad complexes are created when activated Smad2 or Smad3 binds with Smad4. Smad-binding elements (SBE) in the promoter regions of TGF-target genes interact with these activated Smad complexes when they move to the nucleus [82]. Thus, TGF-/Smad signaling directly upregulates ECM genes such as collagens, decorin, fibronectin, and versican. In contrast, the Smad signaling network upregulates TIMPs and downregulates MMPs. This shows that by promoting ECM formation and preventing ECM degradation, the TGF-/Smad signaling route is essential for preserving the mechanical and structural unity of dermal connective tissue. Dermal fibroblasts in aging skin are inhibited from signaling through TGF- by the ROS-induced AP-1. According to several earlier investigations, reduced TGF-signaling may be caused by a particular downregulation of TRII and SMAD3 expression. Impaired TGF-signalling causes decreased neo-collagen production, which lowers the net amount of collagen in the dermis [83].

Interaction Between Fibroblasts and the ECM

Fibroblasts cling to the surrounding healthy ECM, which is primarily made up of type I collagen in young skin [84, 85]. This adhesion enables fibroblasts to spread and keep up a typical extended shape while also applying mechanical pressures to the surrounding ECM. As the ECM degrades over time, fibroblast attachment is hindered in aging skin, leading to smaller fibroblasts with less elongation and collapsed shape [84, 86, 87]. Senescent fibroblasts have reduced size, which is a distinguishing characteristic and is associated with lower levels of ECM component synthesis [72]. Reduced dermal fibroblast cell size and spreading can lead to multiplication in mitochondrial ROS production [88]. TRII is downregulated selectively by the reduction in fibroblast size and mechanical stresses, and this downregulation substantially causes a decrease in TGF-regulated ECM synthesis [86]. Additionally, the diminution of fibroblast size controls ECM deterioration by raising MMP levels. A mechanism has been postulated by which age-related fibroblast size decrease causes activation of AP-1, which then triggers the creation of many Matrix Mellaproteinases as seen in aging human skin. This route may be mediated by fibroblasts with aged characteristics that have elevated ROS levels [73].

TREATMENT

Aging has become a major concern in today's era as age-related conditions are a major cause of death worldwide. Many anti-aging approaches are being studied. Some novel approaches include young blood plasma transfusions, stem cell therapy, senescent cell elimination, *etc.* Table **2** lists some widely used anti-aging drugs. They have different mechanisms ranging from inhibition of autophagy to senescent cell elimination as mentioned earlier to combat aging.

Table 2. Common anti-aging drugs and their mode of action.

Drug	Mode of Action	References
Perifosine	Akt and mTOR axis component inhibition	[89]
RSVA314 and RSVA405	AMPK activation inhibits mTOR and simultaneously increases autophagy and Aβ degradation.	[90]
BRD5631	mTOR-independent pathway causes autophagy, IL-1β decrease, and NPC1.	[91]
PI103	mTOR and selective PI3KC1a inhibitor, Dual ATP-competitive in nature	[92]
Pifithrin-α	p53 inhibitor	[93, 94]
IR-58	Mitochondrial membrane 44 (TIM44)- inhibitor	[95]
Prazosin	Increase in p-AMPK and p53 decrease in Akt/mTOR	[96]
Navitoclax	Targeting Bcl-2 family	[97]
Panobinostat	Decreases Bcl-xL expression and increases acetylation of Histone 3	[98]
Geldanamycin	Reduces HSP90	[99]
Dasatinib	Relates with P53 and inhibits PAI-2	[100]
A1331852	Reduces Bcl-xL	[101]
A1155463	Reduces Bcl-xL	[101]

Natural Products and Their Role in Anti-Aging

Aloe vera

It contains mucopolysaccharides which aid in moisture binding to the skin. It also has a stimulant action on fibroblasts which results in the production of elastin and collagen fibers. This reduces wrinkles and gives elasticity to the skin. It brings softness to the skin *via* its cohesive action on the superficial flaking epidermal cells as well as *via* amino acids [102].

It also inhibits the stimulated granulocyte MMPs and thus further contributing to its anti-aging action. The aloe gel is frequently employed for its use [103].

Curcuma longa

It contains the active constituent of curcumin. It shows its activity *via* multiple mechanisms; one of its primary mechanisms is neutralizing oxidative stress. It does so *via* free radical scavenging, reducing malondialdehyde and also *via* increasing the activity of antioxidant enzymes. It also acts *via* inhibition of MMP-2 expression [103]. Curcumin also shows a positive effect on renal health which contributes to its anti-aging activity [104].

Zingiber officinale

Ginger shows good antioxidant activity when extracted in alcohol [105]. Its antioxidant activity contributes to ginger's delaying the aging of various organs in our body. It reduces inflammation [106], and inhibits elastase derived from fibroblast, which is responsible for breaking down elastin and sometimes collagen too. It also prevents elasticity reduction in the skin [103].

Citrus sinensis

C. sinesis peels have a high content of phenols, flavonoids, and antioxidants [107]. Along with their antioxidant activity, they also reduce MMP 1 expression and improve collagen formation [108]. They also modulate cellular responses like cleavage of procaspase -3, AP-1 translocation, and NF-kB [103].

Piper betel

It shows its activity *via* the prevention of photosensitization-mediated lipid peroxidation as well as inhibitory action on MMP -1, elastase and hyaluronidase [109]. It is recognized in Ayurveda and shows superior free radical scavenging activity along with a radioprotectant activity providing protection from aging caused due to UV light or any other radiation [110].

Curculigo orchioides

Curculigo orchioides is also known as Kali Musli, a rasayana herb native to India. It is used as an anticancer, immunostimulant, antioxidant and antidiabetic agent. Some chemical constituents found in them are phenolic glycosides, mucilage, and saponins. They have shown inhibitory activity against MMP1 in cultured human skin fibroblasts [103, 111].

Prunus dulcis

Prunus dulcis also known as almond is from the Rosaceae family, and it is a source of essential nutrients. Some important chemical constituents present in it are amino acids, carbohydrates, proteins, lipids, fatty acids, and vitamins. It works by reducing the degradative changes induced in the skin upon exposure to UV radiation [112].

Labisia pumila

Labisia pumila shows free radical scavenging activity and its extract markedly inhibited the TNF-α production. Extract of *L. pumila* downregulated enhanced MMP-1 and MMP-9 expression in keratinocytes in a dose-dependent manner which suggests its potential as an antiphotoaging cosmetic ingredient [103].

Aesculus hippocastanum

Aesculus hippocastanum belongs to the family of Hippocastanaceae. It uses fibroblast-populated collagen gels to generate contraction forces by non-muscle (fibroblast) cells. It is pivotal in determining cell morphology, vasoconstriction, and wound healing in non-muscle cells [113]

Significance of *Caenorhabditis elegans*

Around $2/3^{rd}$ of all human disease genes have homologs in the *C. elegans* genome, which makes it a model for studies in aging [114], related disorders, drug screening, and longevity have gained widespread recognition in recent times because of its physiological aging characteristics [115]. Several signaling pathways and associated epigenetic modifications, such as the insulin/IGF-1 signaling (IIS), AMPK, and mTOR were found to be affected by mutations responsible for increasing lifespan in *C. elegans* and were found to delay aging. It is interesting to note that a restricted diet demonstrated a lengthened life span and shielded several metazoans from various age-related diseases. Uncertainty exists regarding the underlying molecular pathways. *C. elegans* has become a popular model system in recent years for high-throughput drug testing [89].

CONCLUSION

The mechanisms established in the different sections of the chapter are of critical significance for future treatments. Many novel treatments nowadays target various aspects. The role of chaperones in our body as a natural defense mechanism is critical. *C. elegans* has a significant contribution to the understanding of all mechanisms due to its simpler nature. The future for anti-aging is becoming brighter with natural bio-actives from terrestrial as well as marine sources.

ABBREVIATIONS

ROS   Reactive Oxygen Species

IsoPs   Isoprostanes

OxLDL   Oxidized LDL

SERCA   Sarcoendoplasmic Reticulum Calcium ATPase

eNOS   Endothelial Nitric Oxide Synthase

ELISA   Enzyme-linked Immunosorbent Assay

MDA   Malondialdehyde

TBAR's   Thiobarbituric Acid Reactive Substances

GSH   Glutathione

COX   Cyclooxygenase

NADH   Nicotinamide Adenine Dinucleotide + H

NADP   Nicotinamide Adenine Dinucleotide Phosphate

SOD   Superoxide Disumutase

GPx   Glutathione Peroxidase

UQ   Ubiquinone

HSP   Heat Shock Protein

ECM   Extracellular Matrix

MMP   Matrix Melloproteinase

TIMP   Tissue Inhibitor of Melloproteinases

TGF   Transforming Growth Factor

SMAD   *Caenorhabditis elegans* Sma Genes and the Drosophila Mad, Mothers Against Decapentaplegic

AP   Activator Protein

Akt-   Protein Kinase B

MTOR   Mechanistic Target of Rapamycin

AMPK   AMP Activated Protein Kinase

IL   Interleukin

NPC   Niemann Pick Disease

Bcl   B-cell Lymphoma

ACKNOWLEDGEMENTS

We acknowledge SVKM's NMIMS and Somaiya Vidyavihar University for providing support while authoring the chapter.

REFERENCES

[1]   Sies H, Berndt C, Jones DP. Oxidative stress. Annu Rev Biochem 2017; 86(1): 715-48.
[http://dx.doi.org/10.1146/annurev-biochem-061516-045037] [PMID: 28441057]

[2]   Rajendran P, Nandakumar N, Rengarajan T, *et al.* Antioxidants and human diseases. Clin Chim Acta 2014; 436: 332-47.
[http://dx.doi.org/10.1016/j.cca.2014.06.004] [PMID: 24933428]

[3]   Sato H, Shibata M, Shimizu T, *et al.* Differential cellular localization of antioxidant enzymes in the trigeminal ganglion. Neuroscience 2013; 248: 345-58.
[http://dx.doi.org/10.1016/j.neuroscience.2013.06.010] [PMID: 23774632]

[4]   Navarro-Yepes J, Zavala-Flores L, Anandhan A, *et al.* Antioxidant gene therapy against neuronal cell death. Pharmacol Ther 2014; 142(2): 206-30.
[http://dx.doi.org/10.1016/j.pharmthera.2013.12.007] [PMID: 24333264]

[5]   Taniyama Y, Griendling KK. Reactive oxygen species in the vasculature: Molecular and cellular mechanisms. Hypertension 2003; 42(6): 1075-81.
[http://dx.doi.org/10.1161/01.HYP.0000100443.09293.4F] [PMID: 14581295]

[6]   Sies H. Hydrogen peroxide as a central redox signaling molecule in physiological oxidative stress: Oxidative eustress. Redox Biol 2017; 11: 613-9.
[http://dx.doi.org/10.1016/j.redox.2016.12.035] [PMID: 28110218]

[7]   Sies H, Jones DP. Reactive oxygen species (ROS) as pleiotropic physiological signalling agents. Nat Rev Mol Cell Biol 2020; 21(7): 363-83.
[http://dx.doi.org/10.1038/s41580-020-0230-3] [PMID: 32231263]

[8]   Dalle-Donne I, Scaloni A, Giustarini D, *et al.* Proteins as biomarkers of oxidative/nitrosative stress in diseases: The contribution of redox proteomics. Mass Spectrom Rev 2005; 24(1): 55-99.
[http://dx.doi.org/10.1002/mas.20006] [PMID: 15389864]

[9]   Morrow JD. Quantification of isoprostanes as indices of oxidant stress and the risk of atherosclerosis in humans. Arterioscler Thromb Vasc Biol 2005; 25(2): 279-86.
[http://dx.doi.org/10.1161/01.ATV.0000152605.64964.c0] [PMID: 15591226]

[10]   Smith KA, Shepherd J, Wakil A, Kilpatrick ES. A comparison of methods for the measurement of 8-isoPGF2a: A marker of oxidative stress. Ann Clin Biochem 2011; 48(2): 147-54.
[http://dx.doi.org/10.1258/acb.2010.010151] [PMID: 21292864]

[11]   Wu T, Rifai N, Roberts LJ II, Willett WC, Rimm EB. Stability of measurements of biomarkers of oxidative stress in blood over 36 hours. Cancer Epidemiol Biomarkers Prev 2004; 13(8): 1399-402.
[http://dx.doi.org/10.1158/1055-9965.1399.13.8] [PMID: 15298964]

[12]   Pai JK, Curhan GC, Cannuscio CC, Rifai N, Ridker PM, Rimm EB. Stability of novel plasma markers associated with cardiovascular disease: Processing within 36 hours of specimen collection. Clin Chem 2002; 48(10): 1781-4.
[http://dx.doi.org/10.1093/clinchem/48.10.1781] [PMID: 12324497]

[13]   Holvoet P, Vanhaecke J, Janssens S, Van de Werf F, Collen D. Oxidized LDL and malondialdehyde-modified LDL in patients with acute coronary syndromes and stable coronary artery disease. Circulation 1998; 98(15): 1487-94.
[http://dx.doi.org/10.1161/01.CIR.98.15.1487] [PMID: 9769301]

[14]   Ehara S, Ueda M, Naruko T, *et al.* Elevated levels of oxidized low density lipoprotein show a positive

relationship with the severity of acute coronary syndromes. Circulation 2001; 103(15): 1955-60.
[http://dx.doi.org/10.1161/01.CIR.103.15.1955] [PMID: 11306523]

[15]   Meisinger C, Baumert J, Khuseyinova N, Loewel H, Koenig W. Plasma oxidized low-density lipoprotein, a strong predictor for acute coronary heart disease events in apparently healthy, middle-aged men from the general population. Circulation 2005; 112(5): 651-7.
[http://dx.doi.org/10.1161/CIRCULATIONAHA.104.529297] [PMID: 16043640]

[16]   Pietta PG. Flavonoids as antioxidants. J Nat Prod 2000; 63(7): 1035-42.
[http://dx.doi.org/10.1021/np9904509] [PMID: 10924197]

[17]   Adachi T, Weisbrod RM, Pimentel DR, *et al.* S-Glutathiolation by peroxynitrite activates SERCA during arterial relaxation by nitric oxide. Nat Med 2004; 10(11): 1200-7.
[http://dx.doi.org/10.1038/nm1119] [PMID: 15489859]

[18]   Chen CA, Wang TY, Varadharaj S, *et al.* S-glutathionylation uncouples eNOS and regulates its cellular and vascular function. Nature 2010; 468(7327): 1115-8.
[http://dx.doi.org/10.1038/nature09599] [PMID: 21179168]

[19]   Rossi R, Dalle-Donne I, Milzani A, Giustarini D. Oxidized forms of glutathione in peripheral blood as biomarkers of oxidative stress. Clin Chem 2006; 52(7): 1406-14.
[http://dx.doi.org/10.1373/clinchem.2006.067793] [PMID: 16690733]

[20]   Meagher EA, FitzGerald GA. Indices of lipid peroxidation *in vivo*: Strengths and limitations. Free Radic Biol Med 2000; 28(12): 1745-50.
[http://dx.doi.org/10.1016/S0891-5849(00)00232-X] [PMID: 10946216]

[21]   Bevan RJ, Durand MF, Hickenbotham PT, *et al.* Validation of a novel ELISA for measurement of MDA-LDL in human plasma. Free Radic Biol Med 2003; 35(5): 517-27.
[http://dx.doi.org/10.1016/S0891-5849(03)00359-9] [PMID: 12927601]

[22]   Walter MF, Jacob RF, Jeffers B, *et al.* Serum levels of thiobarbituric acid reactive substances predict cardiovascular events in patients with stable coronary artery disease. J Am Coll Cardiol 2004; 44(10): 1996-2002.
[http://dx.doi.org/10.1016/j.jacc.2004.08.029] [PMID: 15542282]

[23]   Salonen JT, Nyysso¨nen K, Salonen R, *et al.* Lipoprotein oxidation and progression of carotid atherosclerosis. Circulation 1997; 95(4): 840-5.
[http://dx.doi.org/10.1161/01.CIR.95.4.840] [PMID: 9054740]

[24]   Gaschler MM, Stockwell BR. Lipid peroxidation in cell death. Biochem Biophys Res Commun 2017; 482(3): 419-25.
[http://dx.doi.org/10.1016/j.bbrc.2016.10.086] [PMID: 28212725]

[25]   Wojtunik-Kulesza KA, Oniszczuk A, Oniszczuk T, Waksmundzka-Hajnos M. The influence of common free radicals and antioxidants on development of Alzheimer's Disease. Biomed Pharmacother 2016; 78: 39-49.
[http://dx.doi.org/10.1016/j.biopha.2015.12.024] [PMID: 26898423]

[26]   Gholamian-Dehkordi N, Luther T, Asadi-Samani M, Mahmoudian-Sani MR. An overview on natural antioxidants for oxidative stress reduction in cancers: A systematic review. Immunopathologia Persa 2017; 3(2): e12.
[http://dx.doi.org/10.15171/ipp.2017.04]

[27]   Fang W, Wang C, He Y, Zhou Y, Peng X, Liu S. Resveratrol alleviates diabetic cardiomyopathy in rats by improving mitochondrial function through PGC-1α deacetylation. Acta Pharmacol Sin 2018; 39(1): 59-73.
[http://dx.doi.org/10.1038/aps.2017.50] [PMID: 28770830]

[28]   Lohan SB, Vitt K, Scholz P, Keck CM, Meinke MC. ROS production and glutathione response in keratinocytes after application of β-carotene and VIS/NIR irradiation. Chem Biol Interact 2018; 280: 1-7.

[http://dx.doi.org/10.1016/j.cbi.2017.12.002] [PMID: 29203372]

[29]   Liu X, Chen K, Zhu L, *et al.* Soyasaponin Ab protects against oxidative stress in HepG2 cells *via* Nrf2/HO-1/NQO1 signaling pathways. J Funct Foods 2018; 45: 110-7.
[http://dx.doi.org/10.1016/j.jff.2018.03.037]

[30]   Kovacic P, Somanathan R. Cell signaling and receptors with resorcinols and flavonoids: Redox, reactive oxygen species, and physiological effects. J Recept Signal Transduct Res 2011; 31(4): 265-70.
[http://dx.doi.org/10.3109/10799893.2011.586353] [PMID: 21745156]

[31]   Podda M, Grundmann-Kollmann M. Low molecular weight antioxidants and their role in skin aging. Clin Exp Dermatol 2001; 26(7): 578-82.
[http://dx.doi.org/10.1046/j.1365-2230.2001.00902.x] [PMID: 11696061]

[32]   Pisoschi AM, Pop A. The role of antioxidants in the chemistry of oxidative stress: A review. Eur J Med Chem 2015; 97: 55-74.
[http://dx.doi.org/10.1016/j.ejmech.2015.04.040] [PMID: 25942353]

[33]   Winterbourn CC. Revisiting the reactions of superoxide with glutathione and other thiols. Arch Biochem Biophys 2016; 595: 68-71.
[http://dx.doi.org/10.1016/j.abb.2015.11.028] [PMID: 27095219]

[34]   Farhat Z, Browne RW, Bonner MR, *et al.* How do glutathione antioxidant enzymes and total antioxidant status respond to air pollution exposure? Environ Int 2018; 112: 287-93.
[http://dx.doi.org/10.1016/j.envint.2017.12.033] [PMID: 29324239]

[35]   Lu SC, Mato JM, Espinosa-Diez C, Lamas S. MicroRNA-mediated regulation of glutathione and methionine metabolism and its relevance for liver disease. Free Radic Biol Med 2016; 100: 66-72.
[http://dx.doi.org/10.1016/j.freeradbiomed.2016.03.021] [PMID: 27033954]

[36]   Das A, Majumder D, Saha C. Correlation of binding efficacies of DNA to flavonoids and their induced cellular damage. J Photochem Photobiol B 2017; 170: 256-62.
[http://dx.doi.org/10.1016/j.jphotobiol.2017.04.019] [PMID: 28456117]

[37]   Shokoohinia Y, Rashidi M, Hosseinzadeh L, Jelodarian Z. Quercetin-3-O-β-d-glucopyranoside, a dietary flavonoid, protects PC12 cells from H2O2-induced cytotoxicity through inhibition of reactive oxygen species. Food Chem 2015; 167: 162-7.
[http://dx.doi.org/10.1016/j.foodchem.2014.06.079] [PMID: 25148973]

[38]   Nile SH, Ko EY, Kim DH, Keum YS. Screening of ferulic acid related compounds as inhibitors of xanthine oxidase and cyclooxygenase-2 with anti-inflammatory activity. Rev Bras Farmacogn 2016; 26(1): 50-5.
[http://dx.doi.org/10.1016/j.bjp.2015.08.013]

[39]   Catapano M, Tvrdý V, Karlíčková J, *et al.* The stoichiometry of isoquercitrin complex with iron or copper is highly dependent on experimental conditions. Nutrients 2017; 9(11): 1193.
[http://dx.doi.org/10.3390/nu9111193] [PMID: 29084179]

[40]   Alós E, Rodrigo MJ, Zacarias L. Manipulation of carotenoid content in plants to improve human health InCarotenoids in nature. Cham: Springer 2016; pp. 311-43.

[41]   Joshi YB, Praticò D. Vitamin E in aging, dementia, and Alzheimer's disease. Biofactors 2012; 38(2): 90-7.
[http://dx.doi.org/10.1002/biof.195] [PMID: 22422715]

[42]   Pedersen JZ, Oliveira C, Incerpi S, *et al.* Antioxidant activity of 4-methylcoumarins. J Pharm Pharmacol 2010; 59(12): 1721-8.
[http://dx.doi.org/10.1211/jpp.59.12.0015] [PMID: 18053335]

[43]   Siddiqui K, Bawazeer N, Scaria Joy S. Variation in macro and trace elements in progression of type 2 diabetes. ScientificWorldJournal 2014; 2014: 1-9.
[http://dx.doi.org/10.1155/2014/461591] [PMID: 25162051]

[44] Paliwal C, Ghosh T, George B, *et al.* Microalgal carotenoids: Potential nutraceutical compounds with chemotaxonomic importance. Algal Res 2016; 15: 24-31.
[http://dx.doi.org/10.1016/j.algal.2016.01.017]

[45] Yaroshevich IA, Krasilnikov PM, Rubin AB. Functional interpretation of the role of cyclic carotenoids in photosynthetic antennas *via* quantum chemical calculations. Comput Theor Chem 2015; 1070: 27-32.
[http://dx.doi.org/10.1016/j.comptc.2015.07.016]

[46] Karadas F, Erdoğan S, Kor D, Oto G, Uluman M. The effects of different types of antioxidants (Se, vitamin E and carotenoids) in broiler diets on the growth performance, skin pigmentation and liver and plasma antioxidant concentrations. Rev Bras Cienc Avic 2016; 18(1): 101-16.
[http://dx.doi.org/10.1590/18069061-2015-0155]

[47] Kim JS, Lee WM, Rhee HC, Kim S. Red paprika (Capsicum annuum L.) and its main carotenoids, capsanthin and β-carotene, prevent hydrogen peroxide-induced inhibition of gap-junction intercellular communication. Chem Biol Interact 2016; 254: 146-55.
[http://dx.doi.org/10.1016/j.cbi.2016.05.004] [PMID: 27154496]

[48] Diener A, Rohrmann S. Associations of serum carotenoid concentrations and fruit or vegetable consumption with serum insulin-like growth factor (IGF)-1 and IGF binding protein-3 concentrations in the Third National Health and Nutrition Examination Survey (NHANES III). J Nutr Sci 2016; 5: e13.
[http://dx.doi.org/10.1017/jns.2016.1] [PMID: 27313849]

[49] Llorente B, Martinez-Garcia JF, Stange C, Rodriguez-Concepcion M. Illuminating colors: Regulation of carotenoid biosynthesis and accumulation by light. Curr Opin Plant Biol 2017; 37: 49-55.
[http://dx.doi.org/10.1016/j.pbi.2017.03.011] [PMID: 28411584]

[50] Fiedor J, Burda K. Potential role of carotenoids as antioxidants in human health and disease. Nutrients 2014; 6(2): 466-88.
[http://dx.doi.org/10.3390/nu6020466] [PMID: 24473231]

[51] Pravst I, Žmitek K, Žmitek J. Coenzyme Q10 contents in foods and fortification strategies. Crit Rev Food Sci Nutr 2010; 50(4): 269-80.
[http://dx.doi.org/10.1080/10408390902773037] [PMID: 20301015]

[52] Marreiro D, Cruz K, Morais J, Beserra J, Severo J, de Oliveira A. Zinc and oxidative stress: Current mechanisms. Antioxidants 2017; 6(2): 24.
[http://dx.doi.org/10.3390/antiox6020024] [PMID: 28353636]

[53] Nwachukwu ID, Slusarenko AJ, Gruhlke MC. Sulfur and sulfur compounds in plant defence. Nat Prod Commun 2012; 7(3)
[http://dx.doi.org/10.1177/1934578X1200700323]

[54] Mirończuk-Chodakowska I, Witkowska AM, Zujko ME. Endogenous non-enzymatic antioxidants in the human body. Adv Med Sci 2018; 63(1): 68-78.
[http://dx.doi.org/10.1016/j.advms.2017.05.005] [PMID: 28822266]

[55] May JM, Harrison FE. Role of vitamin C in the function of the vascular endothelium. Antioxid Redox Signal 2013; 19(17): 2068-83.
[http://dx.doi.org/10.1089/ars.2013.5205] [PMID: 23581713]

[56] Quinzii CM, DiMauro S, Hirano M. Human coenzyme Q10 deficiency. Neurochem Res 2007; 32(4-5): 723-7.
[http://dx.doi.org/10.1007/s11064-006-9190-z] [PMID: 17094036]

[57] Fuss JO, Tsai CL, Ishida JP, Tainer JA. Emerging critical roles of Fe-S clusters in DNA replication and repair. Biochim Biophys Acta Mol Cell Res 2015; 1853(6): 1253-71.
[http://dx.doi.org/10.1016/j.bbamcr.2015.01.018] [PMID: 25655665]

[58] Karuppath S, Pillai P, Nair SV, Lakshmanan VK. Comparison and existence of nanotechnology in

traditional alternative medicine: An onset to future medicine. Nanosci Nanotechnol Asia 2018; 8(1): 13-25.
[http://dx.doi.org/10.2174/2210681206666160402004710]

[59]   Soto C. Protein misfolding and disease: Protein refolding and therapy. FEBS Lett 2001; 498(2-3): 204-7.
[http://dx.doi.org/10.1016/S0014-5793(01)02486-3] [PMID: 11412858]

[60]   Nelson R, Sawaya MR, Balbirnie M, Madsen AØ, Riekel C, Grothe R, Eisenberg D. Structure of the cross-β spine of amyloid-like fibrils. Nature. 2005 Jun; 435(7043): 773-8.
Caughey B, Lansbury Jr PT. Protofibrils, pores, fibrils, and neurodegeneration: separating the responsible protein aggregates from the innocent bystanders. Annual review of neuroscience. 2003; 26: 267.

[61]   Glabe CG. Common mechanisms of amyloid oligomer pathogenesis in degenerative disease. Neurobiol Aging 2006; 27(4): 570-5.
[http://dx.doi.org/10.1016/j.neurobiolaging.2005.04.017] [PMID: 16481071]

[62]   Walsh DM. Sel koe DJ Ab oli gomers—a decade of discovery. J Ne u roc hem 2007; 101: 1172-84.

[63]   Soto C, Estrada L, Castilla J. Evidence supporting the prion hypothesis. Trends Biochem Sci 2006; 3(31): 150-5.
[http://dx.doi.org/10.1016/j.tibs.2006.01.002] [PMID: 16473510]

[64]   Huang Y, Zhou J, Luo S, *et al.* Identification of a fluorescent small-molecule enhancer for therapeutic autophagy in colorectal cancer by targeting mitochondrial protein translocase TIM44. Gut 2018; 67(2): 307-19.
[http://dx.doi.org/10.1136/gutjnl-2016-311909] [PMID: 27849558]

[65]   Krisko A, Radman M. Protein damage, aging and age-related diseases. Open Biol 2019; 9(3): 180249.
[http://dx.doi.org/10.1098/rsob.180249] [PMID: 30914006]

[66]   Zhang S, Duan E. Fighting against skin aging: The way from bench to bedside. Cell Transplant 2018; 27(5): 729-38.
[http://dx.doi.org/10.1177/0963689717725755] [PMID: 29692196]

[67]   Quan T, Fisher GJ. Role of age-associated alterations of the dermal extracellular matrix microenvironment in human skin aging: A mini-review. Gerontology 2015; 61(5): 427-34.
[http://dx.doi.org/10.1159/000371708] [PMID: 25660807]

[68]   Yasui T, Yonetsu M, Tanaka R, *et al. In vivo* observation of age-related structural changes of dermal collagen in human facial skin using collagen-sensitive second harmonic generation microscope equipped with 1250-nm mode-locked Cr:Forsterite laser. J Biomed Opt 2012; 18(3): 031108.
[http://dx.doi.org/10.1117/1.JBO.18.3.031108] [PMID: 23212157]

[69]   Verma RP, Hansch C. Matrix metalloproteinases (MMPs): Chemical–biological functions and (Q)SARs. Bioorg Med Chem 2007; 15(6): 2223-68.
[http://dx.doi.org/10.1016/j.bmc.2007.01.011] [PMID: 17275314]

[70]   Pittayapruek P, Meephansan J, Prapapan O, Komine M, Ohtsuki M. Role of matrix metalloproteinases in photoaging and photocarcinogenesis. Int J Mol Sci 2016; 17(6): 868.
[http://dx.doi.org/10.3390/ijms17060868] [PMID: 27271600]

[71]   Nagase H, Visse R, Murphy G. Structure and function of matrix metalloproteinases and TIMPs. Cardiovasc Res 2006; 69(3): 562-73.
[http://dx.doi.org/10.1016/j.cardiores.2005.12.002] [PMID: 16405877]

[72]   Quan T, Little E, Quan H, Qin Z, Voorhees JJ, Fisher GJ. Elevated matrix metalloproteinases and collagen fragmentation in photodamaged human skin: Impact of altered extracellular matrix microenvironment on dermal fibroblast function. J Invest Dermatol 2013; 133(5): 1362-6.
[http://dx.doi.org/10.1038/jid.2012.509] [PMID: 23466932]

[73]   Qin Z, Balimunkwe RM, Quan T. Age-related reduction of dermal fibroblast size upregulates multiple

matrix metalloproteinases as observed in aged human skin *in vivo*. Br J Dermatol 2017; 177(5): 1337-48.
[http://dx.doi.org/10.1111/bjd.15379] [PMID: 28196296]

[74]   Tewari A, Grys K, Kollet J, Sarkany R, Young AR. Upregulation of MMP12 and its activity by UVA1 in human skin: Potential implications for photoaging. J Invest Dermatol 2014; 134(10): 2598-609.
[http://dx.doi.org/10.1038/jid.2014.173] [PMID: 24714202]

[75]   Saibil H. Chaperone machines for protein folding, unfolding and disaggregation. Nat Rev Mol Cell Biol 2013; 14(10): 630-42.
[http://dx.doi.org/10.1038/nrm3658] [PMID: 24026055]

[76]   Yokose U, Hachiya A, Sriwiriyanont P, *et al.* The endogenous protease inhibitor TIMP-1 mediates protection and recovery from cutaneous photodamage. J Invest Dermatol 2012; 132(12): 2800-9.
[http://dx.doi.org/10.1038/jid.2012.204] [PMID: 22718114]

[77]   Stadtman ER. Protein oxidation and aging. Free Radic Res 2006; 40(12): 1250-8.
[http://dx.doi.org/10.1080/10715760600918142] [PMID: 17090414]

[78]   Shin JW, Kwon SH, Choi JY, *et al.* Molecular mechanisms of dermal aging and antiaging approaches. Int J Mol Sci 2019; 20(9): 2126.
[http://dx.doi.org/10.3390/ijms20092126] [PMID: 31036793]

[79]   Vicentini FTMC, He T, Shao Y, *et al.* Quercetin inhibits UV irradiation-induced inflammatory cytokine production in primary human keratinocytes by suppressing NF-κB pathway. J Dermatol Sci 2011; 61(3): 162-8.
[http://dx.doi.org/10.1016/j.jdermsci.2011.01.002] [PMID: 21282043]

[80]   Lee YR, Noh EM, Han JH, *et al.* Brazilin inhibits UVB-induced MMP-1/3 expressions and secretions by suppressing the NF-κB pathway in human dermal fibroblasts. Eur J Pharmacol 2012; 674(2-3): 80-6.
[http://dx.doi.org/10.1016/j.ejphar.2011.10.016] [PMID: 22044921]

[81]   Varga J, Rosenbloom J, Jimenez SA. Transforming growth factor β (TGF β) causes a persistent increase in steady-state amounts of type I and type III collagen and fibronectin mRNAs in normal human dermal fibroblasts. Biochem J 1987; 247(3): 597-604.
[http://dx.doi.org/10.1042/bj2470597] [PMID: 3501287]

[82]   Chen B, Li R, Yan N, *et al.* Astragaloside IV controls collagen reduction in photoaging skin by improving transforming growth factor-β/Smad signaling suppression and inhibiting matrix metalloproteinase-1. Mol Med Rep 2015; 11(5): 3344-8.
[http://dx.doi.org/10.3892/mmr.2015.3212] [PMID: 25591734]

[83]   He T, Quan T, Shao Y, Voorhees JJ, Fisher GJ. Oxidative exposure impairs TGF-β pathway *via* reduction of type II receptor and SMAD3 in human skin fibroblasts. Age 2014; 36(3): 9623.
[http://dx.doi.org/10.1007/s11357-014-9623-6] [PMID: 24550076]

[84]   Fisher GJ, Varani J, Voorhees JJ. Looking older. Arch Dermatol 2008; 144(5): 666-72.
[http://dx.doi.org/10.1001/archderm.144.5.666] [PMID: 18490597]

[85]   Ssnigg H, Dai HM, Ling YY, Stout MB. Identification of a novel senolytic agent, navitoclax, targeting the Bcl-2 family of anti-apoptotic factors Aging Cell 2016; 15: 428-35.

[86]   Fisher GJ, Shao Y, He T, *et al.* Reduction of fibroblast size/mechanical force down-regulates TGF -β type II receptor: Implications for human skin aging. Aging Cell 2016; 15(1): 67-76.
[http://dx.doi.org/10.1111/acel.12410] [PMID: 26780887]

[87]   Fisher GJ, Quan T, Purohit T, *et al.* Collagen fragmentation promotes oxidative stress and elevates matrix metalloproteinase-1 in fibroblasts in aged human skin. Am J Pathol 2009; 174(1): 101-14.
[http://dx.doi.org/10.2353/ajpath.2009.080599] [PMID: 19116368]

[88]   Quan C, Cho MK, Perry D, Quan T. Age-associated reduction of cell spreading induces mitochondrial DNA common deletion by oxidative stress in human skin dermal fibroblasts: Implication for human

skin connective tissue aging. J Biomed Sci 2015; 22(1): 62.
[http://dx.doi.org/10.1186/s12929-015-0167-6] [PMID: 26215577]

[89] Zhang S, Li F, Zhou T, Wang G, Li Z. *Caenorhabditis elegans* as a useful model for studying aging mutations. Front Endocrinol 2020; 11: 554994.
[http://dx.doi.org/10.3389/fendo.2020.554994] [PMID: 33123086]

[90] Fu L, Kim YA, Wang X, *et al.* Perifosine inhibits mammalian target of rapamycin signaling through facilitating degradation of major components in the mTOR axis and induces autophagy. Cancer Res 2009; 69(23): 8967-76.
[http://dx.doi.org/10.1158/0008-5472.CAN-09-2190] [PMID: 19920197]

[91] Vingtdeux V, Chandakkar P, Zhao H, d'Abramo C, Davies P, Marambsud P. Novel synthetic small-molecule activators of AMPK as enhancers of autophagy and amyloid-β peptide degradation. FASEB J 2011; 25(1): 219-31.
[http://dx.doi.org/10.1096/fj.10-167361] [PMID: 20852062]

[92] Kuo SY, Castoreno AB, Aldrich LN, *et al.* Small-molecule enhancers of autophagy modulate cellular disease phenotypes suggested by human genetics. Proc Natl Acad Sci USA 2015; 112(31): E4281-7.
[http://dx.doi.org/10.1073/pnas.1512289112] [PMID: 26195741]

[93] Raynaud FI, Eccles S, Clarke PA, *et al.* Pharmacologic characterization of a potent inhibitor of class I phosphatidylinositide 3-kinases. Cancer Res 2007; 67(12): 5840-50.
[http://dx.doi.org/10.1158/0008-5472.CAN-06-4615] [PMID: 17575152]

[94] Tasdemir E, Maiuri MC, Galluzzi L, *et al.* Regulation of autophagy by cytoplasmic p53. Nat Cell Biol 2008; 10(6): 676-87.
[http://dx.doi.org/10.1038/ncb1730] [PMID: 18454141]

[95] Soto C, Pritzkow S. Protein misfolding, aggregation, and conformational strains in neurodegenerative diseases. Nat Neurosci 2018; 21(10): 1332-40.
[http://dx.doi.org/10.1038/s41593-018-0235-9] [PMID: 30250260]

[96] Blankenberg S, Rupprecht HJ, Bickel C, *et al.* Glutathione peroxidase 1 activity and cardiovascular events in patients with coronary artery disease. N Engl J Med 2003; 349(17): 1605-13.
[http://dx.doi.org/10.1056/NEJMoa030535] [PMID: 14573732]

[97] Cole MA, Quan T, Voorhees JJ, *et al.* Extracellular matrix regulation of fibroblast function: Redefining our perspective on skin aging. J Cell Commun Signal 2018; 12(1): 35-43.
[http://dx.doi.org/10.1007/s12079-018-0459-1] [PMID: 29455303]

[98] Samaraweera L, Adomako A, Rodriguez-Gabin A, McDaid HM. A novel indication for panobinostat as a senolytic drug in NSCLC and HNSCC. Sci Rep 2017; 7(1): 1900.
[http://dx.doi.org/10.1038/s41598-017-01964-1] [PMID: 28507307]

[99] Fuhrmann-Stroissnigg H, Ling YY, Zhao J, *et al.* Identification of HSP90 inhibitors as a novel class of senolytics. Nat Commun 2017; 8(1): 422.
[http://dx.doi.org/10.1038/s41467-017-00314-z] [PMID: 28871086]

[100] Zhu Y, Tchkonia T, Pirtskhalava T, *et al.* The Achilles' heel of senescent cells: From transcriptome to senolytic drugs. Aging Cell 2015; 14(4): 644-58.
[http://dx.doi.org/10.1111/acel.12344] [PMID: 25754370]

[101] Zhu Y, Doornebal EJ, Pirtskhalava T, *et al.* New agents that target senescent cells: The flavone, fisetin, and the BCL-X_L inhibitors, A1331852 and A1155463. Aging (Albany NY) 2017; 9(3): 955-63.
[http://dx.doi.org/10.18632/aging.101202] [PMID: 28273655]

[102] Surjushe A, Vasani R, Saple DG. Aloe vera: A short review. Indian J Dermatol 2008; 53(4): 163-6.
[http://dx.doi.org/10.4103/0019-5154.44785] [PMID: 19882025]

[103] Mukherjee PK, Maity N, Nema NK, Sarkar BK. Bioactive compounds from natural resources against skin aging. Phytomedicine 2011; 19(1): 64-73.
[http://dx.doi.org/10.1016/j.phymed.2011.10.003] [PMID: 22115797]

[104] Benameur T, Soleti R, Panaro MA, *et al.* Curcumin as prospective anti-aging natural compound: Focus on brain. Molecules 2021; 26(16): 4794.
[http://dx.doi.org/10.3390/molecules26164794] [PMID: 34443381]

[105] Shirin APR, Jamuna P. Chemical composition and antioxidant properties of ginger root (*Zingiber officinale*). J Med Plants Res 2010; 4(24): 2674-9.
[http://dx.doi.org/10.5897/JMPR09.464]

[106] Mohd Sahardi NF, Makpol S. Ginger (Zingiber officinale Roscoe) in the prevention of aging and degenerative diseases: Review of current evidence. Evid Based Complementary Altern Med 2019.

[107] Liew SS, Ho WY, Yeap SK, Sharifudin SAB. Phytochemical composition and *in vitro* antioxidant activities of *Citrus sinensis* peel extracts. PeerJ 2018; 6: e5331.
[http://dx.doi.org/10.7717/peerj.5331] [PMID: 30083463]

[108] Amer RI, Ezzat SM, Aborehab NM, *et al.* Downregulation of MMP1 expression mediates the anti-aging activity of *Citrus sinensis* peel extract nanoformulation in UV induced photoaging in mice. Biomed Pharmacother 2021; 138: 111537.
[http://dx.doi.org/10.1016/j.biopha.2021.111537] [PMID: 34311535]

[109] Maity N, Nema NK, Chaudhary SK, Sarkar BK, Mukherjee PK. Hyaluronidase, elastase and matrix metalloproteinase-1 inhibitory activity of standardized extract of piper betel linn. leaf Planta Med 2013; 79(5): 70.
[http://dx.doi.org/10.1055/s-0033-1336512]

[110] Bhattacharya S, Mula S, Gamre S, Kamat JP, Bandyopadhyay SK, Chattopadhyay S. Inhibitory property of Piper betel extract against photosensitization-induced damages to lipids and proteins. Food Chem 2007; 100(4): 1474-80.
[http://dx.doi.org/10.1016/j.foodchem.2005.12.041]

[111] Chauhan NS, Sharma V, Thakur M, Dixit VK. Curculigo orchioides: The black gold with numerous health benefits. J Chin Integr Med 2010; 8(7): 613-23.
[http://dx.doi.org/10.3736/jcim20100703] [PMID: 20619136]

[112] Barreca D, Nabavi SM, Sureda A, *et al.* Almonds (Prunus dulcis Mill. DA webb): A source of nutrients and health-promoting compounds. Nutrients 2020; 12(3): 672.
[http://dx.doi.org/10.3390/nu12030672] [PMID: 32121549]

[113] Fujimura T, Tsukahara K, Moriwaki S, Hotta M, Kitahara T, Takema Y. A horse chestnut extract, which induces contraction forces in fibroblasts, is a potent anti-aging ingredient. J Cosmet Sci 2006; 57(5): 369-76.
[PMID: 17111071]

[114] Brenner S. The genetics of *Caenorhabditis elegans*. Genetics 1974; 77(1): 71-94.
[http://dx.doi.org/10.1093/genetics/77.1.71] [PMID: 4366476]

[115] Moreno-Arriola E, Cárdenas-Rodríguez N, Coballase-Urrutia E, Pedraza-Chaverri J, Carmona-Aparicio L, Ortega-Cuellar D. *Caenorhabditis elegans*: A useful model for studying metabolic disorders in which oxidative stress is a contributing factor. Oxid Med Cell Longev 2014.
[http://dx.doi.org/10.1155/2014/705253]

CHAPTER 3

Therapeutic Scope and Application of Mushroom-Derived Pharmacoactives in Enhancing Health

Sharika Rajasekharan Pillai[1] and **Siriporn Chuchawankul**[1,2,*]

[1] *Immunomodulation of Natural Products Research Unit, Faculty of Allied Health Sciences, Chulalongkorn University, Bangkok 10330, Thailand*

[2] *Department of Transfusion Medicine and Clinical Microbiology, Faculty of Allied Health Sciences, Chulalongkorn University, Bangkok 10330, Thailand*

Abstract: In the present era, the notion that "prevention is better than cure" has gained impetus with increased incidences of infectious and degenerative lifestyle diseases. Recent years have seen many people choosing functional food such as probiotics, plant-based nutritional supplements, and their normal dietary needs. Studies have shown significant health benefits in using these nutraceuticals as they aid in the body's general well-being. Among food varieties, edible mushrooms have also become a functional dietary food. It has been used as a source of nutrition in many parts of the world. Oriental medicine has been using mushrooms as a component in various medicinal concoctions for several decades. Today, with the advent of scientific know-how, around 2,000 edible mushrooms have been identified; among them, 700 possess bioactive compounds. Both *In vitro* and *In vivo* studies have shown immunomodulatory effects *via* the regulation of innate, complement-mediated, and adaptive immunity by enhancing the active mechanisms of immune systems such as the macrophages, IL, TNF-α, IFN-γ, NO, and the complement system. The possibility of modulating these immune system players by the bioactives may pave the way to side-effect-free anticancer and immunosuppressant drugs. Recent studies have also elucidated the neuroprotective effect induced by mushroom-derived compounds through ROS scavenging and antioxidant activity. This chapter highlights the recent findings and the importance of these mushroom-derived compounds and their anti-inflammatory, anti-cancerous antioxidant, and immunomodulatory roles.

Keywords: Antioxidant, Anti-cancer, Functional food, Immunomodulatory, Mushrooms, Therapeutic.

---

* **Corresponding author Siriporn Chuchawankul:** Immunomodulation of Natural Products Research Unit & Department of Transfusion Medicine and Clinical Microbiology, Faculty of Allied Health Sciences, Chulalongkorn University, Bangkok 10330, Thailand; E-mail: siriporn.ch@chula.ac.th

INTRODUCTION

The search for a "Wonder drug" that can cure all diseases efficiently for many populations is a far future, as drugs that can be repurposed to cure many diseases are either less or do not exist. The COVID-19 pandemic caused by the SARS-CoV-2 virus has changed the outlook of drug discovery and forced us to look for options from nature to combat the outbreak [1, 2]. Nature is a diverse repository of bioactives that could be derived from flora and fauna. Human medical knowledge using these has been documented in texts and practices followed from time immemorial but without much scientific evidence to validate the mechanism of action and its effects against diseases [1, 3]. Food habits, health, and disease are interlinked. The primary role of food is to provide sufficient nutrients essential for metabolic processes, health benefits including reduction and prevention of diseases, and mainly to satiate hunger [4].

Mushrooms are known to be treasures of the forest [5] and have been part of many traditional foods and medicines. It has been distinguished and marketed as a superfood due to its functional and nutraceutical importance, becoming a vital part of the human diet for improving health and promoting quality of life [6]. Mushroom extracts and powder-based studies have shown excellent pharmaceutical activities such as neuroprotective, anti-ageing, immunomodulatory, anti-microbial, anti-diabetic, hypocholesteraemia, anti-cancer, and antioxidant activity [6]. The present chapter intends to highlight the recent findings and the importance of these mushroom-derived compounds and their immunomodulatory roles in inflammation and cancer research.

Mushrooms as a Valuable Source of Nutrition and Nutraceuticals

Mushrooms belong to the phyla Basidiomycota, with over 30,000 known species worldwide, and the ones that are of pharmaceutical importance belong to the order Agaricales, Aphyllophorales, Auriculariales, and class Gasteromycetes [7]. Previously, mushrooms were used in the human diet as a culinary delight or a component of traditional medicine. They were forged from the forest by knowledgeable people and were considered expensive and exquisite due to their rarity. Still, with modern agricultural practices, it is possible to optimise the requirements for the growth of desired species of edible mushrooms. Furthermore, various techniques are being used and researched for biomass production through fermentation methods [8]. Current mushroom production has increased five-fold compared to data from the 1990s. With the increase in awareness and appeal for a healthy and clean plant-based diet, mushrooms are a sustainable replacement for meat in terms of protein and essential fatty acids [9]. It is well known that these are rich sources of proteins, unsaturated fatty acids (when compared to a plant-based diet), fibres, carbohydrates (fruiting body contains about 50-60%), water (as moisture content, varying from 70-95%), micronutrients such as vitamins (like vitamin B complex, E, D, and folate) and minerals (including K, P, Na, Ca, Mg, Cu, Fe, Zn, Mo and Cd) [10, 11]. Besides nutritional constituents, the mushroom also comprises compounds that promote health and protect the body against infection and diseases. These are called nutraceutical compounds, namely, lectins, triterpenoids, ganoderic acid, β-glucan, phenolics, flavonoids, hispolon, calcaelin, proteoglycan, lentinan, laccase, nucleoside, nucleotides and ergosterol [11]. In general, the biological activity showed by different mushrooms, such as anti-bacterial, anti-viral, anti-mutagenic, anti-inflammatory, anti-carcinogenic, anti-tumour, anti-obesity, and anti-hypercholesterolemic potential, could be attributed to the presence and interaction of these nutraceuticals with host biochemical processes as shown in Fig. (**1**) [4, 6, 11].

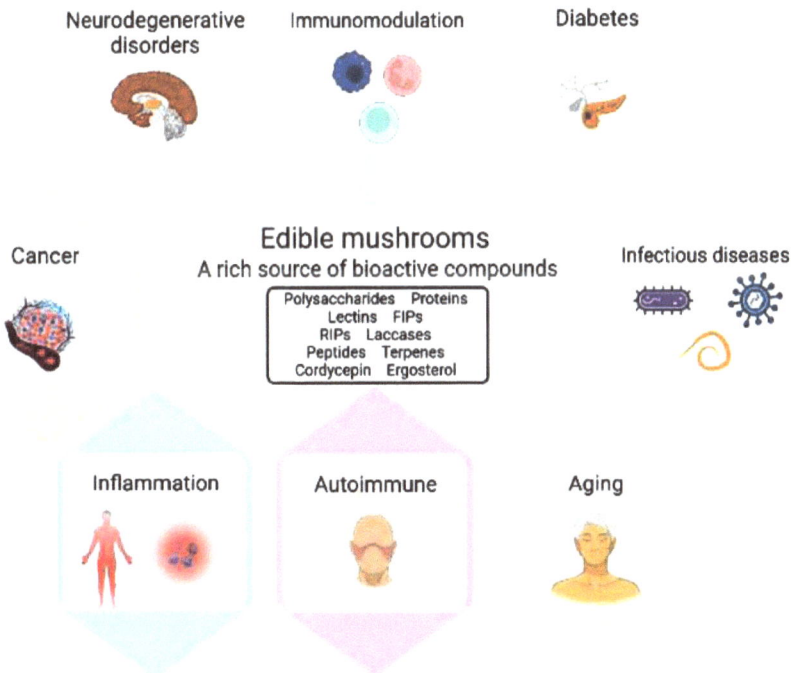

Fig. (1). Functional roles of mushroom-derived bioactive compounds. Due to their pharmaceutical activities, a variety of bioactive compounds in mushrooms have been demonstrated to fight against numerous illnesses including those associated with neurodegenerative disorders, immunomodulation, inflammation, autoimmune, cancer, diabetes, aging and infectious diseases.

Polysaccharides

Mushroom-derived polysaccharides elicit immunomodulatory activity apart from other potent biological properties such as antitumor, antimicrobial, antioxidant, and antiviral activities. These polysaccharides differ in their composition and properties based on the source of the mushroom it is isolated from. For example, some of them are water-soluble, whereas some are not. Some are homopolysaccharides, whereas others are heteropolysaccharides, having moieties such as glucose, galactose, mannose or simple or complex proteins or glucans attached [12 - 14]. The reported health-promoting activities shown by the mushroom-derived polysaccharide are ROS (reactive oxygen species) scavenging, inhibition of lipid peroxidation, and the induction of enzyme-mediated cellular antioxidative process through SOD, CAT, and GPx [15].

β-glucans, commonly present in mushrooms, have been established as one of the most potent therapeutic agents that stimulate the immune system against tumour cells [16]. Glucans comprise glucose polymer, starch, and cellulose and are structural components of the fungal cell wall. It has a β (1-> 3) linkage of glucose polymer. β-glucan exerts immunomodulation *via* the innate immune system, further activating the humoral and cell-mediated adaptive immune system [16]. Most β-glucan are non-digestible polysaccharide moieties and, hence, are known to be an essential prebiotic. Some of the well-studied polysaccharides in this aspect are Krestin (PSK) cultured from *Termetes versicolor*, Lentinan from the fruiting body of *Lentinus edodes,* and Schizophyllan from *Schizhophyllum commune*. Mushroom also contains other polysaccharides such as chitin, hemicellulose, mannose, xylan, α-glucan, and galactose apart from β-glucan [12].

Proteins

Mushrooms are excellent sources of proteins that are not only nutritive but also have potential biological functions and health benefits. Some of the important types are lectins, fungal immunomodulatory proteins (FIPs), ribosome-inactivating proteins (RIP), antimicrobial proteins, ribonucleases, and laccases [17]. Apart from proteins, some peptides exert physiological effects resulting in the promotion of health, these are called bioactive peptides (BPs). These are easily absorbed in the intestine, leading to either local or systemic effects, but most of them remain inactive with their parental protein and only show activity after hydrolysis. Depending on the sequence, they exhibit diverse activities, including anti-microbial, immune-modulatory, opiate-like, antioxidant, anti-thrombotic, hypercholesterolemic, anti-hypertensive, and mineral binding activity [18]. The various functional proteins and peptides are briefly described below.

Lectins

Lectins are ubiquitous and are widely being explored for their capability to interact with cell surface moieties, including insulin [19], fucose [20], galactose [21], lactose [22], and N-acetyl-D-glucosamine [23], hence, have potential biotechnological and therapeutic scope [24]. A variety of intracellular, extracellular, and surface mycelial lectins have been reported to be isolated from various Basidiomycetes including, *Hericium erinaceum*, *Inocybe umberinella*, *Lignosus rhinocerotis*, *Boletus edulis*, *Agrocybe aegerila*, *Marasmius oreades*, *Agaricus bisporus*, *Pholita adipose*, *Pleurotu eous*, *Russula delica*, *Volvariella volvacea*, *Grifola frondose* and *Trametes versiolar* [24]. Reportedly, the molecular weight of these lectins ranges between 12 to 190 kDa and is stable at moderate temperature and pH conditions. However, thermostable lectins that can withstand higher temperatures have been isolated from mushrooms, *Ganoderma carpense*, *Clitocybe nebularis*, *Inocybe umbernella*, *Russula lepida,* and *Agaricus arvensis* [24].

Fungal Immunomodulatory Protein (FIPs)

FIPs are a family of proteins having structural similarity and conserved amino acid sequences, with an average molecular mass of around 12-15 kDa. These proteins are rich in asparagine and valine residues and can interact with carbohydrate moiety, forming glycoproteins that stabilise and increase their biological activity. The first isolated FIP was Ling Zhi-8 from *Ganoderma lucidum*. In the past few decades, over 30 FIPs have been identified from mushrooms and other sources. Reportedly, FIPs exhibit diverse biological activities as they can induce both cell-mediated and humoral responses [24, 25]. The use of FIPs in wound healing, as adjuvants in vaccines, and for promoting neurite outgrowth are some of the other areas under research [25].

Ribosome Inactivating Proteins (RIPs)

RIPs belong to the N-glycosidase family and are well-known for disrupting protein synthesis by rendering the ribosome incapable of binding with the elongation factor by explicitly cleaving the adenine base in the 28S ribosomal RNA subunit. RIPs are widely found in plants, bacteria, and fungi as a defensive mechanism. Ricin was the first RIP to be identified [26, 27]. RIPs are classified into 3 types based on their molecular weight, isoelectric point value, subunit present, and structure type I, II, and III. Type I comprises a single polypeptide chain with a molecular weight of 30 kDa and PI value of around 9.0, sharing a highly conserved active site. Type I lacks a receptor binding chain and enters the cell through endocytosis. One of the RIPs isolated from *Trichosanthes kirilowii* Maxim, TCS, has been reported to self-insert to the membrane by interacting with the negatively charged phospholipid-containing membrane through electrostatic force and hydrophobic interaction as well as be able to bind to lipoprotein receptor protein 1 of trophoblast. On the other hand, type II is a heterodimer consisting of an N-glycosidase A-chain (30kDa) and a lectin-like B-chain (30 KDa). The latter binds to the cell surface receptor, facilitating the cytoplasmic entry of the A-chain. The mannose-containing RIPs bind to mannose receptors of the cell membrane and are then internalised *via* a clathrin-dependent mechanism, whereas others are internalised through a clathrin-independent mechanism. Type III are pro-RIP precursors, having an amino acid-terminal that resembles type I RIPs and a carboxyl-terminal domain that undergoes proteolytic modification, making it an active protein [28]. Several RIPs have been isolated from mushrooms, and some of the potent RIPs that are known to exhibit anti-tumour, anti-cancer, immunomodulatory and anti-viral activities, such as Calcelin from *Calavatia caelata*, Lyophyllin from *Lyophyllum shimeji*, Bolesatine from *Boletus satanas*, RIPs like Flammin, Flammulin, Velin, Velutin from *Flammulina velutipus*, Hypsin from *Hypsizygus marmoreus* and Pleuturegin from *Pleurotus tuber-regium* [29].

Laccases

Fungi commonly produce laccases, but some bacteria, plants, and insects are capable of producing them, Laccases are a group of multi-copper oxidase enzymes that catalyze the oxidation of phenolic compounds. Secreted with a molecular weight of around 60 kDa, these enzymes have an isoelectric point and optimal temperature of around 4.0 and 40-70 °C, respectively, owing to their versatility, stability, and wide range of substrates. Thus, they have potential applications in the food, pharmaceutical, and environmental industries. Studies have reported that various laccases have varying bioactive properties such as anti-proliferative, anti-cancer, anti-neoplastic, anti-inflammatory, anti-viral, anti-microbial, anti-neoplastic, anti-hormonal, hepatoprotective and antioxidant effects [30, 31].

Bioactive Peptides

BPs are peptides isolated from mushrooms with a molecular weight of less than 10 kDa, consisting of a heterogeneous class of compounds that differ in structure and biological function. The length of these peptides varies from 2 to 20 amino acids. The intestine directly absorbs these BPs and causes both local and systemic effects, as well as are considered more stable and less toxic than other bioactives. The major BPs isolated from mushrooms based on literature are several ACE inhibitory peptides from *Agaricus bisporous*, *Grifola frondose*, *Hypsizyus marmoreus*, *Macrocybe gigantea*, *Philiota adiposa,* and *Pleurotus cornucopiae*;

Ubiquitin-like peptide and Agrocybin from *Cyclocybe aegerita*; Cordymin from *Cordyceps militaria*; GLP fraction from *Ganoderma lucidum*, ACE inhibitory peptide from; CULP from *Handkea utiformis*; Eryngin from *Pleurotus eryngii*; POP and Pleurostin from *Pleurotus ostreatus*; Plectin from *Pseudoplectania nigrella*; SU2 peptide from *Russula paludosa*. The various activities exhibited by these BPs are various, such as anti-fungal, mineral binding, antioxidant, anti-biotic, anti-hypertensive, anti-cancer, and anti-microbial [32].

Terpenes and Terpenoids

Terpenoids are modified terpenes, which are simple hydrocarbons containing isoprene units. Many terpenoids are biologically active and are used in treating various diseases. Some of the well-known terpenoids in the market are mostly plant-derived such as paclitaxel, eleutherobin, sarcodictyin A, artemisinin, and excoecariatoxin. Mushroom-isolated terpenoids have been associated with various pharmacological activities like anti-cancer, anti-malarial, anti-cholinesterase, anti-viral, anti-bacterial, and anti-inflammatory activities. Terpenoids are classified depending on the number of carbon units as monoterpenes, sesquiterpenes, diterpenes, triterpenes, and tetraterpenes [8, 33, 34]. Some of the critical bioactives with their pharmacological activities and their mushroom source are mentioned below in Table **1**.

Table 1. List of isolated terpenoids, their pharmacological activity, and parent mushrooms.

Pharmacological Activity	Types of Terpenoids	Mushrooms	References
Anti-microbial	Caprinol- a cuparane type terpenoid	*Coprinus sp.*	[33, 35]
	Lagopodins – a sesquiterpenes	*Coprinus lagopus Coprinus cinereus*	[33, 35]
	Pleuromutilin – a tricyclic diterpenoid	*Clitopilus passeckerianus*	[33, 36]
	Nambinone A-D 1-epinambinone	*Neonothopus nambi*	[33]
	Astraodoric acid A and Astraodoric acid B –lanostane triterpenoids	*Astraeus pteridis and Astraeus odoratus*	[33, 37, 38]
	Ganorbiformins (A-G) –lanostane triterpenoids	*Ganoderma ordbiforme*	[33, 39]
	Hirsutane-type sesquiterpenoids	*Stereum hirsutum*	[33]
	Extracts containing lanostane triterpenoids	*Formitopsis rosea Formitopsis pinicola*	[33]
	Sesquiterpene aryl esters	*Armillaria sp.*	[33, 40]

(Table 1) cont.....

Pharmacological Activity	Types of Terpenoids	Mushrooms	References
	Udasterpurenol A Undalactaranes A and B – a sesquiterpenoids	*Phelbia uda*	[33, 41]
	Merulidial 1 – a sesquiterpene dialdehyde	*Merulius tremellosus*	[33]
Anti-viral	Ganodermadiol, lucidadiol, applanoxidic acid G - triterpenoids	*Ganoderma sp.*	[33]
	Agrocybone – illundane-illundane bis-sesquiterpene	*Agrocybe salicacola*	[33]
	Colossolactones and their variants – a lanlstane triterpenoids	*Ganoderma colosseum*	[33, 42]
	Sterosterin A	*Stereum ostrea*	[33, 43]
Anti-parasitic	Aurisin A Aristolane - a dimeric sesquiterpene	*Neonothopanus nambi*	[33, 44]
	Hypnophillin and Panepoxydone - terpenoids	*Lentius strigosus*	[33, 45]
	Lanostane-type triterpenes 1 and 2	*Asteraeus hygrometicus*	[33, 46 - 48]
Antioxidant	Sesquiterpenoids	*Stereum hirsutum*	[33]
	2,5-cuparadiene-1,4-dione Enokipodin B Enokipidin D	*Flammulina velutipes*	[33]
Anti-inflammatory	Cyathin D, H Neosarcodonin Cyathatriol 11-O-acetylcyanthatriol	*Cyanthus africanus*	[33, 49]
	Cyathin [12R]-11a-epoxy-13a, 14b 15-trihydroxycyath-3-ene Erinacine I	*Cyanthus hookeri*	[33, 50]
	Hericenones Erinacines	*Hericium erinaceus*	[33]
	Labdane diterpenes	*Antrodia camphorata*	[33]
Anti-neurodegenerative disorder	Scabronines Sarcodonins - are Cyanthane diterpenoids	*Sarcodon scabrosus*	[33]
	Cyrnenines A and B – are Cyanthane diterpenoids	*Sarcodon cyrneus*	[33]

(Table 1) cont.....

Pharmacological Activity	Types of Terpenoids	Mushrooms	References
Anti-tumor	Ganoderic acids Lucidimols Ganodermanondiol Ganoderiol F Ganodermanontriol	*Ganoderma sp*	[33, 51]
	Flammulinol A Flammulinolides A-G Sterpuric acid	*Flammulina veluptipes*	[33]
	Formitoside K – a lanostane triterpene glycoside	*Formitopsis nigra*	[33, 52]
	Inonotsuoxides A and B Inonotsulides group A, B, C Inonotsutriols group A-E - are triterpenes	*Inonotus obliques*	[33]
	Astrakurkurone - sesquiterpenoids	*Asteraeus hygrometricus*	[33]
	Antrocin	*Astraeus camphorata*	[33]
	Radiansepenes – a guanacastane-type diterpenoids	*Coperniellus radians*	[33]
	Irofulven – a sesquiterpenoid	*Osmphalotus illudens*	[33, 53]

Cordycepin

Cordycepin is a 3'-deoxyadenosine derived from *Cordyceps militaris*, a mushroom widely used in folk medicine. Studies found that Cordycepin could regulate type II diabetics, inhibit nitric oxide (NO) production in LPS-treated macrophages, be used to treat neurodegenerative disease and induce neuro immunity, suppress T-cell activation, alleviate asthma in mice modal, and protect blood-brain barrier [54].

Ergosterol

Mushrooms are rich in ergosterol, as it is one of the key compounds necessary for maintaining the structure and function of cell membranes. It is the percussor of vitamin D. Hence, it is an important source of vitamin D in the human diet. Also, ergosterol possesses potential activities, such as anti-inflammatory, anti-cancer, hypercholesteraemic, and anti-microbial activity. Ergosterol peroxide is formed by the H_2O_2-dependent enzymatic oxidation of ergosterol to its epi-dioxide and is natively found in mushrooms, yeast, lichens, sponges, and halotolerant algae, it also exhibits immunosuppressive, antioxidant, anti-viral, anti-tumour and anti-inflammatory activity [55].

THERAPEUTIC SCOPE OF MUSHROOM-DERIVED BIOACTIVES

Mushrooms are often considered as functional food, which apart from fulfilling nutritional requirements, also improve overall health when consumed. This could be attributed to various bioactives discussed above, which enhance and protect health. Hence, including mushrooms in daily diet has a tremendous therapeutic value in human health. Furthermore, the isolated compounds have great potential to be developed further into drugs that are non-toxic or have fewer side effects [56]. Here, we focus mainly on the immunomodulatory, anti-cancer, anti-inflammatory, and antioxidant capacity of these bioactives.

Immunomodulatory and Anti-inflammatory Activity

Today's advanced immunotherapy treatments, targeting the immune system in promoting health as well as in preventing or treating disease, have precedent practices, that date back to before the 18th century [57]. Several bio-active have been isolated from the mushrooms that are considered biological response modifiers (BRMs), which can cause cytotoxic effects in cancer cells on one hand and other can enhance the immune system, to attenuate the spread and growth of cancer, hence exhibiting anti-cancer activity [14]. Most of the immunomodulants available are synthetic or semi-synthetic and have side effects. Therefore, the need for natural immunomodulants is increasing. The modulators isolated from mushrooms can mediate its effect through the same or different pathways and are also capable of activating the innate immune system, such as natural killer cells, neutrophils, and macrophages, which produce prostaglandins and cytokines that further activate the adaptive immune system [58].

Polysaccharides are well known to cause immunomodulatory effects in the host. The polysaccharide isolated from *Lentinula edodes*, lentinan, glucans, mannoglucans, and proteoglycans is known to induce non-specific cytotoxic effects in macrophages and enhance cytokine production [58 - 60]. β-d-glucan and β-glucan isolated from *Gymnopus dryophilus* and *Xylaria nigripes* respectively were found to inhibit NO production in macrophages, but peptidoglycans isolated from *Flammulina velutipes*, *Hericium erinaceus*, *Inonotus obliquus*, *Morchella conica*, *Sarcodon assparatus,* and *Tricholoma giganteum* found to enhance NO production [58]. *Agaricus blazei*-derived polysaccharides like heteroglycan, glycoprotein, glucomannan-protein complex, and other glucans tend to stimulate NK cells, macrophages, and dendritic cells, and the induction of Tumor Necrosis factor (TNF), Interferons (IFN) and Interleukin-8 (IL-8) production [61]. Other polysaccharides that stimulate NO, IFN, IL, and TNF were isolated from *Phellinus linteus*, *Tricholoma giganteum*, *Antrodia camphorate*, *Sparassis crispa*, *Sarcodon aspratus*, *Pleurotus ostereatus*, *Ganoderma lucidum* [58].

Lectins from *Agaricus bisporous, Floccularia luteovirens, Boletus edulis, Flammulina velutioes, Ganoderma caspense, Pleurotus eous, Schizophyllum commune* are identified to stimulate mice splenocytes mitogenicity. FIPs isolated from *Taiwanfungus camphoratus, Chroogomphis rutilus, Flammulina velutipes, Ganoderma sp., Trametes versicolor, Volvariella volvacea* were found to enhance the production of IL, IFN TNF, and NO both *in vitro* and *in vivo* [58].

Anti-cancer Activity

Mushroom extracts mainly contain polysaccharides, lectins, and terpenes that are well known for their anticancer activity in cell lines. Since most are isolated from edible mushrooms, these bioactives are non-toxic to humans. A recent review from Panda *et al.*, 2022, discusses the potential of mushrooms in cancer therapy and the ongoing phases of clinical trials where the bioactives are being tested for their activity against breast, colorectal, and prostate cancer. Clinical trial currently focuses on *Lentinula edodes, Coriolus versicolor,* and *Ganoderma lucidium,* species of mushrooms. Several other mushroom varieties such as species belonging to *Agaricus, Antrodia, Clitocybe, Calvatia, Cordyceps, Flammulina, Fomes, Ganoderma, Grifola, Inonotus, Phellinus, Pleurotus, Russula, Sullius, Tramaetes,* and *Xercomus* also show potential anti-cancer activities which are to be taken forward [62].

Lentinan from *Lentinula edodes* enhances the proliferation of CD4$^+$ and CD8$^+$ T cells by activating macrophages, and upregulation of IL-2 and INF-γ also observed [63, 64]. It activates immunogenic death-related proteins in H22 murine hepatocarcinoma cells, which results in cytotoxicity and apoptosis [64, 65]. LNT and oridonin increased their anticancer activity against Hep G2 human hepatoblastoma cells [64, 66]. It causes cytotoxicity by facilitating the uptake of tamofexin and gemcitabine in breast cancer cell lines by stimulating natural killer cells (NK) [64, 67, 68]. Combined with gemcitabine, Lentinan alone induces apoptosis in urothelial bladder cancer cell lines [64, 69]. Lentinan inhibited tumour growth and induced autophagy endoplasmic stress in HT-29 cells and tumour-bearing nonotase diabetics (NON)/ Severe combined immunodeficiency (SCID) mice in colon cancer growth by inducing apoptosis [64, 70]. It causes apoptosis of gastric cell lines BGC823 and Cervical cancer HeLa cells *via* a synergetic effect when combined with docetaxel and cisplatin [64, 71, 72].

Coriolus versicolor is an edible medicinal mushroom with no reported toxicity to humans. Both *in vivo* and *in vitro* studies show its efficacy in targeting various cancer types, including breast, lung, melanoma, colon, leukaemia, cervix, gastric, prostrate, hepatoma, and ovarian cancer. It exhibits immunostimulatory pharmacological activity by activating the innate immune system and adaptive immunity [73]. PSP enhances mitogenic activities, attenuates the induction of IL-1β and IL-6, and increases pro-inflammatory cytokine. Protein-bound polysaccharide (PBP) induces cytotoxicity against MCF-7 cells [73, 74]. PSP reduces cell growth and upregulates TNF-α expression in MCF-7 cell lines [73, 75]. Hot water-extracted polysaccharide stimulated splenocyte proliferation and induced IgM, and IgG1 increased phosphorylation of ERK-1/2 and p38 MAPK, which also enhanced the nuclear translocation of NF-κB p65 subunit [73, 76]. PSK as TLR2 agonist upregulates MHC [class II and CD86] expression on DC/tumor and activates $CD4^+$ and $CD8^+$ T cells to induce IFN-γ in PMBCs [73, 77]. Purified new protein YZP explicitly triggers the differentiation of $CD1d^+$ B cells into IL-10-producing regulatory B cells [73, 77]. Glucan n-home-made purification $-[->6)-\alpha-D-Glcp-(1->]_n$ in sarcoma 180 bearing mice promotes the secretion of IL-2,4,6,10,17 and IFN-α and γ, enhances cytokine production [73, 78]. The aqueous extract increases IL-2,6,12, TNF-α, and IFN-γ from the spleen in mouse mammary carcinoma 4T1 tumour-bearing mice [73, 79].

Lingzhi or *Ganoderma* is a widely used medicinal species across China, America, Japan, Korea, and other countries. Studies show *Ganoderma* can be used as an anti-cancer therapy by its immunomodulatory properties. These effects can be attributed to the presence of FIPS, polysaccharides and terpenoids [80]. The first bioactive to be identified was LZ-8 in 1989, from *G. lucidum*, which showed various pharmacological effects such as the induction of endoplasmic reticulum stress-mediated autophagic death in gastric cancer cell line SGC-7901 [80, 81]. Promotion EGFR mediated anti-proliferative effect and apoptosis induction in lung cancer cell lines [82]. It also enhanced the efficacy of a DNA vaccine against MBT-2 [83]. GMI from *G. microsporum* showed anti-cancer activity against lung cancer cells *via* autophagy induction and inhibited lysosomal degradation [84, 85]. FIP-gts from *G. tsugae* inhibited cell migration in a cervical cancer cell and also could suppress telomerase activity in lung cancer cells [86, 87]. Other bioactives from *G. lucidum* showed NK cell-mediated cytotoxicity through the MAPK signaling pathway. It also increased the IL-1 and IL-6 expression, promoted the cytotoxicity of cytotoxic T-lymphocyte, mediated antitumor activity through complement type 3 receptors, enhancement of antioxidant activity, and reduction of IL-1β, IL-6, and TNF-α. The lipid extract from *G. sinensis* activated immunosuppressive tumor-associated macrophages. *G. artum* was found to activate mitochondrial apoptotic pathways related to host immune response, and induce anti-tumor activity, and TNF-α secretion through the activation of TLR4/ROS/PI3k/Akt/MAPK/NF-κB [80].

Antioxidant Activity

Mushrooms are rich sources of antioxidant compounds such as phenolic, flavonoids, glycosides, polysaccharides, tocopherol, and ergothioneine. Carotenoids and ascorbic acid are derived from the fruiting bodies, mycelium, or as secreted compounds [15, 88]. Some of the mushrooms and their components showing antioxidant activities are listed below Table **2**.

Table 2. Important mushrooms and their antioxidant compounds.

Mushroom Species	Antioxidant Compounds	References
Agaricus sp.	Phenols, gallic acid, flavonoids, tocopherols, p-polysaccharides, hydroxybenzoic acid-derived pyrogallol	[88 - 93]
Auricular auricular	Phenols, glycan	[88, 94]
Antrodia camphorala	Polysaccharides, phenols, ascorbic acid, γ-tocopherol, diterpenes	[88, 95]
Boletus edulus	Organic acids, phenols	[88, 96]
Flammulina veluptis	Phenols, polysaccharides, Flammulin	[88, 97]
Ganoderma sp	Phenols, β-glucans, carboxy-methylated polysaccharides, ganoderio, ganoderic acids, ganodermanontriol	[88, 98]
Hericium erinaceous	Pheonls, steroids, erinacines, hericenone, hericicerins, resorcinol, mono-terpenes, diterpenes	[88, 99]
Lignosus rhinoceros	Phenolic compounds, polysaccharide-proteins	[88, 100]
Pleurotus sp	Heteropolysaccharide acid, laccase, polysaccharide-protein complex, phenols, α-tocopherol, β- carotene, cinnamic acid, flavonoids	[88, 101]
Russula sp.	Tocopherol, catechin, phenol	[88, 102, 103]

The most abundant bioactive components present in mushrooms are phenolic, which could be classified into 1.) hydroxybenzoic acids which are bound to lignin, hydrolyzable tannins, sugars, and organic acids. 2.) Hydroxycinnamic, which is linked to cellulose, lignin, proteins, and tartaric acid. These polyphenolic compounds are known to quench free radicals and promote endogenous antioxidant activities by regulating NRF/ARE in cells. These were also found to activate Sirtuin 1(SIRT1) or NF-κB and others are known to modulate the mitochondrial potential to balance the redox potential. Another important component of mushrooms is flavonoids that promote antioxidant activity in the host. The major flavonoids present in edible mushrooms are myricetin, resveratrol, quercetin, chrysin, catechin, hespertin, naringenin, pyrogall, and kaempferol. Polysaccharides and polysaccharide-protein complexes also play an important role in enhancing the antioxidant property in the host through promoting immuno-stimulation. Other bioactives including ascorbic acid (vitamin

C), tocopherol (vitamin E), ergocalciferol (vitamin D2), and cholecalciferol (vitamin D3) also play an important role as antioxidants [15].

CONCLUSION

Edible mushrooms are a rich source of bioactive compounds which are shown to have promising therapeutic value. The immunomodulatory properties of these compounds could be the key to developing a "wonder drug" that can cure or eradicate the root cause of multiple diseases such as cancer, aging-related neurodegenerative diseases, diabetics, autoimmune disorders, etc. based on the studies, regular uptake of mushrooms can effectively combat and reduce the susceptibility to various diseases and disorders.

ABBREVIATIONS

ACE	Acetylcholinesterase
BPs	Bioactive Peptides
BRMs	Biological Response Modifiers
CAT	Catalase
EGFR	Epidermal Growth Factor Receptor
FIPs	Fungal Immunomodulatory Proteins
GPx	Glutathione Peroxidase
H_2O_2	Hydrogen Peroxide
IFN	Interferon
IL	Interleukin
KDa	Kilodalton
LPS	Lipopolysaccharide
MAPK	Mitogen-activated Protein Kinase
NK cells	Natural Killer cells
NO	Nitric Oxide
PBP	Protein-bound Polysaccharide
PI	Isoelectric Point
PI3k	Phosphoinositide 3-kinase
PBMCs	Peripheral Blood Mononuclear Cells
RIPs	Ribosome-inactivating Proteins
ROS	Reactive Oxygen Species
Rrna	Ribosomal Ribonucleic Acid
TNF	Tumor Necrosis Factor

SIRT1	Sirtuin 1
SOD	Superoxide Dismutase
TLR2	Toll-like Receptor 2
TCS	Tricosanthin

ACKNOWLEDGEMENTS

S.R.P. would like to thank the Second Century Fund (C2F), Chulalongkorn University, Bangkok, Thailand for a postdoctoral fellowship. We are grateful to Dr. James M. Brimson (Research Unit for Innovation & International Affairs, Faculty of Allied Health Sciences) for reviewing and editing the grammar of this manuscript. We sincerely thank Sunita Nilkhet for producing figure using BioRender.

REFERENCES

[1]   Dzobo K. The role of natural products as sources of therapeutic agents for innovative drug discovery. Compr Pharmacol 2022; 408-22.
[http://dx.doi.org/10.1016/B978-0-12-820472-6.00041-4]

[2]   Mathur S, Hoskins C. Drug development: Lessons from nature. Biomed Rep 2017; 6(6): 612-4.
[http://dx.doi.org/10.3892/br.2017.909] [PMID: 28584631]

[3]   Mushtaq S, Abbasi R, Uzair B, Abbasi BH. Natural products as reservoirs of novel therapeutic agents. EXCLI J 2018; 17: 420-51.

[4]   Reis FS, Martins A, Vasconcelos MH, Morales P, Ferreira ICFR. Functional foods based on extracts or compounds derived from mushrooms. Trends Food Sci Technol 2017; 66: 48-62.
[http://dx.doi.org/10.1016/j.tifs.2017.05.010]

[5]   Nowakowski P, Markiewicz-Żukowska R, Bielecka J, Mielcarek K, Grabia M, Socha K. Treasures from the forest: Evaluation of mushroom extracts as anti-cancer agents. Biomed Pharmacother 2021; 143: 112106.
[http://dx.doi.org/10.1016/j.biopha.2021.112106] [PMID: 34482165]

[6]   Morris HJ, Llauradó G, Beltrán Y, Lebeque Y, Bermúdez RC, García N, *et al.* The world of mushrooms nutaceuticals and functional food products: Closing the gap between nutritional research and medical community. 2nd International Conference on Nutraceuticals and Nutrition Supplements. Bangkok, Thailand 2016.

[7]   Rahi DK, Malik D. Diversity of mushrooms and their metabolites of nutraceutical and therapeutic significance. J Mycol 2016; 2016: 1-18.
[http://dx.doi.org/10.1155/2016/7654123]

[8]   Dudekula UT, Doriya K, Devarai SK. A critical review on submerged production of mushroom and their bioactive metabolites. 3 Biotech 2020; 10(8): 1-12.

[9]   You SW, Hoskin RT, Komarnytsky S, Moncada M. Mushrooms as functional and nutritious food ingredients for multiple applications. ACS Food Science & Technology 2022; 2(8): 1184-95.
[http://dx.doi.org/10.1021/acsfoodscitech.2c00107]

[10]   Niego AG, Rapior S, Thongklang N, Raspé O, Jaidee W, Lumyong S, *et al.* Macrofungi as a nutraceutical source: Promising bioactive compounds and market value. Journal of Fungi 2021; 7(5): 397.

[11] Das AK, Nanda PK, Dandapat P, Bandyopadhyay S, Gullón P, Sivaraman GK, *et al.* Edible mushrooms as functional ingredients for development of healthier and more sustainable muscle foods: A flexitarian approach. Molecules 2021; 26(9): 2463.
[http://dx.doi.org/10.3390/molecules26092463]

[12] Singdevsachan SK, Auroshree P, Mishra J, Baliyarsingh B, Tayung K, Thatoi H. Mushroom polysaccharides as potential prebiotics with their antitumor and immunomodulating properties: A review. Bioactive Carbohydrates and Dietary Fibre 2016; 7(1): 1-14.
[http://dx.doi.org/10.1016/j.bcdf.2015.11.001]

[13] Pathak MP, Pathak K, Saikia R, *et al.* Immunomodulatory effect of mushrooms and their bioactive compounds in cancer: A comprehensive review. Biomed Pharmacother 2022; 149: 112901.
[http://dx.doi.org/10.1016/j.biopha.2022.112901] [PMID: 36068771]

[14] Mallard B, Leach DN, Wohlmuth H, Tiralongo J. Synergistic immuno-modulatory activity in human macrophages of a medicinal mushroom formulation consisting of reishi, shiitake and maitake. PLOS ONE 2019; 14(11): e0224740.
[http://dx.doi.org/10.1371/journal.pone.0224740]

[15] Kozarski M, Klaus A, Jakovljevic D, *et al.* Antioxidants of edible mushrooms. Molecules 2015; 20(10): 19489-525.
[http://dx.doi.org/10.3390/molecules201019489] [PMID: 26516828]

[16] Savelkoul HFJ, Chanput W, Wichers HJ. Immunomodulatory effects of mushroom B-glucans. In Calder PC, Yaqoob P, editors, Diet, immunity and inflammation, woodhead publishing series in food science, technology and nutrition no. 232. 2013; pp. 416-34.

[17] Xu X, Yan H, Chen J, Zhang X. Bioactive proteins from mushrooms. Biotechnol Adv 2011; 29(6): 667-74.
[http://dx.doi.org/10.1016/j.biotechadv.2011.05.003] [PMID: 21605654]

[18] Erdmann K, Cheung BWY, Schröder H. The possible roles of food-derived bioactive peptides in reducing the risk of cardiovascular disease. J Nutr Biochem 2008; 19(10): 643-54.
[http://dx.doi.org/10.1016/j.jnutbio.2007.11.010] [PMID: 18495464]

[19] Zhang GQ, Chen QJ, Hua J, *et al.* An inulin-specific lectin with anti-HIV-1 reverse transcriptase, antiproliferative, and mitogenic activities from the edible mushroom *Agaricus bitorquis.* BioMed Res Int 2019; 2019: 1-9.
[http://dx.doi.org/10.1155/2019/1341370] [PMID: 31016184]

[20] Norton P, Comunale MA, Herrera H, *et al.* Development and application of a novel recombinant *Aleuria aurantia* lectin with enhanced core fucose binding for identification of glycoprotein biomarkers of hepatocellular carcinoma. Proteomics 2016; 16(24): 3126-36.
[http://dx.doi.org/10.1002/pmic.201600064] [PMID: 27650323]

[21] Davitashvili E, Kapanadze E, Kachlishvili E, Mikiashvili NA, Elisashvili V. Isolation and characterization of lectins formed by *Cerrena unicolor* (higher basidiomycetes) in solid-state fermentation of sorghum and wheat straw. Int J Med Mushrooms 2015; 17(5): 427-34.
[http://dx.doi.org/10.1615/IntJMedMushrooms.v17.i5.20] [PMID: 26082981]

[22] Wang Y, Wu B, Shao J, *et al.* Extraction, purification and physicochemical properties of a novel lectin from *Laetiporus sulphureus* mushroom. Lebensm Wiss Technol 2018; 91: 151-9.
[http://dx.doi.org/10.1016/j.lwt.2018.01.032]

[23] Machon O, Baldini SF, Ribeiro JP, *et al.* Recombinant fungal lectin as a new tool to investigate *O* - GlcNAcylation processes. Glycobiology 2017; 27(2): 123-8.
[http://dx.doi.org/10.1093/glycob/cww105] [PMID: 27798069]

[24] Singh RS, Walia AK, Kennedy JF. Mushroom lectins in biomedical research and development. Int J Biol Macromol 2020; 151: 1340-50.
[http://dx.doi.org/10.1016/j.ijbiomac.2019.10.180] [PMID: 31751693]

[25]   Ejike UC, Chan CJ, Okechukwu PN, Lim RLH. New advances and potentials of fungal immunomodulatory proteins for therapeutic purposes. Crit Rev Biotechnol 2020; 40(8): 1172-90.
[http://dx.doi.org/10.1080/07388551.2020.1808581] [PMID: 32854547]

[26]   Ng TB, Lam JSY, Wong JH, *et al.* Differential abilities of the mushroom ribosome-inactivating proteins hypsin and velutin to perturb normal development of cultured mouse embryos. Toxicol. *In Vitro* 2010; 24(4): 1250-7.
[http://dx.doi.org/10.1016/j.tiv.2010.02.003] [PMID: 20149862]

[27]   Virgilio M, Lombardi A, Caliandro R, Fabbrini MS. Ribosome-inactivating proteins: From plant defense to tumor attack. Toxins 2010; 2(11): 2699-737.
[http://dx.doi.org/10.3390/toxins2112699] [PMID: 22069572]

[28]   Wang S, Li Z, Li S, Di R, Ho CT, Yang G. Ribosome-inactivating proteins (RIPs) and their important health promoting property. RSC Advances 2016; 6(52): 46794-805.
[http://dx.doi.org/10.1039/C6RA02946A]

[29]   Landi N, Hussain HZF, Pedone PV, Ragucci S, Di Maro A. Ribotoxic proteins, known as inhibitors of protein synthesis, from mushrooms and other fungi according to Endo's fragment detection. Toxins 2022; 14(6): 403.
[http://dx.doi.org/10.3390/toxins14060403] [PMID: 35737065]

[30]   Mayolo-Deloisa K, González-González M, Rito-Palomares M. Laccases in food industry: Bioprocessing, potential industrial and biotechnological applications. Front Bioeng Biotechnol 2020; 8: 222.
[http://dx.doi.org/10.3389/fbioe.2020.00222] [PMID: 32266246]

[31]   Jasim A. Medicinal properties of laccase from Basidiomycetes mushroom: A review. Adv Life Sci Technol 2017; 54: 99-109.

[32]   Landi N, Clemente A, Pedone PV, Ragucci S, Di Maro A. An updated review of bioactive peptides from mushrooms in a well-defined molecular weight range. Toxins 2022; 14(2): 84.
[http://dx.doi.org/10.3390/toxins14020084] [PMID: 35202112]

[33]   Dasgupta A, Acharya K. Mushrooms: An emerging resource for therapeutic terpenoids. 3 Biotech 2019; 9(10).

[34]   Yaoita Y, Kikuchi M, Machida K. Terpenoids and sterols from mushrooms. Studies in Natural Products Chemistry 2015; 44: 1-32.
[http://dx.doi.org/10.1016/B978-0-444-63460-3.00001-8]

[35]   Johansson M, Sterner O, Labischinski H, Anke T. Coprinol, A new antibiotic cuparane from a Coprinus species. Z Naturforsch C J Biosci 2001; 56(1-2): 31-4.
[http://dx.doi.org/10.1515/znc-2001-1-205] [PMID: 11302209]

[36]   Paukner S, Riedl R. Pleuromutilins: Potent drugs for resistant bugs—mode of action and resistance. Cold Spring Harb Perspect Med 2017; 7(1): a027110.
[http://dx.doi.org/10.1101/cshperspect.a027110] [PMID: 27742734]

[37]   Stanikunaite R, Radwan MM, Trappe JM, Fronczek F, Ross SA. Lanostane-type triterpenes from the mushroom *Astraeus pteridis* with antituberculosis activity. J Nat Prod 2008; 71(12): 2077-9.
[http://dx.doi.org/10.1021/np800577p] [PMID: 19067555]

[38]   Arpha K, Phosri C, Suwannasai N, Mongkolthanaruk W, Sodngam S. Astraodoric acids A-D: new lanostane triterpenes from edible mushroom *Astraeus odoratus* and their anti-Mycobacterium tuberculosis H37Ra and cytotoxic activity. J Agric Food Chem 2012; 60(39): 9834-41.
[http://dx.doi.org/10.1021/jf302433r] [PMID: 22957940]

[39]   Isaka M, Chinthanom P, Kongthong S, Srichomthong K, Choeyklin R. Lanostane triterpenes from cultures of the Basidiomycete *Ganoderma orbiforme* BCC 22324. Phytochemistry 2013; 87: 133-9.
[http://dx.doi.org/10.1016/j.phytochem.2012.11.022] [PMID: 23280041]

[40]   Misiek M, Hoffmeister D. Sesquiterpene aryl ester natural products in North American Armillaria species. Mycol Prog 2012; 11(1): 7-15.
[http://dx.doi.org/10.1007/s11557-010-0720-3]

[41]   Schüffler A, Wollinsky B, Anke T, Liermann JC, Opatz T. Isolactarane and sterpurane sesquiterpenoids from the basidiomycete *Phlebia uda*. J Nat Prod 2012; 75(7): 1405-8.
[http://dx.doi.org/10.1021/np3000552] [PMID: 22746380]

[42]   El Dine RS, El Halawany AM, Ma CM, Hattori M. Anti-HIV-1 protease activity of lanostane triterpenes from the vietnamese mushroom *Ganoderma colossum*. J Nat Prod 2008; 71(6): 1022-6.
[http://dx.doi.org/10.1021/np8001139] [PMID: 18547117]

[43]   Isaka M, Srisanoh U, Sappan M, Supothina S, Boonpratuang T. Sterostreins F–O, illudalanes and norilludalanes from cultures of the Basidiomycete *Stereum ostrea* BCC 22955. Phytochemistry 2012; 79: 116-20.
[http://dx.doi.org/10.1016/j.phytochem.2012.04.009] [PMID: 22595359]

[44]   Kanokmedhakul S, Lekphrom R, Kanokmedhakul K, *et al.* Cytotoxic sesquiterpenes from luminescent mushroom *Neonothopanus nambi*. Tetrahedron 2012; 68(39): 8261-6.
[http://dx.doi.org/10.1016/j.tet.2012.07.057]

[45]   Souza-Fagundes EM, Cota BB, Rosa LH, *et al. In vitro* activity of hypnophilin from Lentinus strigosus: A potential prototype for Chagas disease and leishmaniasis chemotherapy. Braz J Med Biol Res 2010; 43(11): 1054-61.
[http://dx.doi.org/10.1590/S0100-879X2010007500108] [PMID: 21088803]

[46]   Mallick S, Dutta A, Dey S, *et al.* Selective inhibition of *Leishmania donovani* by active extracts of wild mushrooms used by the tribal population of India: An *in vitro* exploration for new leads against parasitic protozoans. Exp Parasitol 2014; 138: 9-17.
[http://dx.doi.org/10.1016/j.exppara.2014.01.002] [PMID: 24440295]

[47]   Mallick S, Dey S, Mandal S, *et al.* A novel triterpene from *Astraeus hygrometricus* induces reactive oxygen species leading to death in *Leishmania donovani*. Future Microbiol 2015; 10(5): 763-89.
[http://dx.doi.org/10.2217/fmb.14.149] [PMID: 26000650]

[48]   Mallick S, Dutta A, Chaudhuri A, *et al.* Successful therapy of murine visceral leishmaniasis with astrakurkurone, a triterpene isolated from the mushroom *Astraeus hygrometricus*, involves the induction of protective cell-mediated immunity and TLR9. Antimicrob Agents Chemother 2016; 60(5): 2696-708.
[http://dx.doi.org/10.1128/AAC.01943-15] [PMID: 26883702]

[49]   Han J, Chen Y, Bao L, *et al.* Anti-inflammatory and cytotoxic cyathane diterpenoids from the medicinal fungus *Cyathus africanus*. Fitoterapia 2013; 84: 22-31.
[http://dx.doi.org/10.1016/j.fitote.2012.10.001] [PMID: 23075884]

[50]   Xu Z, Yan S, Bi K, *et al.* Isolation and identification of a new anti-inflammatory cyathane diterpenoid from the medicinal fungus *Cyathus hookeri* Berk. Fitoterapia 2013; 86: 159-62.
[http://dx.doi.org/10.1016/j.fitote.2013.03.002] [PMID: 23500388]

[51]   Shi XW, Liu L, Gao JM, Zhang AL. Cyathane diterpenes from Chinese mushroom *Sarcodon scabrosus* and their neurite outgrowth-promoting activity. Eur J Med Chem 2011; 46(7): 3112-7.
[http://dx.doi.org/10.1016/j.ejmech.2011.04.006] [PMID: 21530015]

[52]   Lee IK, Jung JY, Yeom JH, *et al.* Fomitoside K, a new lanostane triterpene glycoside from the fruiting body of *Fomitopsis nigra*. Mycobiology 2012; 40(1): 76-8.
[http://dx.doi.org/10.5941/MYCO.2012.40.1.076] [PMID: 22783139]

[53]   Ou Y, Li Y, Qian X, Shen Y. Guanacastane-type diterpenoids from *Coprinus radians*. Phytochemistry 2012; 78: 190-6.
[http://dx.doi.org/10.1016/j.phytochem.2012.03.002] [PMID: 22521133]

[54]   Lee CT, Huang KS, Shaw JF, *et al.* Trends in the immunomodulatory effects of *Cordyceps militaris*:

Total extracts, polysaccharides and cordycepin. Front Pharmacol 2020; 11: 575704.
[http://dx.doi.org/10.3389/fphar.2020.575704] [PMID: 33328984]

[55]   Nowak R, Nowacka-Jechalke N, Pietrzak W, Gawlik-Dziki U. A new look at edible and medicinal mushrooms as a source of ergosterol and ergosterol peroxide - UHPLC-MS/MS analysis. Food Chem 2022; 369: 130927.
[http://dx.doi.org/10.1016/j.foodchem.2021.130927] [PMID: 34461517]

[56]   Chaturvedi VK, Agarwal S, Gupta KK, Ramteke PW, Singh MP. Medicinal mushroom: Boon for therapeutic applications. 3 Biotech 2018; 8: 1-20.

[57]   Bucktrout SL, Bluestone JA, Ramsdell F. Recent advances in immunotherapies: From infection and autoimmunity, to cancer, and back again. Genome Medicine 2018; 10(1): 1-10.

[58]   Zhao S, Gao Q, Rong C, *et al.* Immunomodulatory effects of edible and medicinal mushrooms and their bioactive immunoregulatory products. J Fungi 2020; 6(4): 269.
[http://dx.doi.org/10.3390/jof6040269] [PMID: 33171663]

[59]   Bisen PS, Baghel RK, Sanodiya BS, Thakur GS, Prasad GBKS. *Lentinus edodes*: A macrofungus with pharmacological activities. Curr Med Chem 2010; 17(22): 2419-30.
[http://dx.doi.org/10.2174/092986710791698495] [PMID: 20491636]

[60]   Morales D, Rutckeviski R, Villalva M, *et al.* Isolation and comparison of α- and β-D-glucans from shiitake mushrooms (*Lentinula edodes*) with different biological activities. Carbohydr Polym 2020; 229: 115521.
[http://dx.doi.org/10.1016/j.carbpol.2019.115521] [PMID: 31826486]

[61]   Firenzuoli F, Gori L, Lombardo G. The medicinal mushroom *Agaricus blazei Murrill*: Review of literature and pharmaco-toxicological problems. Evid Based Complement Alternat Med 2008; 5(1): 3-15.
[http://dx.doi.org/10.1093/ecam/nem007] [PMID: 18317543]

[62]   Panda SK, Sahoo G, Swain SS, Luyten W. Anticancer activities of mushrooms: A neglected source for drug discovery. Pharmaceuticals 2022; 15(2): 176.
[http://dx.doi.org/10.3390/ph15020176] [PMID: 35215289]

[63]   Chen S, Liu C, Huang X, *et al.* Comparison of immunomodulatory effects of three polysaccharide fractions from *Lentinula edodes* water extracts. J Funct Foods 2020; 66: 103791.
[http://dx.doi.org/10.1016/j.jff.2020.103791]

[64]   Trivedi S, Patel K, Belgamwar V, Wadher K. Functional polysaccharide lentinan: Role in anti-cancer therapies and management of carcinomas. Pharmacological Research-Modern Chinese Medicine. 2022 Jan 10:100045.

[65]   Wang W, Yang X, Li C, Li Y, Wang H, Han X. Immunogenic cell death (ICD) of murine H22 cells induced by lentinan. Nutr Cancer 2022; 74(2): 640-9.
[http://dx.doi.org/10.1080/01635581.2021.1897632] [PMID: 33715541]

[66]   Sun Z, Han Q, Duan L, Yuan Q, Wang H. Oridonin increases anticancer effects of lentinan in HepG2 human hepatoblastoma cells. Oncol Lett 2018; 15(2): 1999-2005.
[PMID: 29434900]

[67]   Yi W, Zhang P, Hou J, *et al.* Enhanced response of tamoxifen toward the cancer cells using a combination of chemotherapy and photothermal ablation induced by lentinan-functionalized multi-walled carbon nanotubes. Int J Biol Macromol 2018; 120(Pt B): 1525-32.
[http://dx.doi.org/10.1016/j.ijbiomac.2018.09.085] [PMID: 30227209]

[68]   Zhang P, Yi W, Hou J, Yoo S, Jin W, Yang Q. A carbon nanotube-gemcitabine-lentinan three-component composite for chemo-photothermal synergistic therapy of cancer. Int J Nanomedicine 2018; 13: 3069-80.
[http://dx.doi.org/10.2147/IJN.S165232] [PMID: 29872294]

[69]   Sun M, Zhao W, Xie Q, Zhan Y, Wu B. Lentinan reduces tumor progression by enhancing

gemcitabine chemotherapy in urothelial bladder cancer. Surg Oncol 2015; 24(1): 28-34.
[http://dx.doi.org/10.1016/j.suronc.2014.11.002] [PMID: 25434982]

[70]   Zhang Y, Liu Y, Zhou Y, *et al.* Lentinan inhibited colon cancer growth by inducing endoplasmic reticulum stress-mediated autophagic cell death and apoptosis. Carbohydr Polym 2021; 267: 118154.
[http://dx.doi.org/10.1016/j.carbpol.2021.118154] [PMID: 34119128]

[71]   Zhao L, Xiao Y, Xiao N. Effect of lentinan combined with docetaxel and cisplatin on the proliferation and apoptosis of BGC823 cells. Tumour Biol 2013; 34(3): 1531-6.
[http://dx.doi.org/10.1007/s13277-013-0680-8] [PMID: 23404406]

[72]   Yan B. DI S, Wang G, Zhang J. Effect of lentinan on cisplatin's inhibition effects on cervical cancer Hela cell line. Chinese Journal of Biochemical Pharmaceutics 2014; 49-50.

[73]   Habtemariam S. *Trametes versicolor* (Synn. *Coriolus versicolor*) polysaccharides in cancer therapy: Targets and efficacy. Biomedicines 2020; 8(5): 135.
[http://dx.doi.org/10.3390/biomedicines8050135] [PMID: 32466253]

[74]   Pawlikowska M, Jędrzejewski T, Piotrowski J, Kozak W. Fever-range hyperthermia inhibits cells immune response to protein-bound polysaccharides derived from *Coriolus versicolor* extract. Mol Immunol 2016; 80: 50-7.
[http://dx.doi.org/10.1016/j.molimm.2016.10.013] [PMID: 27825050]

[75]   Kowalczewska M, Piotrowski J, Jędrzejewski T, Kozak W. Polysaccharide peptides from *Coriolus versicolor* exert differential immunomodulatory effects on blood lymphocytes and breast cancer cell line MCF-7 *in vitro*. Immunol Lett 2016; 174: 37-44.
[http://dx.doi.org/10.1016/j.imlet.2016.04.010] [PMID: 27091479]

[76]   Yang S, Zhuang T, Si Y, Qi K, Zhao J. *Coriolus versicolor* mushroom polysaccharides exert immunoregulatory effects on mouse B cells *via* membrane Ig and TLR-4 to activate the MAPK and NF-κB signaling pathways. Mol Immunol 2015; 64(1): 144-51.
[http://dx.doi.org/10.1016/j.molimm.2014.11.007] [PMID: 25480394]

[77]   Koido S, Homma S, Okamoto M, *et al.* Combined TLR2/4-activated dendritic/tumor cell fusions induce augmented cytotoxic T lymphocytes. PLoS One 2013; 8(3): e59280.
[http://dx.doi.org/10.1371/journal.pone.0059280] [PMID: 23555011]

[78]   Awadasseid A, Eugene K, Jamal M, *et al.* Effect of *Coriolus versicolor* glucan on the stimulation of cytokine production in sarcoma-180-bearing mice. Biomed Rep 2017; 7(6): 567-72.
[http://dx.doi.org/10.3892/br.2017.999] [PMID: 29188061]

[79]   Luo KW, Yue GGL, Ko CH, *et al. In vivo* and *in vitro* anti-tumor and anti-metastasis effects of *Coriolus versicolor* aqueous extract on mouse mammary 4T1 carcinoma. Phytomedicine 2014; 21(8-9): 1078-87.
[http://dx.doi.org/10.1016/j.phymed.2014.04.020] [PMID: 24856767]

[80]   Cao Y, Xu X, Liu S, Huang L, Gu J. Ganoderma: A cancer immunotherapy review. Front Pharmacol 2018; 9: 1217.
[http://dx.doi.org/10.3389/fphar.2018.01217] [PMID: 30410443]

[81]   Liang C, Li H, Zhou H, *et al.* Recombinant Lz-8 from *Ganoderma lucidum* induces endoplasmic reticulum stress-mediated autophagic cell death in SGC-7901 human gastric cancer cells. Oncol Rep 2012; 27(4): 1079-89.
[http://dx.doi.org/10.3892/or.2011.1593] [PMID: 22179718]

[82]   Lin TY, Hsu HY, Sun WH, Wu TH, Tsao SM. Induction of Cbl-dependent epidermal growth factor receptor degradation in Ling Zhi-8 suppressed lung cancer. Int J Cancer 2017; 140(11): 2596-607.
[http://dx.doi.org/10.1002/ijc.30649] [PMID: 28198003]

[83]   Lin CC, Yu YL, Shih CC, *et al.* A novel adjuvant Ling Zhi-8 enhances the efficacy of DNA cancer vaccine by activating dendritic cells. Cancer Immunol Immunother 2011; 60(7): 1019-27.
[http://dx.doi.org/10.1007/s00262-011-1016-4] [PMID: 21499904]

[84]   Hsin IL, Ou CC, Wu MF, *et al.* GMI, an immunomodulatory protein from *Ganoderma microsporum*, potentiates cisplatin-induced apoptosis *via* autophagy in lung cancer cells. Mol Pharm 2015; 12(5): 1534-43.
[http://dx.doi.org/10.1021/mp500840z] [PMID: 25811903]

[85]   Hsin IL, Sheu GT, Jan MS, *et al.* Inhibition of lysosome degradation on autophagosome formation and responses to GMI, an immunomodulatory protein from *Ganoderma microsporum*. Br J Pharmacol 2012; 167(6): 1287-300.
[http://dx.doi.org/10.1111/j.1476-5381.2012.02073.x] [PMID: 22708544]

[86]   Liao CH, Hsiao YM, Sheu GT, *et al.* Nuclear translocation of telomerase reverse transcriptase and calcium signaling in repression of telomerase activity in human lung cancer cells by fungal immunomodulatory protein from *Ganoderma tsugae*. Biochem Pharmacol 2007; 74(10): 1541-54.
[http://dx.doi.org/10.1016/j.bcp.2007.07.025] [PMID: 17720143]

[87]   Wang G, Zhao J, Liu J, Huang Y, Zhong JJ, Tang W. Enhancement of IL-2 and IFN-γ expression and NK cells activity involved in the anti-tumor effect of ganoderic acid Me *in vivo*. Int Immunopharmacol 2007; 7(6): 864-70.
[http://dx.doi.org/10.1016/j.intimp.2007.02.006] [PMID: 17466920]

[88]   Mwangi RW, Macharia JM, Wagara IN, Bence RL. The antioxidant potential of different edible and medicinal mushrooms. Biomed Pharmacother 2022; 147: 112621.
[http://dx.doi.org/10.1016/j.biopha.2022.112621] [PMID: 35026489]

[89]   Dogan A, Dalar A, Sadullahoglu C, *et al.* Investigation of the protective effects of horse mushroom (*Agaricus arvensis* Schaeff.) against carbon tetrachloride-induced oxidative stress in rats. Mol Biol Rep 2018; 45(5): 787-97.
[http://dx.doi.org/10.1007/s11033-018-4218-4] [PMID: 29931536]

[90]   Liu J, Jia L, Kan J, Jin C. *In vitro* and *in vivo* antioxidant activity of ethanolic extract of white button mushroom (*Agaricus bisporus*). Food Chem Toxicol 2013; 51: 310-6.
[http://dx.doi.org/10.1016/j.fct.2012.10.014] [PMID: 23099505]

[91]   Mourão F, Umeo SH, Takemura OS, Linde GA, Colauto NB. Antioxidant activity of *Agaricus brasiliensis basidiocarps* on different maturation phases. Braz J Microbiol 2011; 42(1): 197-202.
[http://dx.doi.org/10.1590/S1517-83822011000100024] [PMID: 24031621]

[92]   Pereira E, Barros L, Martins A, Ferreira ICFR. Towards chemical and nutritional inventory of Portuguese wild edible mushrooms in different habitats. Food Chem 2012; 130(2): 394-403.
[http://dx.doi.org/10.1016/j.foodchem.2011.07.057]

[93]   Kosani M, Rankovi B, Ran A, i , Stanojkovi T. Evaluation of metal contents and bioactivity of two edible mushrooms *Agaricus campestris* and *Boletus edulis*. Emir J Food Agric 2017; 29(2): 98-103.
[http://dx.doi.org/10.9755/ejfa.2016-06-656]

[94]   Qiu J, Zhang H, Wang Z. Ultrasonic degradation of Polysaccharides from *Auricularia auricula* and the antioxidant activity of their degradation products. Lebensm Wiss Technol 2019; 113: 108266.
[http://dx.doi.org/10.1016/j.lwt.2019.108266]

[95]   Hseu YC, Chen SC, Yech YJ, Wang L, Yang HL. Antioxidant activity of *Antrodia camphorata* on free radical-induced endothelial cell damage. J Ethnopharmacol 2008; 118(2): 237-45.
[http://dx.doi.org/10.1016/j.jep.2008.04.004] [PMID: 18486375]

[96]   Jaworska G, Pogoń K, Skrzypczak A, Bernaś E. Composition and antioxidant properties of wild mushrooms *Boletus edulis* and *Xerocomus badius* prepared for consumption. J Food Sci Technol 2015; 52(12): 7944-53.
[http://dx.doi.org/10.1007/s13197-015-1933-x] [PMID: 26604366]

[97]   Liu Y, Zhang B, Ibrahim SA, Gao SS, Yang H, Huang W. Purification, characterization and antioxidant activity of polysaccharides from *Flammulina velutipes* residue. Carbohydr Polym 2016; 145: 71-7.

[http://dx.doi.org/10.1016/j.carbpol.2016.03.020] [PMID: 27106153]

[98] Kozarski M, Klaus A, Nikšić M, *et al.* Antioxidative activities and chemical characterization of polysaccharide extracts from the widely used mushrooms *Ganoderma applanatum, Ganoderma lucidum, Lentinus edodes* and *Trametes versicolor*. J Food Compos Anal 2012; 26(1-2): 144-53.
[http://dx.doi.org/10.1016/j.jfca.2012.02.004]

[99] Han ZH, Ye JM, Wang GF. Evaluation of *in vivo* antioxidant activity of *Hericium erinaceus* polysaccharides. Int J Biol Macromol 2013; 52: 66-71.
[http://dx.doi.org/10.1016/j.ijbiomac.2012.09.009] [PMID: 23000690]

[100] Lau BF, Abdullah N, Aminudin N, Lee HB, Tan PJ. Ethnomedicinal uses, pharmacological activities, and cultivation of *Lignosus* spp. (tiger's milk mushrooms) in Malaysia – A review. J Ethnopharmacol 2015; 169: 441-58.
[http://dx.doi.org/10.1016/j.jep.2015.04.042] [PMID: 25937256]

[101] He P, Li F, Huang L, Xue D, Liu W, Xu C. Chemical characterization and antioxidant activity of polysaccharide extract from spent mushroom substrate of *Pleurotus eryngii*. J Taiwan Inst Chem Eng 2016; 69: 48-53.
[http://dx.doi.org/10.1016/j.jtice.2016.10.017]

[102] Gursoy N, Sarikurkcu C, Tepe B, Halil Solak M. Evaluation of antioxidant activities of 3 edible mushrooms: *Ramaria flava* (Schaef.: Fr.) Quél., *Rhizopogon roseolus* (Corda) T.M. Fries., and *Russula delica* Fr. Food Sci Biotechnol 2010; 19(3): 691-6.
[http://dx.doi.org/10.1007/s10068-010-0097-8]

[103] Li H, Wang X, Xiong Q, Yu Y, Peng L. Sulfated modification, characterization, and potential bioactivities of polysaccharide from the fruiting bodies of *Russula virescens*. Int J Biol Macromol 2020; 154: 1438-47.
[http://dx.doi.org/10.1016/j.ijbiomac.2019.11.025] [PMID: 31733257]

CHAPTER 4

Natural Products as Antioxidant Adjunct Therapy for Blood Parasitic Infections

Paweena Pradniwat[1,2,*]

[1] *Department of Clinical Microscopy, Faculty of Allied Health Sciences, Chulalongkorn University, Bangkok, Thailand*

[2] *Immunomodulation of Natural Products Research Unit, Chulalongkorn University, Bangkok, Thailand*

Abstract: Human blood protozoa infections cause oxidative stresses from the parasites, host's defense systems, and administered drugs. Oxidative stress is an important tool to eliminate parasites from the host's body. However, the host's cells, tissues, and even organs would be damaged along with parasites. Many pathologies such as cerebral malaria, and renal or hepatic failures are a result of the unbalanced oxidative condition. Many medicinal plant extracts show both anti-protozoa and antioxidant activities simultaneously. Therefore, the administration of medicinal plant extracts in combination with chemical drugs should be beneficial for patients with blood-protozoa infection, by both eradicating the parasites and alleviating the oxidative stress. In addition, the combination might also help prevent parasite resistance to chemical drugs as the extract and chemical drugs aim at different targets simultaneously. In this chapter, the properties and benefits of medicinal plant extracts are discussed.

Keywords: Acute respiratory distress syndrome (ARDS), Aldo-keto reductase (AKR), Anti-plasmodial, Antimalaria, Anti-babesia, Anti-leishmania, Anti-oxidant, Antioxidant adjunct therapy, Catalase, Glutathione (GSH), Malondialdehyde (MDA), Natural product, Nicotinamide adenine dinucleotide phosphate reduced (NADPH) oxidase, Nitric oxide synthase (NOS), Oxidative burst, Oxidative enzyme, Oxidative stress, Reactive oxygen species (ROS), Superoxide dismutase (SOD), Xanthine oxidase (XO), 2,2-Diphenyl-1-picrylhydrazyl (DPPH).

INTRODUCTION

Human blood protozoans continue to cause serious parasitic diseases around the globe. According to World Health Orgainisation (WHO), Malaria infections were

---
[*] **Corresponding author Paweena Pradniwat:** Department of Clinical Microscopy, Faculty of Allied Health Sciences, Chulalongkorn University, Bangkok, Thailand and Immunomodulation of Natural Products Research Unit, Chulalongkorn University, Bangkok, Thailand; Tel: +(66) 22181545; E-mail: paweena.p@chula.ac.th

Pardeep Kaur, Tewin Tencomnao, Robin and Rajendra G. Mehta (Eds.)

241 million cases and 627000 deaths in 2020 [1]. Malaria infections remained endemic in impoverished countries with transmission-suitable climates [2]. Despite the general waning trend of *Plasmodium falciparum* malaria in Africa, from 40% (1910–1929) to 24% (2010–2015), a new rising trend was reported in 2016 compared to that of 2015 by WHO [2]. Five species of human *Plasmodium* parasites are *Plasmodium falciparum*, *P. vivax*, *P. ovale*, *P. malariae*, and *P. knowlesi* [3]. Malaria causes fever and flu-like maladies, such as shaking chills, headache, muscle aches, tiredness, nausea, vomiting, diarrhea, anemia, and jaundice [3].

In addition to numerous species of *Babesia* reported to infect wild and domestic animals including livestock, six species have up till now been established as human parasites: *Babesia crassa*-like agent, *Babesia divergens*, *Babesia duncani*, *Babesia microti*, *Babesia motasi*, and *Babesia venatorum* [4]. Human babesiosis is acquired mainly in the temperate zone. The predominant *B. microti* was endemic in the northern United States and southwestern China [4]. Even with the low global prevalence of human *Babesia spp.* infection of 2.23%, the increasing cases of immunocompetent patients are alarming. Approximately half of the infections are commonly asymptomatic or mistaken for malaria [5]. The usual symptoms are fever and hemolytic anemia. However, in immunocompromised persons, *Babesia spp.* triggers hemolytic anemia, intravascular coagulopathy, hepatomegaly, and splenomegaly, and results in respiratory distress syndrome, heart failure, inflammation of the central nervous system, and death [5].

700,000 to 1 million *Leishmania* new cases are estimated per year [6]. Visceral leishmaniasis (VL), otherwise known as kala-azar, has an estimated 50,000 to 90,000 new cases worldwide per annum. Above 90% of VL new cases reported in 2020, were from Brazil, China, Ethiopia, Eritrea, India, Kenya, Somalia, South Sudan, Sudan, and Yemen. VL is lethal in 95% of untreated cases. The symptoms are irregular fever sessions, weight loss, spleen and liver enlargement, and anemia. Most cases were reported in Brazil, East Africa, and India. VL is still one of the leading parasitic ailments with a high potential for outbreak and mortality. The most common cutaneous leishmaniasis (CL) has an estimated new case of 600,000 to 1 million worldwide annually. Roughly 95% of the cases take place in the Americas, the Mediterranean basin, the Middle East, and Central Asia. In 2020, above 85% of new CL cases were in Afghanistan, Algeria, Brazil, Colombia, Iraq, Libya, Pakistan, Peru, the Syrian Arab Republic, and Tunisia. Mucocutaneous leishmaniasis (ML) causes skin lesions, developing into fractional or entire damage of mucous membranes, such as in the nose, mouth, and throat. More than 90% of ML cases were in the Plurinational State of Bolivia, Brazil, Ethiopia, and Peru [6].

The life-threatening human African trypanosomiasis predominantly impacts poor people and travelers in rural endemic areas. Since the WHO's reinforced control and surveillance program in 2001, human African trypanosomiasis infections diminished significantly to less than 1,000 cases in 2019, with 2.5 million people screened yearly [7]. However, the disease is considered fatal if not treated [7].

These parasites cause enormous economic expenditure and remain one of the major causes of death. Therefore, new anti-parasite agents are still urgently and persistently explored.

Natural products from medicinal plants and fruits hold great potential for fighting against parasites as well as the free radicals produced during infections. Natural products have more possibility than artificial compounds to contain multiple and/or novel targets, owing to their structural features: multiple stereocenters, flexible conformations, and heteroatom presences [2].

OXIDATIVE STRESS IN BLOOD PARASITE INFECTIONS

Oxidative stress is a consequence of the broken balance between oxidizing species and antioxidants. Blood protozoa usually have many stages inside hosts, such as erythrocytic, hepatic, or muscle stages. Protozoa, host defense system, and antimicrobial drugs are responsible for oxidative burdens inside host cells and tissues. The high oxidative stress during malarial infection is accountable for both tissue and systemic oxidative damages, involving crucial organs like the brain and lungs. Consequences of the most life-threatening cerebral malaria, brain parenchyma lesion, leading to physical and cognitive impairments are thus possible [8, 9].

Janka, *et al.* [10] described the oxidative stress affecting the myocardial wall and causing high pulmonary pressure in children with severe malaria. This cardiopulmonary effect was initiated by intravascular hemolysis and a decreased nitric oxide (NO) generation [10].

Also, in an experimental malaria study, oxidative damage markers linked to kidney acute tubular damage, 4-hydroxynonenal (4-HNE), and heme oxygenase-1 (HO-1), were found to be increasingly expressed [11].

Percário *et al.* [12] proposed that oxidative stress induction in malaria is a result of various factors. These considerations are: 1) the consumption of hemoglobin producing free radical assembly *via* Fenton and Haber–Weiss reactions, 2) the host's immune response against the parasites, 3) microvascular cytoadherence and anemia leading to ischemia and reperfusion syndrome, 4) free radicals directly created by the parasites, and 5) anti-parasite drugs used. At least some of these aspects should be veritable for other parasites, especially those with the intra-erythrocytic stage as well. Fig. (**1**) depicts the causes of oxidative stress occurring during blood protozoa infections. Although, oxidative mechanism is intended to slay the parasites, it causes damage to the host cells and organs [13].

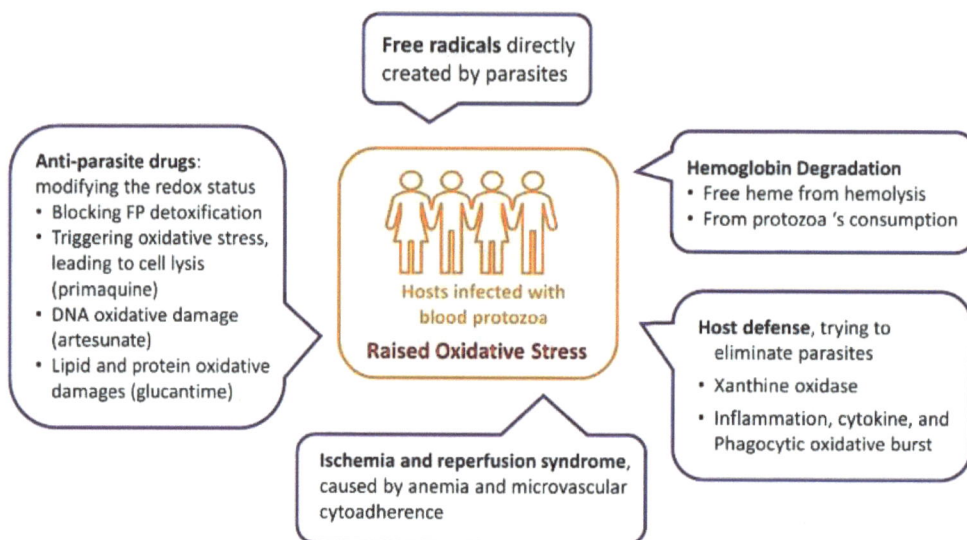

Fig. (1). Causes of oxidative stress occurring during blood protozoa infections. Oxidative stress induced by blood protozoa infections is a result of 1) hemoglobin degradation, 2) the host's immune response, 3) ischemia and reperfusion syndrome, 4) free radicals produced by parasites, and 5) anti-parasite drugs.

Malarial Infection

Plasmodium-Induced Oxidative Stress in the Host

There are many sources of oxidative stress during malarial infections, from the parasite, host, or medication. The oxidant species are either from the host's attempt to get rid of the protozoa or the *Plasmodium's* high growing and multiplying rates. The malarial infection causes oxidative stress in different stages of infection. This oxidative stress can be destructive or favorable, depending on the disease stages [14].

For malaria, the oxidative stress biomarker malondialdehyde (MDA) was reportedly increased in patients with oxidative stress such as in pediatric complicated malaria infections [15], and in the *P. falciparum*-infected uncomplicated sickle cell disease patients [16]. Therefore, MDA was used as a biomarker for oxidative stresses in malarial infection as well as other infections and diseases.

The severe acute respiratory distress syndrome (ARDS) is distinguished by pulmonary edema as a result of increased vascular permeability. Similarly, Anidi *et al.* [17] showed that lung-sequestered erythrocytes generated ROS/RNS (Reactive Oxygen Species/Reactive Nitrogen Species), responsible for the said vascular permeability.

The brain-existed *Plasmodium* raising oxidative stress, along with blood flow blockade from the erythrocyte-vessel adhesions, causes ischemia and reperfusion syndrome. Also, the high oxidative stress inside the central nervous system is related to the deteriorating degree of the disease [18]. Moreover, long-term physical and cognitive dysfunctions are likely to occur in *P. berghei*-infected mice after brain oxidative damage [8, 9].

Scaccabarozzi *et al.* [19] reported an excess oxidative stress response and reduced antioxidant defenses in *P. berghei* NK65-infected C57BL/6J mice with high parasitemia, concurrently developing lethal ARDS. The overwhelmed oxidative responses were demonstrated by the alteration of liver antioxidant enzymes (lower levels of catalase activity and total glutathione), increased MDA levels, and triglyceride accumulation. On the other hand, with a self-limiting *P. chabaudi* AS infection, the infected mice exhibited hepatopathy, but not leading to lipid alterations or antioxidant enzyme (catalase, superoxide dismutase activities, and glutathione) reductions. The *P. chabaudi* AS-infected mice were more likely to progress to inflammation and cytokine burst, possibly assisting parasite clearance [20].

Even though the study was performed *in vivo* in mouse *Plasmodium spp.* infections, it could be applied to human malarial infections as well. In the liver phase, infections with high parasitemia might lead to excess oxidative stress and ARDS. If the intervention therapy to reduce the blood parasite number can be administered, patients would have fewer symptoms and a better recovery.

Hemoglobin Degradation Induces Oxidative Stress

Heme is a highly toxic oxidative compound, damaging both protozoa and the host. *Plasmodium falciparum* consumes more or less 75% of erythrocyte hemoglobin [21 - 23], its major food source in red blood cells. During this intra-erythrocytic phase, harmful free heme and ROS are released and hemozoin is formed [21, 24, 25]. Hydroxyl radicals are produced by heme irons, *via* the Fenton reaction [12].

To keep the cells safe, this free, highly toxic heme is kept in harmless heme-interlinked crystalline forms, hemozoin, or malaria pigment [25 - 27], or undergoes the neutralization processes. Such processes are free heme degradation [22, 28], glutathione reaction [29], and the bound form with free heme-binding proteins [30, 31].

Still, if only a minute quantity as 0.5% of free heme escaped, damage to host proteins and membranes (including red blood cells), as well as *Plasmodium spp.* would occur [32]. In addition, usually occurring in *Plasmodium spp.* infections, the red blood cell hemolysis either infected or not, is likewise the source of free heme [32].

Host's Xanthine Oxidase Induces Oxidative Stress

Xanthine oxidase (XO) is the host oxidative enzyme responsible for breaking down hypoxanthine to xanthine and eventually uric acid [33]. This reaction creates reactive oxygen species, for instance, superoxide ($O_2\cdot-$) and hydrogen peroxide (H_2O_2) [33]. In both mice [34] and humans [35, 36], XO levels were raised in *Plasmodium* infections. Patients with severe cerebral malaria showed greater XO levels than those with uncomplicated malaria [35, 36]. XO is both protecting and damaging the host during malarial infections. XO defensive activity functions by competitively consuming hypoxanthine, thus depriving the parasite of the material for purine synthesis [37]. Likewise, ROS generated by XO also harms the *Plasmodium* parasites. For example, when compared to controls, the lower parasitemia levels in mice injected with XO pre-treated *P. yoelii* indicated that the parasites lost the efficiency to multiply in a murine host. Conversely, in the presence of the antioxidant enzyme catalase, XO pre-treated *P. yoelii* successfully re-established its virulence [13]. On the other hand, XO-derived extracellular ROS causes inflammation in malaria patients, especially in concert with infected red blood cell (iRBC) lysate. This combination could stimulate monocyte-derived macrophages and dendritic cells *in vitro*, leading to inflammatory cytokine productions, such as interleukin-1beta (IL-1b), interleukin-8 (IL-8), C-C Motif Chemokine Ligand 5 (CCL5), and C-C Motif Chemokine Ligand 2 (CCL2) [36, 38]. Furthermore, XO helps promote both dendritic cell and T cell responses to *Plasmodium* infection. XO amplifies the ability of *P. falciparum*–activated dendritic cells, which in turn increases T cell proliferation [38].

Phagocytic Oxidative Burst from Host Defense Mechanism

One of the host's attempts to get rid of *Plasmodium* parasites is to activate phagocytes. These innate immune cells such as neutrophils and monocytes, consequently, create enormous quantities of ROS and RNS, or oxidative burst in these cells after phagocytosing *P. falciparum* merozoites [39, 40]. Nicotinamide adenine dinucleotide phosphate reduced (NADPH) oxidase is activated to produce high ROS amounts inside the phagosome, leading to the parasite's death [41].

Despite the benefits of killing parasites, the phagocytosis of *Plasmodium* antigens lowers the oxidative capacity of phagocytic cells. Schwarzer and Arese [42], showed that after a phagocytosis of purified hemozoin, macrophages had decreased NADPH oxidase activity. Also, neutrophils isolated from *P. falciparum*-infected Gambian children showed diminished oxidative burst capacity, compared to neutrophils from uninfected controls [43]. These studies suggested that *Plasmodium* infection could lessen the host's oxidative burst.

Largely, the phagocytic oxidative burst downregulation may be favorable as it diminishes the host's oxidative stress, however, the waning oxidative stress would also allow the replication and thriving of the parasites [14, 21].

Antimalarial Drugs

The current antimalarial drugs depend on many mechanisms to eliminate parasite infections.

The four drug classifications presently available for malarial treatments are quinoline-related compounds, antifolates, artemisinin derivatives, and antimicrobials [44]. These drugs are always in combination as no single medicine can exterminate all forms of *Plasmodium* parasites. The regimens are assigned according to the *Plasmodium* species, the disease severity, and the parasites' drug-resistant abilities [44].

Artemisinin combination therapies (ACTs) currently have the best efficacy and the first-line treatment for uncomplicated falciparum malaria [45].

Hydroxychloroquine or chloroquine phosphate, in combination with primaquine phosphate, is ideal in case of uncomplicated infections caused by chloroquine-sensitive *P. falciparum* [46, 47].

With a similar mechanism as hydroxychloroquine, chloroquine phosphate kills the *P. vivax* or *P. ovale* hypnozoites by assembling in the parasite acid vesicles and increasing the pH. Proguanil inhibits deoxythymidylate synthesis by restraining dihydrofolate reductase *via* parasite mitochondrial electron transport arrest [48, 49].

Quinidine gluconate mainly kills schizonts that reside in red blood cells, with only a slight effect on sporozoites or extra-erythrocytic parasites [46, 47].

Usually, in combination with chloroquine or atovaquone, proguanil is used for the treatment and prevention of malarial infections, since the combination can inhibit parasite replications and kill blood schizonts. Quinidine can kill gametocytes of *P. vivax* and *P. malariae*, but not *P. falciparum* [49].

Antifolate drugs hinder the *Plasmodium* folate metabolism, an essential pathway for malarial persistence [50]. Despite the antifolate-resistant *Plasmodium spp.*, antifolate drugs continue to be first-line treatments against chloroquine-resistant parasites in many sub-Saharan African countries [50]. To augment the antifolate drug effectiveness in addition to preventing the growth of resistant *Plasmodium* strains, using antifolates in combination with drugs attacking different targets should be considered [50].

For chloroquine-resistant *P. falciparum* treatment, artemether-lumefantrine is the first-line medication for inhibiting nucleic acid and protein synthesis. The second option for chloroquine-resistant *P. falciparum* is quinine sulfate along with doxycycline, tetracycline, or clindamycin. The parasites' replication and transcription are disrupted as quinine inserts itself into the *Plasmodium* DNA [49].

The quinoline-related compound, intra-erythrocytic schizonticide, quinidine gluconate is the drug of choice for severe malaria. Along with quinidine gluconate, combinations with clindamycin, doxycycline, or tetracycline are usually included in the treatment of patients with severe malaria either by intravenous (IV) or oral form [51]. The quinine-clindamycin combination is safe and effective against multidrug-resistant *P. falciparum* malaria, especially in children and pregnant women in which tetracycline is prohibited [52].

A synthetic derivative of tetracycline, doxycycline can kill blood schizonts in a slow-acting fashion. When in combination with the fast-acting schizonticide quinine, this therapy is greatly successful for malaria remedy [53].

Anti-malarial Drugs Interfering with Oxidative Stress

Commonly used antimalarials, artemisinin, artesunate, chloroquine, coartem, and quinine, could induce oxidative stress by modifying the redox status in both healthy and ill persons [21, 54].

As *Plasmodium spp.* is susceptible to oxidative species, numerous antimalarial medications are relying on oxidative stress to eradicate the parasite. Many antimalarial drugs are interfering with oxidative stress. The 4-aminoquinoline antimalarials, like chloroquine, quinolones and amodiaquine, block detoxification of ferriprotoporphyrin (FP) [55]. As the intermediate hemozoin dimer cannot be formed, the nontoxic hemozoin crystal formation is therefore impossible. Subsequently, the accumulation of oxidative-free FP probably injures membranes and enzymes due to its detergent-like properties in addition to its contribution to harmful redox reactions [24, 56, 57]. Intriguingly, Srivastava *et al.* [58] reported the increased antioxidant enzyme glutathione-S-transferase activity in the chloroquine-resistant strains of *P. falciparum, P. yoelii, and P. berghei*, compared to the counterpart chloroquine-sensitive strains.

The only drug clinically approved for *Plasmodium vivax* exoerythrocytic infections is 8-aminoquinoline (primaquine) [21]. However, its mechanism of action is still not well apprehended [21]. Possibly, primaquine is converted into an active quinone metabolite by the liver, and acts by interfering with the mitochondrial function of the exoerythrocytic parasites [59, 60].

Still, the primaquine hydroxylated metabolites might cause hemolytic side effects as its redox cycling triggers significant oxidative stress on the erythrocyte. In those with compromised antioxidative systems, such as G6PDH deficient patients, the cell's ability to detoxify ROS lessens, resulting in cell lysis [61].

The endoperoxide antimalarials, such as artemisinin, dihydroartemisinin, and artesunate, are in more use owing to the rise of drug-resistant *Plasmodium spp.*. The active endoperoxide groups, gathered in the cytosol and membrane of a parasite, interact with the reduced heme (FP-FeII) [62, 63], forming a cytotoxic carbon-centered radical intermediate that later reacts with parasite lipids and enzymes [63 - 66]. Interestingly, the antioxidant N-acetylcysteine (NAC) was reported to thwart the anti-parasitic activity of artesunate against *P. falciparum* [67].

Even though oxidative stress intensifying is an efficacious mechanism for parasite eradication, it may also harm the host. The cellular DNA oxidative damage caused by artesunate was found in the human *in vitro* study [67] and in mice [68].

Besides, Akanbi *et al.* [69] described that malaria patients receiving anti-malarial drugs possessed greater lipid peroxidation levels and lesser antioxidant levels, compared to non-treated patients. This emphasizes that the host's increased oxidative stress is instigated by anti-malarial drugs. The use of antioxidants, like quercetin, in combination with chloroquine was proposed to balance the drug's oxidative effects in the host [70].

Babesia spp. Infection

Similar to malaria infections, *Babesia spp.* infections cause oxidative alterations inside hosts.

Since the enzyme aldo-keto reductase (AKR) was believed to be a key antioxidant element, Huang *et al.* [71] studied AKR in *B. microti*-infected KM mice and proposed that BmAKR (*B. microti* aldo-keto reductase) protein expression was promoted by *B. microti* to thwart oxidative stress. They found that the *Bmakr* mRNA expression level in *B. microti*-infected red blood cells (iRBCs) was raised threefold after 150 μM H_2O_2 treatment, compared to that of untreated iRBCs. Also, *Bmakr* mRNA relative expression levels of iRBCs were significantly upregulated after 24-hour treatments with the drugs robenidine and atovaquone, but not artemisinin or quinine.

Many studies have revealed that AKRs were also recognized in *B. bovis* [72], *T. cruzi* [73], and *L. donovani* [74].

Kucukkurt, *et al.* [75] reported the result from a study of 10 Anatolian black goats naturally infected with *B. ovis*. The results of the oxidative stress markers, whole blood MDA (9.59±0.63 nmol/ml), DNA damage by alkaline comet assay (95.32±7.65 AU), protein carbonyl: PCO (1.38±0.05 nmol/mg protein), and plasma nitrite/nitrate products: NOx (1.56±0.13 μmol/L) levels were significantly higher than those of the control group. On the other hand, the antioxidant markers reduced glutathione: GSH (19.53±1.73 g/dl), serum total antioxidant activity: AOA (1.56±0.13 mmol/L) were significantly lower than those of the control group [75].

A large amount of ROS and NOx occurred inside the host's cells infected with *Babesia spp.*, in so doing causing cell and tissue injuries [75, 76]. The oxidation of polyunsaturated fatty acids by ROS led to the production of lipid peroxidation (LP) products such as MDA [77]. Kucukkurt *et al.* [75] proposed that increased LP biomarker MDA level might indicate the elevated level of DNA damage caused by oxidative free radical generation. Likewise, Koçyiğit *et al.* [78] revealed the DNA damage induced by free radical production from polymorphonuclear cells in cutaneous leishmaniasis infection. Furthermore, the increased plasma PCO level of infected goats hinted that the alterations of protein structure and function were caused by *Babesia* infection [78].

Clindamycin and quinine are the usual medications given to *Babesia*-infected patients [79]. However, in case of immunosuppressed patients, this combination proved to be unsatisfactory. The administration of atovaquone plus azithromycin is then recommended. Regularly used antimalarials might induce oxidative stress in both healthy and infected persons by changing the redox status [54]. Since the anti-babesia and antimalarial drugs are quite similar, they cause the alike oxidative stress effects in both patient groups [54].

Trypanosoma spp. Infection

When infected by *Trypanosoma cruzi*, the host's cell responds by oxidative burst. *T. cruzi* infection also stimulates oxidative stress, inducing protein oxidation and DNA damage in human cells [80, 81]. Therefore, *T. cruzi* must endure both endogenous oxidative metabolic by-products from its aerobic metabolism and the host's defense system (the superoxide anions and ROS productions). Interestingly, trypanosomatids lack catalase and classical selenium-containing glutathione peroxidases, hence the limited ability to cope with ROS [81]. To survive, *T. cruzi* has developed complicated anti-oxidative processes, such as ROS detoxification pathways, DNA repair pathways, and specialized polymerases, to guard its genome against oxidative damage [81]. These also promote the genetic diversity of the parasite. Many studies also hinted that oxidative setting might be favorable for parasites as it aided in the parasite's iron mobilization from the host's storage [81]. During infection, both oxidative stress and DNA damage induction in host cells occurs. The equilibrium of these two pathways might help promote the process of infection. By interfering with these processes, we might be able to impede *T. cruzi* [80].

As a result, antioxidant therapy might be helpful in *Trypanosoma*-infected patients. A report showed that when host cells were treated with glutathione precursor, *i.e.*, NAC, NRF2 activator (sulforaphane), and benznidazole (BNZ), the parasites busted and the host cells' DNA damages were reduced significantly [80].

Leishmania spp. Infection

Similar to *Trypanosoma spp.* infection, oxidative stress occurs in CL patients from the parasite metabolism and host's defense system. In contrast, the host-produced ROS and RNS may augment the leishmanicidal activity in CL patients [78].

In contrast, Acestor *et al.* [82] found that the metastatic (M^+) *L. (V.) guyanensis* clones have produced a higher amount of the distinct cytoplasmic peroxiredoxin (PXN) dimers, formed after treatments with hydrogen peroxide or heat shock, than that of nonmetastatic (M^-) ones. As the 2-Cys dimerization of PXN is obligatory for the hydrogen peroxide (H_2O_2) detoxification, M^+ promastigotes showed significantly higher neutralization activity than that in M^- parasites, when treated with amplifying concentrations of H_2O_2. This might be a verification that the *Leishmania* promastigote microbicidal resistance is connected to peroxiredoxin conformation. With this more stable PXN dimer, the parasite could survive and live better in the host's cells, resulting in metastatic disease development [82].

Glucantime, is a pentavalent antimonial meglumine antimoniate used to treat *Leishmania* infection. Still, glucantime is well-known for its toxic effects, for example, its ability to cause oxidative damage to lipids and proteins [83], described as the oxidative stress-derived DNA damage caused by meglumine antimoniate. Its mutagenic ability is through the oxidation of DNA bases. Nonetheless, the reducing compounds, such as ascorbic acid and isoflavone genistein, could reduce this mutagenic damage [83].

Nevertheless, the free radical intermediates not only induce the destruction of the parasites but also generate oxidative damage in non-infected cells. For this reason, *Leishmania*-infected patients should be treated quickly to neutralize the oxidative DNA damage to their cells and tissues. With high resistance M^+L. *(V.) guyanensis*, careful oxidative stress management should be ensured as the low oxidative level might not be beneficial in killing parasites, while the high oxidative level could cause great damage to the host's cells.

NATURAL PRODUCTS FOR BLOOD PROTOZOA TREATMENTS

Numerous antioxidative pathways are used to protect the body from free radical species. The three major classes of antioxidant enzymes are catalases, superoxide dismutases (SOD), and glutathione peroxidases (GPX) hold great responsibilities in maintaining cellular homeostasis [84]. Nevertheless, with exposure to diseases and environmental pollutants, the body's antioxidative defenses are often unsatisfactory [85]. As a result, antioxidant treatments to boost the host's antioxidant capability, while not undermining the anti-parasite mechanisms are under intense study.

Antioxidant natural products show advantages in blood protozoa infections by helping avert or minimize oxidative damages occurring during parasitic infections. They also show favorable advantages in malarial and other blood protozoa infections.

Blood protozoa infections cause symptoms and pathologies, at least in part by oxidative stress either by the parasites themself, parasite-related mechanisms, or host defensive responses. Accordingly, many studies focused on antioxidant management along with anti-parasite medications. Many antioxidants were used to help fight against the free radicals increased during the infection and therapy. These supplements are vitamin A, vitamin C, vitamin D, vitamin E, NAC, zinc, and selenium [86 - 101]. The combination, like vitamin A and zinc supplementation, was used in pregnant women to prevent placental malaria [99]. Moreover, the high activity of the antioxidant such as tempol demonstrated a more effective activity in reducing oxidative and inflammatory damages, therefore increasing animal embryo survival [102]. Additionally, green tea extract was also revealed to reduce plasma BUN and creatinine levels during *Plasmodium berghei* ANKA (PbANKA) infection in ICR mice [103].

The treatments for infected patients must be appropriately balanced for both anti-parasite and antioxidative stress. Since one of the host's responses and drug mechanisms to eliminate the parasites is the increased oxidative stress to the protozoa, the medications to lower such conditions might decrease the anti-parasite competency. However, the high oxidative condition either from the host's defense system or the anti-parasite drug is dangerous for hosts as it can lead to inflammation and tissue damage.

Numerous medicinal plant extracts were reported to show anti-protozoa and antioxidant effects simultaneously. Fig. (**2**) describes the activities of natural products beneficial to hosts during blood protozoa infections. Likewise, some medicinal plants that possess both anti-protozoa and antioxidant effects are described and listed Table **1** here.

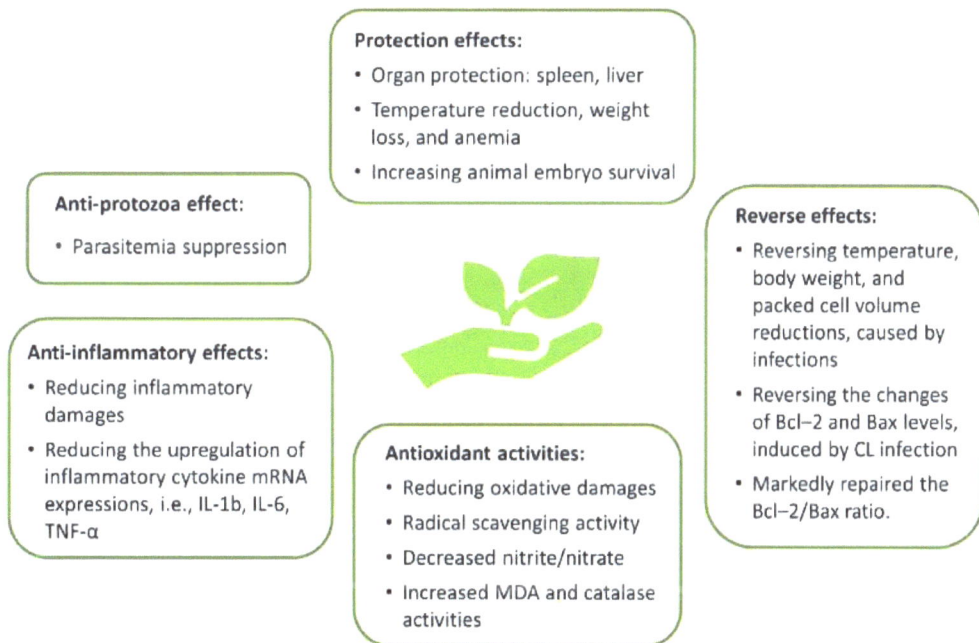

Protection effects:
- Organ protection: spleen, liver
- Temperature reduction, weight loss, and anemia
- Increasing animal embryo survival

Anti-protozoa effect:
- Parasitemia suppression

Anti-inflammatory effects:
- Reducing inflammatory damages
- Reducing the upregulation of inflammatory cytokine mRNA expressions, i.e., IL-1b, IL-6, TNF-α

Antioxidant activities:
- Reducing oxidative damages
- Radical scavenging activity
- Decreased nitrite/nitrate
- Increased MDA and catalase activities

Reverse effects:
- Reversing temperature, body weight, and packed cell volume reductions, caused by infections
- Reversing the changes of Bcl–2 and Bax levels, induced by CL infection
- Markedly repaired the Bcl–2/Bax ratio.

Fig. (2). The natural product activities beneficial to hosts during blood protozoa infections. Natural products are beneficial for patients with blood protozoa infections by showing various activities: 1) anti-protozoa effect, 2) antioxidant effect, 3) anti-inflammatory effect, 4) reversing damages triggered by protozoa, and 5) cell and organ protection effect.

Table 1. The natural plant extracts containing both antioxidants and anti-protozoa activity.

Botanical Name	Family	Anti-protozoa Activities	Part Used	References
Acanthus polystachyus Delile	Acanthaceae	antioxidant anti-plasmodial	leaf	[112, 131]
Achillea millefolium L.	Asteraceae	antioxidant anti-plasmodial anti-babesia anti-trypanosoma anti-leishmania	whole plant	[105 - 110]
Ageratum conyzoides L.	Asteraceae	antioxidant anti-plasmodial anti-babesia anti-trypanosoma anti-leishmania	whole plant	[105, 132]
Aloysia citrodora	Verbenaceae	antioxidant anti-plasmodial anti-trypanosoma anti-leishmania	oil	[133 - 135]
Alpinia galanga	Zingiberaceae	antioxidant anti-plasmodial anti-trypanosoma anti-leishmania	rhizome	[136 - 142]
Anthocleista djalonensis A. Chev	Gentianaceae	antioxidant anti-plasmodial	stem bark	[130]
Azadirachta indica Juss.	Meliaceae	antioxidant anti-plasmodial anti-babesia anti-trypanosoma	leaves	[105, 143 - 150]
Baecked frutenscen L.	Myrtaceae	antioxidant anti-plasmodial anti-babesia anti-trypanosoma anti-leishmania	leaves	[105, 107, 151 - 154]
Blumea balsamifera L.DC.	Asteraceae	antioxidant anti-plasmodial anti-babesia anti-Trypanosoma anti-leishmania	leaf	[105, 155 - 158]
Brucea javanica (L.) Merr.	Simaroubaceae	antioxidant anti-plasmodial anti-babesia	bark	[105, 159 - 163]

(Table 1) cont.....

Botanical Name	Family	Anti-protozoa Activities	Part Used	References
Cassia fistula L.	Fabaceae	antioxidant anti-plasmodial anti-babesia anti-leishmania	pods	[105, 164 - 166]
Catharanthus roseus L.	Apocynaceae	antioxidant anti-plasmodial anti-babesia anti-trypanosoma	aerial part	[105, 167 - 170]
Clerodendrum violaceum	Labiatae	antioxidant anti-plasmodial	leaf	[111]
Curcuma aeruginosa Roxb.	Zingiberaceae	antioxidant anti-plasmodial anti-babesia	rhizomes	[105, 171 - 172]
Curcuma xanthorrhiza Roxb.	Zingiberaceae	antioxidant anti-plasmodial anti-babesia	rhizomes	[105, 173 - 175]
Erythrina burttii	Umbelliferae	antioxidant anti-plasmodial	root bark	[119]
Foeniculum vulgare Mill.	Umbelliferae	antioxidant anti-plasmodial anti-babesia anti-leishmania	seeds	[105, 176 -180]
Gardenia ternifolia	Rubiaceae	antioxidant anti-plasmodial	leaf	[123, 124]
Lansium domesticum Corr.	Meliaceae	antioxidant anti-plasmodial anti-babesia anti-trypanosoma anti-leishmania (in silico)	bark	[105, 181 - 183]
Lippia multiflora	Verbenaceae	antioxidant anti-plasmodial anti-trypanosoma anti-leishmania	leaf	[113, 184]
Morinda citrifolia L.	Rubiaceae	antioxidant anti-plasmodial anti-babesia anti-trypanosoma anti-leishmania	fruit	[105, 185 - 187]
Moringa oleifera Lam.	Moringaceae	antioxidant anti-plasmodial anti-trypanosoma anti-leishmania	leaf	[115, 118, 188-192]

(Table 1) cont.....

Botanical Name	Family	Anti-protozoa Activities	Part Used	References
Nigella sativa	Ranunculaceae	antioxidant anti-plasmodial anti-babesia anti-trypanosoma anti-leishmania	seed	[193 - 198]
Ocimum sanctum	low antimalaria	antioxidant anti-plasmodial anti-leishmania	whole plant	[199 - 201]
Piper retrofractum Vahl.	Piperaceae	antioxidant anti-plasmodial anti-babesia	fruit	[105, 202]
Piper sarmentosum	Piperaceae	antioxidant anti-plasmodial	leaf	[140, 203-205]
Rouvolfia serpentina (L.) Benth.	Apocynaceae	antioxidant anti-plasmodial anti-babesia	bark	[105, 206, 207]
Strychnos lucida R.Br.	Loganiaceae	antioxidant anti-plasmodial anti-babesia	wood	[105, 208]
Swietenia macrophylla King.	Meliaceae	antioxidant anti-plasmodial anti-babesia	seeds	[105, 209, 210]
Tinospora crispa Miers.	Menispermaceae	antioxidant anti-plasmodial anti-babesia	stem	[105, 211 - 213]
Uncaria gambir Roxb.	Rubiaceae	antioxidant anti-plasmodial anti-babesia	leaves	[105, 140, 214 - 216]
Vitis trifolia L.	Vitaceae	antioxidant anti-plasmodial anti-babesia	leaves	[105, 217]
Zingiber aromaticum Valeton	Zingiberaceae	antioxidant anti-plasmodial anti-babesia	rhizomes	[105, 218]

Achillea millefolium Aerial Part Decoction and Essential Oil

Lidiya *et al.* [104] described that *A. millefolium* decoction was rich in phenolic acids, *i.e.*, caffeoylquinic and dicaffeoylquinic acids derivatives. In addition, hyperoside, rutin, kaempferol, gallic acid, and luteolin were also found in the extract. These components were likely the source of *A. millefolium* antioxidative activity (IC50 = 51.0 µg/mL). However, *A. millefolium* essential oil showed moderate antimalarial and weak anti-protozoa activities against *Babesia spp.*, and *Trypanosoma spp* [105 - 110].

Clerodendrum violaceum Leaf Methanolic Extract

Compared with ethyl acetate and hexane extracts, the methanolic extract of *Clerodendrum violaceum* leaf contained the highest amounts of phenols, flavonoids, vitamin C, vitamin E, and selenium. Also, the *Clerodendrum violaceum* leaf methanolic extract exhibited 88.75% DPPH radical scavenging activity and 72% hydrogen peroxide scavenging activity in a concentration-dependent manner [111]. These results showed enzyme activities neighboring those of the standard antioxidant butylated hydroxytoluene (BHT) [111].

The *in vivo* antioxidant study was performedby investigating chloroquine-sensitive *Plasmodium berghei* NK65-infected adult Swiss albino mice. The erythrocytic and hepatic enzymes, superoxide dismutase, and catalase activities of infected mice were significantly increased ($p < 0.05$) while the counterpart glutathione peroxidase activities were significantly reduced ($p < 0.05$), compared to untreated infected controls [111]. Notably, the high concentration, *i.e.*, 500 mg/kg, of *Clerodendrum violaceum* leaf methanolic extract could better bring the enzyme activities closer to those of the normal uninfected and chloroquine-treated infected controls [111].

Acanthus polystachyus Leaf Hydro-methanolic Extract

The *Acanthus polystachyus* leaf hydro-methanolic extract contains flavonoids, saponins, tannins, glycosides, phenols, terpenoids, and anthraquinones [112]. The extract showed a concentration-dependent free radical scavenging activity by *in vitro* diphenyl-2-picrylhydrazyl (DPPH) scavenging assay, with ascorbic acid as a standard antioxidant [112]. At 1,000 μg/mL concentrations, the percentage inhibitions of the extract and ascorbic acid were 82.54% and 96.83%, respectively [112].

When compared with the negative control group, all tested *A. polystachyus* extract concentrations (100, 200, and 400 mg/kg) displayed significant parasitemia suppression. The highest 49.25% parasitemia suppression ability of *A. polystachyus* extracts was presented at the highest tested dose of 400 mg/kg [112].

Also, Rane's (curative) test was performed by monitoring parasitemia levels daily from day 3 to day 7, using Giemsa-stained thin blood films. All doses of the extract demonstrated a significant curative action on day 7 [112]. The mean survival time in the curative test was also significantly extended in the *A. polystachyus* extract-treated group as compared to the negative control [112].

Besides, A. polystachyus extract is quite safe with the median lethal dose (LD50) of >2gm/kg orally taken [112].

Lippia multiflora Leaf Extract and *Lippia sidoides* Essential Oils

Lippia multiflora leaf ethanolic extract presented ≥40% increased SOD and robust antiplasmodial activities compared to the control, which was as good as the positive control corosolic acid [113]. The extract contained a very low total phenolic content but possessed saponins, tannins, and flavonoids, which might be accountable for its strong antioxidant activity [113]. Additionally, *Lippia multiflora* leaf ethanolic extract displayed a weak cytotoxic effect with cell survival >50% on human RBCs and HL-60 leukemia cells at the highest concentration of 200 μg/mL [113].

The essential oil from *Lippia sidoides* (LSEO) was used in a study by de Medeiros *et al.* [114]. Its major component was thymol (78.37%), which might be responsible for trypanocidal and leishmanicidal activities. The IC50/48-hour values of LSEO against *L. amazonensis* promastigote and amastigote were 44.38 and 34.4 μg/mL, respectively [114]. Moreover, the essential oil displayed low toxicity against macrophages, whereas thymol showed higher toxicity [114].

Moringa oleifera Lam Extract

Different parts of *Moringa oleifera* Lam showed many important activities [115, 116]. The leaves are stated to display antihypertensive, antioxidant, hypocholesterolemic, antifungal, radioprotective, antinociceptive and wound-healing activities [115, 116]. The roots and barks have diuretic, central inhibitory, antispasmodic, and antiepileptic effects. Additionally, the seeds present antipyretic and anti-inflammatory activities. The ethanolic extract of *M. oleifera* Lam contains saponins, glycosides, and some phenolics [116].

No physical or behavioral signs of acute toxicity were observed in Swiss albino mice treated with acetone *M. oleifera* extracts. The lethal dose (LD50) was at least above 2,000 mg/kg body weight [115].

One study was performed in chloroquine-sensitive *P. berghei*-infected Swiss albino mice, with chloroquine as a standard treatment and the infected untreated mice as a negative control [115]. The extract showed dose-dependent parasitemia suppression, mean survival time, and prophylactic and curative activities. These activities were significantly raised at all treatment doses, compared to negative control mice. The highest parasitemia suppression (77%), mean survival time (25.8 ± 1.90 days) and prophylactic (82.5%) activities were from the highest tested dose of 600 mg/kg, closer to those of the chloroquine-treated group. The curative activity of 600 mg/kg *M. oleifera* extract displayed a significantly lower parasitemia number than that of negative control ($p < 0.05$) [115]. In addition, the *M. Oleifera* leaf ethanolic extract by pressurized liquid extraction (PLE) method showed the DPPH scavenging activity (50% Effective Concentration: EC50) of 21 ± 3 µg/mL [117].

El-Khadragy *et al.* [118] investigated the properties of the biosynthesized silver nanoparticles (Ag-NPs) with *M. oleifera* leaf extract treatment, which revealed a beneficial effect by diminishing silver nanoparticle toxicity. The extract contained phenols 9.466 mg eq. Gallic acid/g sample, flavonoids 0.609 mg eq. Rutin/g sample. Also, the extract displayed a strong free radical scavenging power (DPPH) of 36.%. In addition, BALB/c female mice were subcutaneously injected with 0.1 mL *L. major* (10^6 promastigotes). The result showed that mice treated with Ag-NPs with *M. oleifera* leaf extract reversed the alterations of Bcl–2 and Bax levels, induced by CL during infection, and markedly repaired the Bcl–2/Bax ratio. Fascinatingly, all CL-induced noxious events were prevented by *M. oleifera* leaf extract.

Erythrina burttii Acetone Root-bark Extract

The acetone root-bark extract of *Erythrina burttii* showed radical scavenging activity (EC50 value) against DPPH of 12.0 µg/mL. For *in vitro* antimalarial activity, *E. burttii* acetone extract displayed the IC50 values of 0.97 ± 0.2 and 1.73 ± 0.5 g/mL against chloroquine-sensitive (D6) and chloroquine-resistant (W2) *Plasmodium falciparum* strains, respectively [119]. The most vigorous antiplasmodial compounds with two free phenolic groups were isoflav-3-enes burttinol-A and burttinol-C, and the burttinol-D (2-arylbenzofuran derivative) with IC50 < 10 µM and free radical scavenging EC50 around 10 µM, compared with the reported quercetin (EC50 = 5.0 M) in radical scavenging activity, and antiplasmodial activity (IC50 = 10 µM) [120]. The *E. burttii* acetone extract at a concentration of 800 mg/kg/day given to *Plasmodium berghei* ANKA-infected male Swiss albino mice, showed *in vivo* antimalarial activity of 52% parasitemia suppression at day 4 [119].

Indigofera oblongifolia Leaf Extract

Lubbad *et al.* [121] reported the antimalarial and antioxidant activities and host spleen protection effect of *I. oblongifolia* leaf methanolic extract from *P. chabaudi*-induced injuries. The study was performed in healthy female C57BL/6 mice, intraperitoneally injected with $10^6 P.$ *chabaudi*-parasitized erythrocytes.

I. oblongifolia leaf extract (IOLE) could significantly decrease the parasitemia percentage. The most effective 100 mg IOLE/kg dose could reduce parasitemia from 38% to 12% [121].

The *P. chabaudi* infection induced spleen injury, manifesting spleen white and red pulp disorganization, hemozoin granules, and infected erythrocytes. Also, the nitrite/nitrate, MDA, and catalase levels were significantly changed by the *Plasmodium* infection causing increased spleen oxidative damage [121]. IOLE treatment could significantly improve these conditions, *i.e.*, decrease nitrite/nitrate levels, and increase MDA, and catalase activities. In addition, the inflammatory cytokine mRNA expressions such as IL-1b, IL-6, and tumor necrosis factor-alpha (TNF-α) upregulation from *P. chabaudi* infection, were reduced after IOLE treatment [121].

Argania spinosa Fruit Ethyl Acetate Extract, and Decoction

The *Argania spinosa* (L.) Skeels, fruit ethyl acetate (EA) extract, and decoction contain flavonoids, polyphenols, tannins, and anthocyanins [122]. The antioxidant activities were tested by DPPH and ABTS assays. The half maximal inhibitory concentrations (IC50) of EA extract by DPPH, and ABTS radical scavenging assay were 32.3±1.1 µg/mL and 27.6±1.1 µg/mL, respectively. For the argan decoction, the IC50 by DPPH, and ABTS radical scavenging assay were 78.8±4.0 µg/mL and 11.9±0.6 µg/mL, respectively [122]. The amount of anthocyanins was in good correlation with the potential antioxidant (R^2 = 0.9867) and antimalarial (R^2 = 0.8175) activities [122]. Furthermore, the antimalarial activity (IC50 = 35 to >100 µg/mL) was reported, with the reference antimalarial (chloroquine) standard against *P. falciparum* strains, presented IC50 = 0.1 (FcB1-Columbia strain) and 0.28 µg/mL (FcM29-Cameroon strain) [122].

Gardenia ternifolia

Gardenia ternifolia leaf acetone extract has four flavonoids, *i.e.*, [1] 3,5,3'-trihydroxy-7,4'-dimethoxyflavone [2], 5,7-trihydroxy-4'-methoxyflavone [3], 5,7-dihydroxy-3,4'-dimethoxyflavone [4], 5,4'-dihydroxy-7-methoxyflavanone and two triterpenoids (β-sitosterol and stigmasterol). By DPPH assay, the 3,5,3'-trihydroxy-7,4'-dimethoxyflavone showed the highest antioxidant activity with IC50 = 40.3± 1.55 µM. substantially lower than quercetin (IC50 = 20.1±1.34 µM) [123].

Gardenia ternifolia root bark crude methanolic extract showed a 30-59% parasitemia suppressive effect. 600 mg/kg butanol, chloroform, and aqueous fractions created parasitemia suppression of 51.33%, 40.73%, and 25.75%, respectively [124].

The alkaloids, flavonoids, saponins, and terpenoids in butanol and chloroform fractions might be accountable for their high antiplasmodial activity as the lower activity aqueous fraction contains only anthocyanins and saponins [124].

The crude extract's curative and prophylactic properties were 36-63% and 24-37%, respectively. The infected mice's survival time with the crude extract treatment was significantly prolonged, compared to *P. berghei* infected control without the crude extract treatment. The crude extract protected hosts from weight loss, temperature reduction, and anemia while butanol and chloroform fractions showed temperature, body weight, and packed cell volume reverse reductions [124].

The acute toxicity study indicated that the extract LD50 was greater than 2,000 mg/kg, with no visible signs of overt toxicity observed by physical and behavioral alterations [124].

Furthermore, *G. ternifolia* leaf surface exudates showed *in vitro* antiplasmodial activities (IC50 values of 1.06 and 0.94 µg/mL) against chloroquine-resistant (W2) and chloroquine-sensitive (D6) *Plasmodium falciparum*, respectively [125].

Ziziphus mauritiana

Yahia *et al.* [126] reported the LC-ESI-MS analysis of *Ziziphus spp.* extracts from all plant parts, which showed 28 bioactive compounds, with a high proportion of quinic acid and rutin. *Z. mauritiana* leaf methanolic extracts displayed the highest total antioxidant capacity (30~31 mg GAE/g DW), owing to its greatest quantity in phenolic compounds including tannins and flavonoids [126 - 128]. By DPPH assay, the fruits and seeds of *Z. lotus* from Bengardane and Oued Esseder, Tunisia, showed antioxidant activities though IC50 of 12.16 and 11.41 µg/mL, respectively [126].

Phytochemical investigation of *Z. mauritiana* root methanolic extract brought about the isolation of two 4(14)-type and three 5(13)-type cyclopeptide alkaloids. Four compounds were reported to have strong antiplasmodial activities, *i.e.*, mauritine M (IC50 = 3.7 µM), nummularine H (IC50 = 3.7 µM), hemsine A (IC50 = 7.3 µM) and nummularine B (IC50 = 10.3 µM), compared to dihydroartemisinin, the standard antiplasmodial compound (IC50 = 4.2 nM) [129].

In one study by Attemene, *et al.* [130], the antiplasmodial activity was assessed against the K1, multidrug-resistant *P. falciparum*. The IC50 was specified by the *in vitro* uptake of 3[H]-hypoxanthine by *P. falciparum*. *Ziziphus mauritiana* Lam hydroethanolic (HZm) extract showed dose-dependent activities of parasitemia inhibition and mean survival time. The parasitemia inhibition was 88.97% at a dose of 600 mg/kg body weight, significantly reduced parasitemia in *Plasmodium berghei*-infected Swiss mice compared to negative control ($p < 0.001$). Notably, chloroquine showed 99.92% inhibition [130].

Moreover, HZm showed an elevating inhibitory curative activity at experimental doses. The mean survival time at 600 mg/kg dose was 20.6 days, which statistically increased compared to distilled water as negative control (8 days). Remarkably, the mean survival time in the chloroquine treatment group was 30 days [130].

The comparatively high antiplasmodial activity could probably be owing to the existence of hydroxyproline elements in the macrocycle ring and the terminal N-methylated or N, N-dimethylated amino acid residues [129].

Anthocleista djalonensis

The phytochemical screening of HAd (*Anthocleista djalonensis* A. Chev stem bark hydroethanolic extract) disclosed that many phytocompounds such as alkaloids and terpenoids are present [130]. The HAd showed dose-dependent activities of parasitemia inhibition and mean survival time. The parasitemia inhibition percentage was 70.55% (600 mg/kg body weight), while chloroquine showed 99.92% inhibition. The mean survival time at 600 mg/kg dose was 18.2 days, which statistically increased compared to distilled water as a negative control (8 days). Notably, the mean survival time in the chloroquine treatment group was 30 days [130]. As for the curative activity, HAd showed a Dose-dependent inhibitory activity at investigational doses [130].

CONCLUSION

Medicinal plants contain many bioactive compounds such as phenolic compounds, flavonoids, terpenoids, alkaloids, *etc.* These compounds give the plant its activities against protozoans and free-radical species. Other than the ability to stop the parasite's proliferation and growth, the plant extract can help with the host's homeostasis. Their antioxidant property could be valuable for adjunctive treatment in malaria and other blood protozoa management. Accordingly, many studies focused on antioxidant management along with anti-parasite medications. Many antioxidants were used to fight against free radicals during the infection and therapy. The medicinal plant extracts used with careful management for patients with blood protozoa infections should be beneficial in eliminating the parasites as well as in reducing damage caused by oxidative stress.

ABBREVIATIONS

4-HNE	4-Hydroxynonenal
ABTS	2,2'-Azino-bis-(3-ethylbenzothiazoline-6 sulfonic) acid
ACTs	Artemisinin Combination Therapies
Ag-NP	Silver Nanoparticles
AKR	Aldo-keto Reductase
AOA	Antioxidant Activity
ARDS	Acute Respiratory Distress Syndrome
Bax	B-cell Lymphoma Protein 2 (Bcl-2)-associated X
Bcl-2	B-cell Lymphoma Protein 2
BmAKR/Bmakr	*B. microti* Aldo-keto Reductase
BNZ	Benznidazole
BUN	Blood Urea Nitrogen
CCL2	C-C Motif Chemokine Ligand 2
CCL5	C-C Motif Chemokine Ligand 5
CL	Cutaneous Leishmaniasis
DPPH	2,2-Diphenyl-1-picrylhydrazyl
EA	Ethyl Acetate
EC50	Effective Concentration 50
FP	Ferriprotoporphyrin
G6PDH	Glucose-6-phosphate Dehydrogenase, Reduced form
GPX	Glutathione Peroxidase
GSH	Glutathione, Reduced form
HAd	Hydroethanolic extracts of *Anthocleista djalonensis* A. Chev stem bark
HO-1	Heme Oxygenase-1
IC50	Half-maximal Inhibitory Concentration, Inhibitory Concentration 50
IL-1b	Interleukin 1 Beta
IL-8	Interleukin 8
iRBC	Infected Red Blood Cell
LC-ESI-MS	Liquid Chromatography Electrospray Ionization Tandem Mass Spectrometry
LD50	Lethal Dose 50
LP	Lipid Peroxidation
LSEO	Essential Oils from *Lippia sidoides*
MDA	Malondialdehyde

ML	Mucocutaneous Leishmaniasis
mRNA	Messenger Ribonucleic Acid
NAC	N-acetylcysteine
NADPH	Nicotinamide Adenine Dinucleotide Phosphate, Reduced form
NO	Nitric Oxide
NOS	Nitric Oxide Synthase
NOx	Nitrite/Nitrate Products
NRF2	Nuclear Factor Erythroid 2-related Factor 2
PCO	Protein Carbonyl
PLE	Pressurized Liquid Extraction
PXN	Peroxiredoxin
RBC	Red Blood Cell
ROS/RNS	Reactive Oxygen Species/Reactive Nitrogen Species
SOD	Superoxide Dismutase
TNF-α	Tumor Necrosis Factor-alpha
VL	Visceral Leishmaniasis
WHO	World Health Organization
XO	Xanthine Oxidase

REFERENCES

[1]   World malaria report 2021. Geneva: World Health Organization 2021.

[2]   Tajuddeen N, Van Heerden FR. Antiplasmodial natural products: An update. Malar J 2019; 18(1): 404.
[http://dx.doi.org/10.1186/s12936-019-3026-1] [PMID: 31805944]

[3]   CDC. CDC - Malaria - about malaria - faqs . Centers for Disease Control and Prevention. Centers for Disease Control and Prevention 2022. Available from: https://www.cdc.gov/malaria/about/faqs.html

[4]   Kumar A, O'Bryan J, Krause P. The global emergence of human babesiosis. Pathogens 2021; 10(11): 1447.
[http://dx.doi.org/10.3390/pathogens10111447] [PMID: 34832603]

[5]   Karshima SN, Karshima MN, Ahmed MI. Global meta-analysis on *Babesia* infections in human population: Prevalence, distribution and species diversity. Pathog Glob Health 2022; 116(4): 220-35.
[http://dx.doi.org/10.1080/20477724.2021.1989185] [PMID: 34788196]

[6]   Leishmaniasis 2022. Available from: https://www.who.int/news-room/fact-sheets/detail/leishmaniasis

[7]   Trypanosomiasis, human African (sleeping sickness) World Health Organization 2022. Available from: https://www.who.int/news-room/fact-sheets/detail/trypanosomiasis-human-african-(sleeping-sickness)

[8]   Reis PA, Comim CM, Hermani F, *et al.* Cognitive dysfunction is sustained after rescue therapy in experimental cerebral malaria, and is reduced by additive antioxidant therapy. PLoS Pathog 2010; 6(6): e1000963.
[http://dx.doi.org/10.1371/journal.ppat.1000963] [PMID: 20585569]

[9]   Imai T, Iwawaki T, Akai R, *et al.* Evaluating experimental cerebral malaria using oxidative stress

indicator OKD48 mice. Int J Parasitol 2014; 44(10): 681-5.
[http://dx.doi.org/10.1016/j.ijpara.2014.06.002] [PMID: 24995619]

[10]   Janka JJ, Koita OA, Traoré B, *et al.* Increased pulmonary pressures and myocardial wall stress in children with severe malaria. J Infect Dis 2010; 202(5): 791-800.
[http://dx.doi.org/10.1086/655225] [PMID: 20662718]

[11]   Na-Ek P, Punsawad C. Expression of 4-Hydroxynonenal (4-HNE) and Heme Oxygenase-1 (HO-1) in the Kidneys of *Plasmodium berghei*-Infected Mice. J Trop Med 2020; 2020: 1-7.
[http://dx.doi.org/10.1155/2020/8813654] [PMID: 33149743]

[12]   Percário S, Moreira D, Gomes B, *et al.* Oxidative stress in malaria. Int J Mol Sci 2012; 13(12): 16346-72.
[http://dx.doi.org/10.3390/ijms131216346] [PMID: 23208374]

[13]   Dockrell HM, Playfair JH. Killing of *Plasmodium yoelii* by enzyme-induced products of the oxidative burst. Infect Immun 1984; 43(2): 451-6.
[http://dx.doi.org/10.1128/iai.43.2.451-456.1984] [PMID: 6546375]

[14]   Gomes ARQ, Cunha N, Varela ELP, *et al.* Oxidative stress in malaria: Potential benefits of antioxidant therapy. Int J Mol Sci 2022; 23(11): 5949.
[http://dx.doi.org/10.3390/ijms23115949] [PMID: 35682626]

[15]   Nsiah K, Bahaah B, Oppong Afranie B, Koffie S, Akowuah E, Donkor S. Oxidative stress and hemoglobin level of complicated and uncomplicated malaria cases among children: A cross-sectional study in kumasi metropolis, Ghana. J Trop Med 2019; 1-6.
[http://dx.doi.org/10.1155/2019/8479076] [PMID: 31360173]

[16]   Atiku SM, Louise N, Kasozi DM. Severe oxidative stress in sickle cell disease patients with uncomplicated *Plasmodium falciparum* malaria in Kampala, Uganda. BMC Infect Dis 2019; 19(1): 600.
[http://dx.doi.org/10.1186/s12879-019-4221-y] [PMID: 31288760]

[17]   Anidi IU, Servinsky LE, Rentsendorj O, Stephens RS, Scott AL, Pearse DB. CD36 and Fyn kinase mediate malaria-induced lung endothelial barrier dysfunction in mice infected with *Plasmodium berghei* PLoS One 2013; 8(8): e71010.
[http://dx.doi.org/10.1371/journal.pone.0071010] [PMID: 23967147]

[18]   Bartoloni A, Zammarchi L. Clinical aspects of uncomplicated and severe malaria. Mediterr J Hematol Infect Dis 2012; 4(1): e2012026.
[http://dx.doi.org/10.4084/mjhid.2012.026] [PMID: 22708041]

[19]   Scaccabarozzi D, Deroost K, Corbett Y, *et al.* Differential induction of malaria liver pathology in mice infected with *Plasmodium chabaudi* AS or *Plasmodium berghei* NK65. Malar J 2018; 17(1): 18.
[http://dx.doi.org/10.1186/s12936-017-2159-3] [PMID: 29316914]

[20]   Deroost K, Lays N, Pham TT, *et al.* Hemozoin induces hepatic inflammation in mice and is differentially associated with liver pathology depending on the *Plasmodium strain*. PLoS One 2014; 9(11): e113519.
[http://dx.doi.org/10.1371/journal.pone.0113519] [PMID: 25419977]

[21]   Becker K, Tilley L, Vennerstrom JL, Roberts D, Rogerson S, Ginsburg H. Oxidative stress in malaria parasite-infected erythrocytes: Host–parasite interactions. Int J Parasitol 2004; 34(2): 163-89.
[http://dx.doi.org/10.1016/j.ijpara.2003.09.011] [PMID: 15037104]

[22]   Loria P, Miller S, Foley M, Tilley L. Inhibition of the peroxidative degradation of haem as the basis of action of chloroquine and other quinoline antimalarials. Biochem J 1999; 339(2): 363-70.
[http://dx.doi.org/10.1042/bj3390363] [PMID: 10191268]

[23]   Krugliak M, Zhang J, Ginsburg H. Intraerythrocytic *Plasmodium falciparum* utilizes only a fraction of the amino acids derived from the digestion of host cell cytosol for the biosynthesis of its proteins. Mol Biochem Parasitol 2002; 119(2): 249-56.

[http://dx.doi.org/10.1016/S0166-6851(01)00427-3] [PMID: 11814576]

[24]   Tilley L, Loria P, Foley M. Chloroquine and other quinoline antimalarials. In: Totowa RPJ, Ed. Antimalarial chemotherapy. Totowa: Humana Press 2001; pp. 87-122.
[http://dx.doi.org/10.1385/1-59259-111-6:87]

[25]   Vasquez M, Zuniga M, Rodriguez A. Oxidative stress and pathogenesis in Malaria. Front Cell Infect Microbiol 2021; 11: 768182.
[http://dx.doi.org/10.3389/fcimb.2021.768182] [PMID: 34917519]

[26]   Egan TJ, Combrinck JM, Egan J, *et al.* Fate of haem iron in the malaria parasite *Plasmodium falciparum*. Biochem J 2002; 365(2): 343-7.
[http://dx.doi.org/10.1042/bj20020793] [PMID: 12033986]

[27]   Slater AFG, Cerami A. Inhibition by chloroquine of a novel haem polymerase enzyme activity in malaria trophozoites. Nature 1992; 355(6356): 167-9.
[http://dx.doi.org/10.1038/355167a0] [PMID: 1729651]

[28]   Zhang F, Schmidt WG, Hou Y, Williams AF, Jacobson K. Spontaneous incorporation of the glycosyl-phosphatidylinositol-linked protein Thy-1 into cell membranes. Proc Natl Acad Sci USA 1992; 89(12): 5231-5.
[http://dx.doi.org/10.1073/pnas.89.12.5231] [PMID: 1351678]

[29]   Ginsburg H, Famin O, Zhang J, Krugliak M. Inhibition of glutathione-dependent degradation of heme by chloroquine and amodiaquine as a possible basis for their antimalarial mode of action. Biochem Pharmacol 1998; 56(10): 1305-13.
[http://dx.doi.org/10.1016/S0006-2952(98)00184-1] [PMID: 9825729]

[30]   Harwaldt P, Rahlfs S, Becker K. Glutathione S-transferase of the malarial parasite *Plasmodium falciparum*: Characterization of a potential drug target. Biol Chem 2002; 383(5): 821-30.
[http://dx.doi.org/10.1515/BC.2002.086] [PMID: 12108547]

[31]   Campanale N, Nickel C, Daubenberger CA, *et al.* Identification and characterization of heme-interacting proteins in the malaria parasite, *Plasmodium falciparum*. J Biol Chem 2003; 278(30): 27354-61.
[http://dx.doi.org/10.1074/jbc.M303634200] [PMID: 12748176]

[32]   Haldar K, Mohandas N. Malaria, erythrocytic infection, and anemia. Hematology (Am Soc Hematol Educ Program) 2009; (1): 87-93.
[http://dx.doi.org/10.1182/asheducation-2009.1.87] [PMID: 20008186]

[33]   Battelli MG, Polito L, Bortolotti M, Bolognesi A. Xanthine oxidoreductase-derived reactive species: Physiological and pathological effects. Oxid Med Cell Longev 2016; 1-8.
[http://dx.doi.org/10.1155/2016/3527579] [PMID: 26823950]

[34]   Tubaro E, Lotti B, Cavallo G, Croce C, Borelli G. Liver xanthine oxidase increase in mice in three pathological models. Biochem Pharmacol 1980; 29(13): 1939-43.
[http://dx.doi.org/10.1016/0006-2952(80)90107-0] [PMID: 6994748]

[35]   Iwalokun BA, Bamiro SB, Ogunledun A. Levels and interactions of plasma xanthine oxidase, catalase and liver function parameters in Nigerian children with *Plasmodium falciparum* infection. Acta Pathol Microbiol Scand Suppl 2006; 114(12): 842-50.
[http://dx.doi.org/10.1111/j.1600-0463.2006.apm_457.x] [PMID: 17207084]

[36]   Ty MC, Zuniga M, Götz A, Kayal S, Sahu PK, Mohanty A, *et al.* Malaria inflammation by xanthine oxidase-produced reactive oxygen species. EMBO Mol 2019; 11(8)
[http://dx.doi.org/10.15252/emmm.201809903]

[37]   Berman PA, Human L, Freese JA. Xanthine oxidase inhibits growth of *Plasmodium falciparum* in human erythrocytes *in vitro*. J Clin Invest 1991; 88(6): 1848-55.
[http://dx.doi.org/10.1172/JCI115506] [PMID: 1752946]

[38]   Götz A, Ty MC, Rodriguez A. Oxidative stress enhances dendritic cell responses to *Plasmodium*

falciparum. Immunohorizons 2019; 3(11): 511-8.
[http://dx.doi.org/10.4049/immunohorizons.1900076] [PMID: 31690559]

[39]   Kharazmi A, Jepsen S, Andersen BJ. Generation of reactive oxygen radicals by human phagocytic cells activated by *Plasmodium falciparum*. Scand J Immunol 1987; 25(4): 335-41.
[http://dx.doi.org/10.1111/j.1365-3083.1987.tb02198.x] [PMID: 3033817]

[40]   Aitken EH, Alemu A, Rogerson SJ. Neutrophils and Malaria. Front Immunol 2018; 9: 3005.
[http://dx.doi.org/10.3389/fimmu.2018.03005] [PMID: 30619354]

[41]   Forman HJ, Torres M. Reactive oxygen species and cell signaling: Respiratory burst in macrophage signaling. Am J Respir Crit Care Med 2002; 166(12 Pt 2) (Suppl. 1): S4-8.
[http://dx.doi.org/10.1164/rccm.2206007] [PMID: 12471082]

[42]   Schwarzer E, Arese P. Phagocytosis of malarial pigment hemozoin inhibits NADPH-oxidase activity in human monocyte-derived macrophages. Biochim Biophys Acta Mol Basis Dis 1996; 1316(3): 169-75.
[http://dx.doi.org/10.1016/0925-4439(96)00021-X] [PMID: 8781535]

[43]   Cunnington AJ, Njie M, Correa S, Takem EN, Riley EM, Walther M. Prolonged neutrophil dysfunction after *Plasmodium falciparum* malaria is related to hemolysis and heme oxygenase-1 induction. J Immunol 2012; 189(11): 5336-46.
[http://dx.doi.org/10.4049/jimmunol.1201028] [PMID: 23100518]

[44]   Herchline TE, Simon RQ. Malaria medication 2020. Available from: https://emedicine.medscape.com/article/221134-medication

[45]   Mutabingwa TK. Artemisinin-based combination therapies (ACTs): Best hope for malaria treatment but inaccessible to the needy! Acta Trop 2005; 95(3): 305-15.
[http://dx.doi.org/10.1016/j.actatropica.2005.06.009] [PMID: 16098946]

[46]   Naß J, Efferth T. The activity of Artemisia spp. And their constituents against Trypanosomiasis. Phytomedicine 2018; 47: 184-91.
[http://dx.doi.org/10.1016/j.phymed.2018.06.002] [PMID: 30166103]

[47]   Pinheiro LCS, Feitosa LM, Silveira FFD, Boechat N. Current antimalarial therapies and advances in the development of semi-synthetic artemisinin derivatives. An Acad Bras Cienc 2018; 90(1 suppl 2) (Suppl. 2): 1251-71.
[http://dx.doi.org/10.1590/0001-3765201820170830] [PMID: 29873667]

[48]   Cottrell G, Musset L, Hubert V, Le Bras J, Clain J. Emergence of resistance to atovaquone-proguanil in malaria parasites: insights from computational modeling and clinical case reports. Antimicrob Agents Chemother 2014; 58(8): 4504-14.
[http://dx.doi.org/10.1128/AAC.02550-13] [PMID: 24867967]

[49]   Hill SR, Thakur RK, Sharma GK. Antimalarial Medications. StatPearls 2022. Available from: https://www.ncbi.nlm.nih.gov/books/NBK470158/

[50]   Gregson A, Plowe CV. Mechanisms of resistance of malaria parasites to antifolates. Pharmacol Rev 2005; 57(1): 117-45.
[http://dx.doi.org/10.1124/pr.57.1.4] [PMID: 15734729]

[51]   Jain A, Jack J. StatPearls 2022. Available from: https://www.ncbi.nlm.nih.gov/books/NBK542193/

[52]   Pukrittayakamee S, Chantra A, Vanijanonta S, Clemens R, Looareesuwan S, White NJ. Therapeutic responses to quinine and clindamycin in multidrug-resistant falciparum malaria. Antimicrob Agents Chemother 2000; 44(9): 2395-8.
[http://dx.doi.org/10.1128/AAC.44.9.2395-2398.2000] [PMID: 10952585]

[53]   Tan KR, Magill AJ, Arguin PM, Parise ME. Doxycycline for malaria chemoprophylaxis and treatment: report from the CDC expert meeting on malaria chemoprophylaxis. Am J Trop Med Hyg 2011; 84(4): 517-31.
[http://dx.doi.org/10.4269/ajtmh.2011.10-0285] [PMID: 21460003]

[54] Muhammad A, Ibrahim MA, Mohammed HA, *et al.* Alteration of redox status by commonly used antimalarial drugs in the north-western region of Nigeria. Hum Exp Toxicol 2017; 36(2): 176-83.
[http://dx.doi.org/10.1177/0960327116641735] [PMID: 27037298]

[55] Kavishe RA, Koenderink JB, Alifrangis M. Oxidative stress in malaria and artemisinin combination therapy: Pros and Cons. FEBS J 2017; 284(16): 2579-91.
[http://dx.doi.org/10.1111/febs.14097] [PMID: 28467668]

[56] Pandey AV, Bisht H, Babbarwal VK, Srivastava J, Pandey KC, Chauhan VS. Mechanism of malarial haem detoxification inhibition by chloroquine. Biochem J 2001; 355(2): 333-8.
[http://dx.doi.org/10.1042/bj3550333] [PMID: 11284719]

[57] Sullivan DJ. Theories on malarial pigment formation and quinoline action. Int J Parasitol 2002; 32(13): 1645-53.
[http://dx.doi.org/10.1016/S0020-7519(02)00193-5] [PMID: 12435449]

[58] Srivastava P, Puri SK, Kamboj KK, Pandey VC. Glutathione-S-transferase activity in malarial parasites. Trop Med Int Health 1999; 4(4): 251-4.
[http://dx.doi.org/10.1046/j.1365-3156.1999.00387.x] [PMID: 10320651]

[59] Beaudoin RL, Aikawa M. Primaquine-induced changes in morphology of exoerythrocytic stages of malaria. Science 1968; 160(3833): 1233-4.
[http://dx.doi.org/10.1126/science.160.3833.1233] [PMID: 5648260]

[60] Aikawa M, Beaudoin RL. Morphological effects of 8-aminoquinolines on the exoerythrocytic stages of *Plasmodium fallax*. Mil Med 1969; 134(9): 986-99.
[http://dx.doi.org/10.1093/milmed/134.9.986] [PMID: 4987076]

[61] Bolchoz LJC, Morrow JD, Jollow DJ, McMillan DC. Primaquine-induced hemolytic anemia: Effect of 6-methoxy-8-hydroxylaminoquinoline on rat erythrocyte sulfhydryl status, membrane lipids, cytoskeletal proteins, and morphology. J Pharmacol Exp Ther 2002; 303(1): 141-8.
[http://dx.doi.org/10.1124/jpet.102.036921] [PMID: 12235244]

[62] Paitayatat S, Tarnchompoo B, Thebtaranonth Y, Yuthavong Y. Correlation of antimalarial activity of artemisinin derivatives with binding affinity with ferroprotoporphyrin IX. J Med Chem 1997; 40(5): 633-8.
[http://dx.doi.org/10.1021/jm960767v] [PMID: 9057849]

[63] Meshnick SR. Artemisinin: Mechanisms of action, resistance and toxicity. Int J Parasitol 2002; 32(13): 1655-60.
[http://dx.doi.org/10.1016/S0020-7519(02)00194-7] [PMID: 12435450]

[64] Olliaro PL, Haynes RK, Meunier B, Yuthavong Y. Possible modes of action of the artemisinin-type compounds. Trends Parasitol 2001; 17(3): 122-6.
[http://dx.doi.org/10.1016/S1471-4922(00)01838-9] [PMID: 11286794]

[65] Posner GH, Meshnick SR. Radical mechanism of action of the artemisinin-type compounds. Trends Parasitol 2001; 17(6): 266-7.
[http://dx.doi.org/10.1016/S1471-4922(01)02001-3] [PMID: 11378030]

[66] Borstnik K, Paik I, Shapiro TA, Posner GH. Antimalarial chemotherapeutic peroxides: Artemisinin, yingzhaosu A and related compounds. Int J Parasitol 2002; 32(13): 1661-7.
[http://dx.doi.org/10.1016/S0020-7519(02)00195-9] [PMID: 12435451]

[67] Berdelle N, Nikolova T, Quiros S, Efferth T, Kaina B. Artesunate induces oxidative DNA damage, sustained DNA double-strand breaks, and the ATM/ATR damage response in cancer cells. Mol Cancer Ther 2011; 10(12): 2224-33.
[http://dx.doi.org/10.1158/1535-7163.MCT-11-0534] [PMID: 21998290]

[68] Singh S, Giri A, Giri S. The antimalarial agent artesunate causes sperm DNA damage and hepatic antioxidant defense in mice. Mutat Res Genet Toxicol Environ Mutagen 2015; 777: 1-6.
[http://dx.doi.org/10.1016/j.mrgentox.2014.11.001] [PMID: 25726169]

[69] Akanbi OM, Odaibo AB, Afolabi KA, Ademowo OG. Effect of self-medication with antimalarial drugs on malaria infection in pregnant women in South-Western Nigeria. Med Princ Pract 2005; 14(1): 6-9.
[http://dx.doi.org/10.1159/000081915] [PMID: 15608474]

[70] Kumar Mishra S, Singh P, Rath SK. Protective effect of quercetin on chloroquine-induced oxidative stress and hepatotoxicity in mice. Malar Res Treat 2013; 2013: 1-10.
[http://dx.doi.org/10.1155/2013/141734] [PMID: 23607047]

[71] Huang Q, Cao J, Zhou Y, *et al. Babesia microti* Aldo-keto reductase-like protein involved in antioxidant and anti-parasite response. Front Microbiol 2017; 8: 2006.
[http://dx.doi.org/10.3389/fmicb.2017.02006] [PMID: 29075254]

[72] Dalrymple BP, Peters JM, Vuocolo T. Characterisation of genes encoding two novel members of the aldo-keto reductase superfamily. Biochem Int 1992; 28(4): 651-7.
[PMID: 1482401]

[73] Garavaglia PA, Cannata JJB, Ruiz AM, *et al.* Identification, cloning and characterization of an aldo-keto reductase from *Trypanosoma cruzi* with quinone oxido-reductase activity. Mol Biochem Parasitol 2010; 173(2): 132-41.
[http://dx.doi.org/10.1016/j.molbiopara.2010.05.019] [PMID: 20595031]

[74] Rath J, Gowri VS, Chauhan SC, Padmanabhan PK, Srinivasan N, Madhubala R. A glutathione-specific aldose reductase of *Leishmania donovani* and its potential implications for methylglyoxal detoxification pathway. Gene 2009; 429(1-2): 1-9.
[http://dx.doi.org/10.1016/j.gene.2008.09.037] [PMID: 18983902]

[75] Kucukkurt I, Cigerci IH, Ince S, *et al.* The effects of babesiosis on oxidative stress and DNA damage in anatolian black goats naturally infected with babesia ovis. Iran J Parasitol 2014; 9(1): 90-8.https://www.ncbi.nlm.nih.gov/pmc/articles/PMC4289885/
[PMID: 25642264]

[76] Ince S, Kozan E, Kucukkurt I, Bacak E. The effect of levamisole and levamisole+vitamin C on oxidative damage in rats naturally infected with *Syphacia muris*. Exp Parasitol 2010; 124(4): 448-52.
[http://dx.doi.org/10.1016/j.exppara.2009.12.017] [PMID: 20045691]

[77] Serarslan G, Yilmaz HR, Söğüt S. Serum antioxidant activities, malondialdehyde and nitric oxide levels in human cutaneous leishmaniasis. Clin Exp Dermatol 2005; 30(3): 267-71.
[http://dx.doi.org/10.1111/j.1365-2230.2005.01758.x] [PMID: 15807687]

[78] Kocyigit A, Keles H, Selek S, Guzel S, Celik H, Erel O. Increased DNA damage and oxidative stress in patients with cutaneous leishmaniasis. Mutat Res Genet Toxicol Environ Mutagen 2005; 585(1-2): 71-8.
[http://dx.doi.org/10.1016/j.mrgentox.2005.04.012] [PMID: 16005255]

[79] Drugs B. Encyclopedia of Parasitology. 4th ed. Berlin: Springer 2016; pp. 275-85.

[80] Florentino PTV, Mendes D, Vitorino FNL, Martins DJ, Cunha JPC, Mortara RA, *et al.* DNA damage and oxidative stress in human cells infected by *Trypanosoma cruzi*. PLOS Pathogens. McCulloch R, editor 2021; 17: p. (4)e1009502.
[http://dx.doi.org/10.1371/journal.ppat.1009502]

[81] Machado-Silva A, Cerqueira PG, Grazielle-Silva V, Gadelha FR, Peloso Ede F, Teixeira SM, *et al.* How *Trypanosoma cruzi* deals with oxidative stress: Antioxidant defence and DNA repair pathways. Mut Res/Rev in Mutat Res 2016; 767: 8-22. Available from: https://www.sciencedirect.com/science/article/abs/pii/S1383574215300089

[82] Acestor N, Masina S, Ives A, Walker J, Saravia NG, Fasel N. Resistance to oxidative stress is associated with metastasis in mucocutaneous leishmaniasis. J Infect Dis 2006; 194(8): 1160-7.
[http://dx.doi.org/10.1086/507646] [PMID: 16991092]

[83] De Jesus LCL, Soares REP, Moreira VR, Pontes RL, Castelo-Branco PV, Pereira SRF. Genistein and

ascorbic acid reduce oxidative stress-derived DNA damage induced by the antileishmanial meglumine antimoniate. Antimicrob Agents Chemother 2018; 62(9): e00456-18.
[http://dx.doi.org/10.1128/AAC.00456-18] [PMID: 29941649]

[84] Krishnamurthy P, Wadhwani A. Antioxidant enzymes and human health. Antioxidant enzyme. In: El-Missiry MA, Ed. Antioxidant Enzyme. London: IntechOpen 2012.
[http://dx.doi.org/10.5772/48109]

[85] Poljsak B, Šuput D, Milisav I. Achieving the balance between ROS and antioxidants: when to use the synthetic antioxidants. Oxid Med Cell Longev 2013; 1-11.
[http://dx.doi.org/10.1155/2013/956792] [PMID: 23738047]

[86] Yakoob MY, Qadir M, Hany O, Vitamin A. Vitamin A supplementation for prevention and treatment of malaria during pregnancy and childhood: A systematic review and meta-analysis. J Epidemiol Glob Health 2018; 8(1-2): 20-8.
[http://dx.doi.org/10.2991/j.jegh.2018.04.104] [PMID: 30859783]

[87] Achan J, Mpimbaza A. Editorial: Vitamin A as adjunct therapy for cerebral malaria: what is the evidence? Afr Health Sci 2012; 12(2): 87-8.
[http://dx.doi.org/10.4314/ahs.v12i2.1] [PMID: 23056010]

[88] Serghides L, Kain KC. Mechanism of protection induced by vitamin A in falciparum malaria. Lancet 2002; 359(9315): 1404-6.
[http://dx.doi.org/10.1016/S0140-6736(02)08360-5] [PMID: 11978340]

[89] Shi X, Wei M, Xu Z, *et al.* Vitamin C inhibits blood-stage *plasmodium* parasites *via* oxidative stress. Front Cell Dev Biol 2021; 9: 639944.
[http://dx.doi.org/10.3389/fcell.2021.639944] [PMID: 34046404]

[90] Marwaha N. Ascorbic acid co-administration with artemisinin based combination therapies in falciparum malaria. Indian J Med Res 2016; 143(5): 539-41.
[http://dx.doi.org/10.4103/0971-5916.187100] [PMID: 27487995]

[91] Ebohon O, Irabor F, Omoregie ES. Ascorbic acid coadministration with artesunate–amodiaquine, up-regulated antioxidant enzymes gene expression in bone marrow cells and elicited biochemical changes in *Plasmodium berghei*-infected mice. SN Applied Sciences 2021; 3(1): 6.
[http://dx.doi.org/10.1007/s42452-020-04063-5]

[92] Setto JM, Libonati RMF, Ventura AMRS, *et al.* Association between vitamin D serum levels and clinical, laboratory, and parasitological parameters in patients with malaria from an endemic area of the Amazon. Rev Soc Bras Med Trop 2022; 55: e0077-2021.
[http://dx.doi.org/10.1590/0037-8682-0077-2021] [PMID: 35416868]

[93] Herbas MS, Okazaki M, Terao E, Xuan X, Arai H, Suzuki H. α-Tocopherol transfer protein inhibition is effective in the prevention of cerebral malaria in mice. Am J Clin Nutr 2010; 91(1): 200-7.
[http://dx.doi.org/10.3945/ajcn.2009.28260] [PMID: 19923370]

[94] Levander OA, Fontela R, Morris VC, Ager AL Jr. Protection against murine cerebral malaria by dietary-induced oxidative stress. J Parasitol 1995; 81(1): 99-103.
[http://dx.doi.org/10.2307/3284013] [PMID: 7876987]

[95] Treeprasertsuk S, Krudsood S, Tosukhowong T, *et al.* N-acetylcysteine in severe falciparum malaria in Thailand. Southeast Asian J Trop Med Public Health 2003; 34(1): 37-42.
[PMID: 12971512]

[96] Charunwatthana P, Faiz MA, Ruangveerayut R, *et al.* N-acetylcysteine as adjunctive treatment in severe malaria: A randomized, double-blinded placebo-controlled clinical trial. Crit Care Med 2009; 37(2): 516-22.
[http://dx.doi.org/10.1097/CCM.0b013e3181958dfd] [PMID: 19114891]

[97] Quadros Gomes BA, Da Silva LFD, Quadros Gomes AR, *et al.* N-acetyl cysteine and mushroom *Agaricus sylvaticus* supplementation decreased parasitaemia and pulmonary oxidative stress in a mice

model of malaria. Malar J 2015; 14(1): 202.
[http://dx.doi.org/10.1186/s12936-015-0717-0] [PMID: 25971771]

[98]   Ekeh FN, Ekechukwu NE, Chukwuma CF, *et al.* Mixed vitamin C and zinc diet supplements co-administered with artemether drug improved haematological profile and survival of mice infected with *Plasmodium berghei.* Food Sci Hum Wellness 2019; 8(3): 275-82.
[http://dx.doi.org/10.1016/j.fshw.2019.05.003]

[99]   Darling AM, Mugusi FM, Etheredge AJ, *et al.* Vitamin A and Zinc supplementation among pregnant women to prevent placental malaria: A randomized, double-blind, placebo-controlled trial in tanzania. Am J Trop Med Hyg 2017; 96(4): 16-0599.
[http://dx.doi.org/10.4269/ajtmh.16-0599] [PMID: 28115667]

[100] Suradji EW, Hatabu T, Kobayashi K, *et al.* Selenium-induced apoptosis-like cell death in *Plasmodium falciparum.* Parasitology 2011; 138(14): 1852-62.
[http://dx.doi.org/10.1017/S0031182011001399] [PMID: 21854677]

[101] Gamain B, Arnaud J, Favier A, Camus D, Dive D, Slomianny C. Increase in glutathione peroxidase activity in malaria parasite after selenium supplementation. Free Radic Biol Med 1996; 21(4): 559-65.
[http://dx.doi.org/10.1016/0891-5849(96)00120-7] [PMID: 8886808]

[102] Sarr D, Cooper CA, Bracken TC, Martinez-Uribe O, Nagy T, Moore JM. Oxidative stress: A potential therapeutic target in placental malaria. Immunohorizons 2017; 1(4): 29-41.
[http://dx.doi.org/10.4049/immunohorizons.1700002] [PMID: 28890952]

[103] Somsak V, Jaihan U, Srichairatanakool S, Uthaipibull C. Protection of renal function by green tea extract during *Plasmodium berghei* infection. Parasitol Int 2013; 62(6): 548-51.
[http://dx.doi.org/10.1016/j.parint.2013.08.004] [PMID: 23988625]

[104] Lidiya G, Gadjalova A, Mihaylova D, Pavlov A. *Achillea millefolium* L. - Phytochemical profile and *in vitro* antioxidant activity. Int Food Res J 2015; 22: 1347-52.

[105] Murnigsih T, Subeki , Matsuura H, *et al.* Evaluation of the inhibitory activities of the extracts of Indonesian traditional medicinal plants against *Plasmodium falciparum* and *Babesia gibsoni.* J Vet Med Sci 2005; 67(8): 829-31.
[http://dx.doi.org/10.1292/jvms.67.829] [PMID: 16141673]

[106] Abou Baker DH. *Achillea millefolium* L. ethyl acetate fraction induces apoptosis and cell cycle arrest in human cervical cancer (HeLa) cells. Ann Agric Sci 2020; 65(1): 42-8.
[http://dx.doi.org/10.1016/j.aoas.2020.03.003]

[107] Guz L, Adaszek Ł, Wawrzykowski J, Ziętek J, Winiarczyk S. *In vitro* antioxidant and antibabesial activities of the extracts of Achillea millefolium. Pol J Vet Sci 2019; 22(2): 369-76.
[PMID: 31269341]

[108] Luize PS, Tiuman TS, Morello LG, *et al.* Effects of medicinal plant extracts on growth of *Leishmania* (L.) *Amazonensis* and *Trypanosoma cruzi.* RBCF Rev Bras Cienc Farm 2005; 41(1): 85-94.
[http://dx.doi.org/10.1590/S1516-93322005000100010]

[109] Santoro GF, Cardoso MG, Guimarães LGL, Mendonça LZ, Soares MJ. Trypanosoma cruzi: Activity of essential oils from *Achillea millefolium* L., *Syzygium aromaticum* L. and *Ocimum basilicum* L. on epimastigotes and trypomastigotes. Exp Parasitol 2007; 116(3): 283-90.
[http://dx.doi.org/10.1016/j.exppara.2007.01.018] [PMID: 17349626]

[110] Trumbeckaite S, Benetis R, Bumblauskiene L, *et al.* *Achillea millefolium* L. s.l. herb extract: Antioxidant activity and effect on the rat heart mitochondrial functions. Food Chem 2011; 127(4): 1540-8.
[http://dx.doi.org/10.1016/j.foodchem.2011.02.014]

[111] Balogun EA, Zailani AH, Adebayo JO. Augmentation of antioxidant system: Contribution to antimalarial activity of *Clerodendrum violaceum* leaf extract TANG 2014; 4(4): 1-9.

[112] Kifle ZD, Atnafie SA. Anti-oxidant potential and antimalarial effects of *Acanthus polystachyus* delile

(acanthaceae) against *Plasmodium berghei*: Evidence for *in vivo* Antimalarial Activity. J Exp Pharmacol 2020; 12: 575-87.
[http://dx.doi.org/10.2147/JEP.S282407] [PMID: 33343202]

[113] Appiah-Opong R, Agyemang K, Dotse E, *et al.* Anti-plasmodial, cytotoxic and antioxidant activities of selected ghanaian medicinal plants. J Evid Based Integr Med 2022. 2515690X211073709

[114] De Medeiros MGF, Da Silva AC, Citó AMGL, *et al. In vitro* antileishmanial activity and cytotoxicity of essential oil from *Lippia sidoides* Cham. Parasitol Int 2011; 60(3): 237-41.
[http://dx.doi.org/10.1016/j.parint.2011.03.004] [PMID: 21421075]

[115] Upadhye KP, Rangari VD, Mathur VB. Evaluation of antinociceptive activities of fresh leaf juice and ethanolic extract of *Moringa oleifera* lam. Asian J Pharm Clin Res 2011; 4(1): 114-6.

[116] Mulisa E, Girma B, Tesema S, Yohannes M, Zemene E, Amelo W. Evaluation of *in vivo* antimalarial activities of leaves of *Moringa oleifera* against *Plasmodium berghei* in mice. Jundishapur J Nat Pharm Prod 2018.
[http://dx.doi.org/10.5812/jjnpp.60426]

[117] Rodríguez-Pérez C, Gilbert-López B, Mendiola JA, Quirantes-Piné R, Segura-Carretero A, Ibáñez E. Optimization of microwave-assisted extraction and pressurized liquid extraction of phenolic compounds from *Moringa oleifera* leaves by multiresponse surface methodology. Electrophoresis 2016; 37(13): 1938-46.
[http://dx.doi.org/10.1002/elps.201600071] [PMID: 27122439]

[118] El-khadragy M, Alolayan E, Metwally D, *et al.* Clinical efficacy associated with enhanced antioxidant enzyme activities of silver nanoparticles biosynthesized using *Moringa oleifera* leaf extract, against cutaneous leishmaniasis in a murine model of *Leishmania major*. Int J Environ Res Public Health 2018; 15(5): 1037.
[http://dx.doi.org/10.3390/ijerph15051037] [PMID: 29786651]

[119] Yenesew A, Akala HM, Twinomuhwezi H, *et al.* The antiplasmodial and radical scavenging activities of flavonoids of *Erythrina burttii*. Acta Trop 2012; 123(2): 123-7.
[http://dx.doi.org/10.1016/j.actatropica.2012.04.011] [PMID: 22575309]

[120] Gupta AK, Saxena S, Saxena M. Integrated ligand and structure based studies of flavonoids as fatty acid biosynthesis inhibitors of *Plasmodium falciparum*. Bioorg Med Chem Lett 2010; 20(16): 4779-81.
[http://dx.doi.org/10.1016/j.bmcl.2010.06.120] [PMID: 20637612]

[121] Lubbad MY, Al-Quraishy S, Dkhil MA. Antimalarial and antioxidant activities of Indigofera oblongifolia on *Plasmodium chabaudi*-induced spleen tissue injury in mice. Parasitol Res 2015; 114(9): 3431-8.
[http://dx.doi.org/10.1007/s00436-015-4568-y] [PMID: 26109255]

[122] El Babili F, Bouajila J, Fouraste I, Valentin A, Mauret S, Moulis C. Chemical study, antimalarial and antioxidant activities, and cytotoxicity to human breast cancer cells (MCF7) of *Argania spinosa*. Phytomedicine 2010; 17(2): 157-60.
[http://dx.doi.org/10.1016/j.phymed.2009.05.014] [PMID: 19576744]

[123] Awas E, Omosa LK, Midiwo JO, Ndakala A, Mwaniki J. Antioxidant activities of flavonoid aglycones from Kenyan gardenia ternifolia schum and Thonn. IOSR J Pharm Biol Sci 2016; 11(3): 136-41.

[124] Nureye D, Assefa S, Nedi T, Engidawork E. *In vivo* antimalarial activity of the 80% methanolic root bark extract and solvent fractions of *Gardenia ternifolia* Schumach. & Thonn. (Rubiaceae) against *Plasmodium berghei*. Evid Based Complement Alternat Med 2018; 2018: 1-10.
[http://dx.doi.org/10.1155/2018/9217835] [PMID: 30008788]

[125] Ochieng CO, Ogweno Mid J, Okinda Owu P. Anti-plasmodial and larvicidal effects of surface exudates of *Gardenia ternifolia* aerial parts. Res J Pharm 2010; 4(2): 45-50.
[http://dx.doi.org/10.3923/rjpharm.2010.45.50]

[126] Yahia Y, Benabderrahim MA, Tlili N, Bagues M, Nagaz K. Bioactive compounds, antioxidant and antimicrobial activities of extracts from different plant parts of two *Ziziphus Mill.* species. PLoS One 2020; 15(5): e0232599.
[http://dx.doi.org/10.1371/journal.pone.0232599] [PMID: 32428000]

[127] Esteki T, Urooj A. Antioxidant components and activity in the peel of *Ziziphus jujuba Mill.* J Pharma Res 2012; 5: 2705-9.

[128] Abalaka ME, Mann A, Adeyemo SO. Studies on *in-vitro* antioxidant and free radical scavenging potential and phytochemical screening of leaves of *Ziziphus mauritiana* L. and *Ziziphus spina-christi* L. compared with Ascorbic acid. J Med Genet Genomics 2011; 3(2): 28-34.

[129] Panseeta P, Lomchoey K, Prabpai S, *et al.* Antiplasmodial and antimycobacterial cyclopeptide alkaloids from the root of *Ziziphus mauritiana.* Phytochemistry 2011; 72(9): 909-15.
[http://dx.doi.org/10.1016/j.phytochem.2011.03.003] [PMID: 21450320]

[130] Attemene SDD, Beourou S, Tuo K, *et al.* Antiplasmodial activity of two medicinal plants against clinical isolates of *Plasmodium falciparum* and *Plasmodium berghei* infected mice. J Parasit Dis 2018; 42(1): 68-76.
[http://dx.doi.org/10.1007/s12639-017-0966-7] [PMID: 29491562]

[131] Nahrevanian H, Sheykhkanlooye Milan B, Kazemi M, Hajhosseini R, Soleymani Mashhadi S, Nahrevanian S. Antimalarial effects of iranian flora *Artemisia sieberi* on *Plasmodium berghei in vivo* in mice and phytochemistry analysis of its herbal extracts. Malar Res Treat 2012; 1-8.
[http://dx.doi.org/10.1155/2012/727032] [PMID: 22315701]

[132] Nour AMM, Khalid SA, Kaiser M, Brun R, Abdalla WE, Schmidt TJ. The antiprotozoal activity of methylated flavonoids from *Ageratum conyzoides* L. J Ethnopharmacol 2010; 129(1): 127-30.
[http://dx.doi.org/10.1016/j.jep.2010.02.015] [PMID: 20219663]

[133] SUNA S, INCEDAYI B, Tamer C, Ozcan Sinir G, Çopur Ö. Lemon verbena (*Lippia citriodora Kunth*) beverages: Physicochemical properties, contents of total phenolics and minerals, and bioaccessibility of antioxidants. Ital J Food Sci 2019; 31: 40-53.

[134] Jaradat N, Hawash M, Abualhasan MN, Qadi M, Ghanim M, Massarwy E, *et al.* Spectral characterization, antioxidant, antimicrobial, cytotoxic, and cyclooxygenase inhibitory activities of *Aloysia citriodora* essential oils collected from two Palestinian regions. BMC complement med ther 2021; 21(1)
[http://dx.doi.org/10.1186/s12906-021-03314-1]

[135] Rojas J, Palacios O, Ronceros S. Efecto del aceite esencial de Aloysia triphylla britton (cedrón) sobre el *Trypanosoma cruzi* en ratones. Rev Peru Med Exp Salud Publica 2012; 29(1): 61-8.
[http://dx.doi.org/10.1590/S1726-46342012000100009] [PMID: 22510908]

[136] Al-Adhroey AH, Nor ZM, Al-Mekhlafi HM, Mahmud R. Median lethal dose, antimalarial activity, phytochemical screening and radical scavenging of methanolic *Languas galanga* rhizome extract. Molecules 2010; 15(11): 8366-76.
[http://dx.doi.org/10.3390/molecules15118366] [PMID: 21081857]

[137] Mohd Abd Razak MR, Afzan A, Ali R, *et al.* Effect of selected local medicinal plants on the asexual blood stage of chloroquine resistant *Plasmodium falciparum.* BMC Complement Altern Med 2014; 14(1): 492.
[http://dx.doi.org/10.1186/1472-6882-14-492] [PMID: 25510573]

[138] Mahae N, Chaiseri S. Antioxidant activities and antioxidative components in extracts of *Alpinia galanga* (L.) Sw. Witthayasan Kasetsat Witthayasat 2009; 43: 358-69.

[139] Kaur A, Singh R, Dey CS, Sharma SS, Bhutani KK, Singh IP. Antileishmanial phenylpropanoids from *Alpinia galanga* (Linn.) Willd. Indian J Exp Biol 2010; 48(3): 314-7.
[PMID: 21046987]

[140] An NTG, Huong LT, Satyal P, *et al.* Mosquito larvicidal activity, antimicrobial activity, and chemical

compositions of essential oils from four species of myrtaceae from central vietnam. Plants 2020; 9(4): 544.
[http://dx.doi.org/10.3390/plants9040544] [PMID: 32331486]

[141] Uchiyama N. Antichagasic activities of natural products against *Trypanosoma cruzi*. J Health Sci 2009; 55(1): 31-9.
[http://dx.doi.org/10.1248/jhs.55.31]

[142] Roshan Jahn MS, Getha K, Mohd-Ilham A & Norhayati I, Muhammad Haffiz J, Amyra AS. *In vitro* anti-leismanial activity of malaysian medicinal and forest plant species. J Trop For Sci 2018; 30(2): 234-41.
[http://dx.doi.org/10.26525/jtfs2018.30.2.234241]

[143] Habila N, Humphrey NC, Abel AS. Trypanocidal potentials of *Azadirachta indica* seeds against *Trypanosoma evansi*. Vet Parasitol 2011; 180(3-4): 173-8.
[http://dx.doi.org/10.1016/j.vetpar.2011.03.037] [PMID: 21524857]

[144] Wanzala EN, Gikonyo NK, Murilla G, Githua M, Hassanali A. *In vitro* and *in vivo* anti-trypanosomal activities of methanol extract of *Azadirachta indica* stem-bark. Afr J Tradit Complement Altern Med 2017; 14(6): 72-7.
[http://dx.doi.org/10.21010/ajtcam.v14i6.8]

[145] Fahrimal Y, Aliza D, Fitriani A. Erina, Azhar A. Protective Effect of Neem (*Azadirachta Indica*) Leaf Extract on Liver of *Trypanosoma evansi* Infected Rats (*Rattus norvegicus*). Proceedings of the 2nd Syiah Kuala International Conference on Medicine and Health Sciences (SKIC-MHS 2018). Banda Aceh, Indonesia. 2018; 172-7.

[146] Gupta N, Srivastva N, Bubber P, Puri S. The antioxidant potential of *Azadirachta indica* ameliorates cardioprotection following diabetic mellitus-induced microangiopathy. Pharmacogn Mag 2016; 12(46) (Suppl. 3): 371.
[http://dx.doi.org/10.4103/0973-1296.185772] [PMID: 27563227]

[147] Alzohairy MA. Therapeutics role of *Azadirachta indica* (Neem) and their active constituents in diseases prevention and treatment. Evid Based Complement Alternat Med 2016; 2016: 1-11.
[http://dx.doi.org/10.1155/2016/7382506] [PMID: 27034694]

[148] Nagano MS, Batalini C. Phytochemical screening, antioxidant activity and potential toxicity of *Azadirachta indica* A. Juss (neem) leaves. Rev Colomb Cienc Quím Farm 2021; 50(1): 29-47.

[149] Tauheed AM, Mamman M, Ahmed A, Suleiman MM, Balogun EO. Partially purified leaf fractions of *Azadirachta indica* inhibit trypanosome alternative oxidase and exert antitrypanosomal effects on *Trypanosoma congolense*. Acta Parasitol 2022; 67(1): 120-9.
[http://dx.doi.org/10.1007/s11686-021-00437-w] [PMID: 34156634]

[150] Ngure RM, Ongeri B, Karori SM, Wachira W, Maathai RG, Kibugi JK, *et al*. Anti-trypanosomal effects of *Azadiracta indica* (neem) extract on *Trypanosoma brucei* rhodesiense-infected mice. East J Med 2013; 14(1): 2-9.

[151] Kamarazaman IS, Mohamad Ali NA, Abdullah F, *et al*. *In vitro* wound healing evaluation, antioxidant and chemical profiling of *Baeckea frutescens* leaves ethanolic extract. Arab J Chem 2022; 15(6): 103871.
[http://dx.doi.org/10.1016/j.arabjc.2022.103871]

[152] Nisa K, Nurhayati S, Apriyana W, Indrianingsih AW. Investigation of total phenolic and flavonoid contents, and evaluation of antimicrobial and antioxidant activities from *Baeckea frutescens* extracts. IOP Conf Ser Earth Environ Sci 2017; 101: 012002.
[http://dx.doi.org/10.1088/1755-1315/101/1/012002]

[153] Quang TH, Cuong NX, Van Minh C, Van Kiem P. New flavonoids from *Baeckea Frutescens* and their antioxidant activity. Nat Prod Commun 2008; 3(5): 1934578X0800300.
[http://dx.doi.org/10.1177/1934578X0800300515]

[154] Norhayati I, Getha K, Haffiz JM, Ilham AM, Sahira HL, Syarifah MM, *et al. In vitro* antitrypanosomal activity of Malaysian plants. J Trop For Sci 2013; 25: 52-9.

[155] Putri SD, Rusdi , Asra R. A review: Antioxidant activities of sembung leaves (*Blumea balsamifera* (L.) DC). EAS Journal of Pharmacy and Pharmacology 2020; 2(5): 166-72.
[http://dx.doi.org/10.36349/easjpp.2020.v02i05.001]

[156] Ginting B, Maulana I, Karnila I. Biosynthesis copper nanoparticles using *Blumea balsamifera* leaf extracts: Characterization of its antioxidant and cytotoxicity activities. Surf Interfaces 2020; 21: 100799.
[http://dx.doi.org/10.1016/j.surfin.2020.100799]

[157] Kusumawati IGA, Wisnu APIM, Yogeswara IBA. Antioxidant and antihypertensive activity of Loloh Sembung (*Blumea balsamifera*) Proceedings 2017. Available from: https://www.researchgate.net/publication/334251496_Antioxidant_and_antihypertensive_activity_of_Loloh_Sembung_Blumea_balsamifera

[158] Liana D, Rungsihirunrat K. Phytochemical screening, antimalarial activities, and genetic relationship of 16 indigenous Thai Asteraceae medicinal plants: A combinatorial approach using phylogeny and ethnobotanical bioprospecting in antimalarial drug discovery. J Adv Pharm Technol Res 2021; 12(3): 254-60.
[http://dx.doi.org/10.4103/japtr.JAPTR_238_21] [PMID: 34345604]

[159] Ablat A, Mohamad J, Awang K, Shilpi JA, Arya A. Evaluation of antidiabetic and antioxidant properties of *Brucea javanica* seed. Sci World J 2014; 2014: 1-8.
[http://dx.doi.org/10.1155/2014/786130] [PMID: 24688431]

[160] Risnadewi WN, Muliasari H, Hamdin CD, Andayani Y. Comparative antioxidant activity of *Brucea javanica* (L) Merr seed extract derived from maceration and soxhletation method 2019.

[161] Simamora A, Timotius KH, Santoso AW. Antidiabetic, antibacterial and antioxidant activities of different extracts from *Brucea javanica* (L.) merr seeds. Pharmacogn J 2019; 11(3): 479-85.
[http://dx.doi.org/10.5530/pj.2019.11.76]

[162] Sidek HJ, Abd Karim HA, Mahmud Z. Phytochemical screening, antioxidant activity and phenolic content of different plant parts of *Brucea javanica* (L.). Jurnal Intelek 2019; 14(2): 33-43.
[http://dx.doi.org/10.24191/ji.v14i2.215]

[163] Raeisi M, Mirkarimi K, Jannat B, *et al. In vitro* effect of some medicinal plants on *Leishmania major* strain MRHO/IR/75/ER. Medical Laboratory Journal 2020; 14(4): 46-52.
[http://dx.doi.org/10.29252/mlj.14.4.46]

[164] Kaur S, Kumar A, Thakur S, *et al.* Antioxidant, antiproliferative and apoptosis-inducing efficacy of fractions from *Cassia fistula* L. leaves. Antioxidants 2020; 9(2): 173.
[http://dx.doi.org/10.3390/antiox9020173] [PMID: 32093300]

[165] Thabit S, Handoussa H, Roxo M, El Sayed NS, Cestari de Azevedo B, Wink M. Evaluation of antioxidant and neuroprotective activities of *Cassia fistula* (L.) using the *Caenorhabditis elegans* model. PeerJ 2018; 6: e5159.
[http://dx.doi.org/10.7717/peerj.5159] [PMID: 30023139]

[166] Mwangi RW, Macharia JM, Wagara IN, Bence RL. The medicinal properties of *Cassia fistula* L: A review. Biomed Pharmacother 2021; 144: 112240.
[http://dx.doi.org/10.1016/j.biopha.2021.112240] [PMID: 34601194]

[167] Sampathkumar K, Keerthana S, Mahalakshmi S, Ramesh B, Sivaraj C, Pramodh A. Antioxidant and anticancer activities of roots of *Catharanthus roseus* (L.) G.Don. Res J Chem Environ 2021; 25: 158-65.

[168] Mir M. Phytochemical analysis and antioxidant properties of the various extracts of *Catharanthus roseus*. J Chem Pharm Res 2018; 10: 1-10.

[169] Mardani-Nejad S, Khavari-Nejad RA, Saadatmand S, Najafi F, Aberoomand Azar P. Potent antioxidant properties of rolB-transformed *Catharanthus roseus* (L.) G. Don. Iran J Pharm Res 2016; 15(2): 537-50.
[PMID: 27642325]

[170] Barrales-Cureño HJ, Reyes CR, García IV. Valdez LG L, De Jesús AG, Ruíz JAC, Herrera LMS, Caballero MCC, Magallón JAS, Perez JE, Montoya JM. Alkaloids of pharmacological importance in *Catharanthus roseus*. In: Kurek J, Ed. Alkaloids - Their Importance in Nature and Human Life. London: IntechOpen 2019.
[http://dx.doi.org/10.5772/intechopen.82006]

[171] Simoh S, Sew YS, Abd Rahim F, Ahmad MA, Zainal A. Comparative analysis of metabolites and antioxidant potentials from different plant parts of *Curcuma aeruginosa* Roxb. Sains Malays 2018; 47(12): 3031-41.
[http://dx.doi.org/10.17576/jsm-2018-4712-13]

[172] Nurcholis W, Khumaida N, Syukur M, Bintang M. Variability of total phenolic and flavonoid content and antioxidant activity among 20 *Curcuma aeruginosa* Roxb. Accessions of Indonesia. Asian Journal of Biochemistry 2016; 11(3): 142-8.
[http://dx.doi.org/10.3923/ajb.2016.142.148]

[173] Setiawan PYB, Kertia N, Nurrochmad A, Wahyuono S. Synergistic anti-inflammatory effects of *Curcuma xanthorrhiza* rhizomes and *Physalis angulata* herb extract on lipopolysaccharide-stimulated RAW 264.7 cells. J Appl Pharm 2022; 88-98.

[174] Rahmat E, Lee J, Kang Y. Javanese turmeric (*Curcuma xanthorrhiza* roxb.): ethnobotany, phytochemistry, biotechnology, and pharmacological activities. Zarrelli A, eds. In: Evid-based CAM, Ed. Evid-based Complement Altern Med. 2021; pp. 1-15.

[175] Jantan I, Saputri FC, Qaisar MN, Buang F. Correlation between Chemical Composition of *Curcuma domestica* and *Curcuma xanthorrhiza* and Their Antioxidant Effect on Human Low-Density Lipoprotein Oxidation. Evid Based Complement Alternat Med 2012; 1-10.
[http://dx.doi.org/10.1155/2012/438356] [PMID: 23243446]

[176] Rather MA, Dar BA, Sofi SN, Bhat BA, Qurishi MA. *Foeniculum vulgare*: A comprehensive review of its traditional use, phytochemistry, pharmacology, and safety. Arab J Chem 2016; 9: S1574-83.
[http://dx.doi.org/10.1016/j.arabjc.2012.04.011]

[177] Ahmed AF, Shi M, Liu C, Kang W. Comparative analysis of antioxidant activities of essential oils and extracts of fennel (*Foeniculum vulgare* Mill.) seeds from Egypt and China. Food Sci Hum Wellness 2019; 8(1): 67-72.
[http://dx.doi.org/10.1016/j.fshw.2019.03.004]

[178] Kalleli F, Bettaieb Rebey I, Wannes WA, *et al.* Chemical composition and antioxidant potential of essential oil and methanol extract from Tunisian and French fennel (*Foeniculum vulgare* Mill.) seeds. J Food Biochem 2019; 43(8): e12935.
[http://dx.doi.org/10.1111/jfbc.12935] [PMID: 31368565]

[179] Badgujar SB, Patel VV, Bandivdekar AH. *Foeniculum vulgare* Mill: A review of its botany, phytochemistry, pharmacology, contemporary application, and toxicology. BioMed Res Int 2014; 2014: 1-32.
[http://dx.doi.org/10.1155/2014/842674] [PMID: 25162032]

[180] Mostafa G, Nahid J, Javad SS, Alireza D, Ebrahim SS. Effect of *Foeniculum vulgare* aqueous and alcoholic seed extract against zoonotic cutaneous leishmaniasis. Ethiop J Health Sci 2021; 31(2): 401-8.
[PMID: 34158792]

[181] Yapp DTT, Yap SY. Lansium domesticum: Skin and leaf extracts of this fruit tree interrupt the lifecycle of *Plasmodium falciparum*, and are active towards a chloroquine-resistant strain of the parasite (T9) *in vitro*. J Ethnopharmacol 2003; 85(1): 145-50.

[http://dx.doi.org/10.1016/S0378-8741(02)00375-6] [PMID: 12576213]

[182] Subandrate S, Sinulingga S, Wahyuni S, Altiyan MF, Fatmawati F. Antioxidant potential of lansium domesticum corr. Seed extract in white male rat (*Rattus novergicus*) induced by alcohol. Molekul 2016; 11(1): 1.
[http://dx.doi.org/10.20884/1.jm.2016.11.1.189]

[183] Abdallah HM, Mohamed GA, Ibrahim SRM. *Lansium domesticum*—A fruit with multi-benefits: traditional uses, phytochemicals, nutritional value, and bioactivities. Nutrients 2022; 14(7): 1531.
[http://dx.doi.org/10.3390/nu14071531] [PMID: 35406144]

[184] Ohashi M, Amoa-Bosompem M, Kwofie KD, *et al. In vitro* antiprotozoan activity and mechanisms of action of selected G hanaian medicinal plants against *Trypanosoma*, *Leishmania*, and *Plasmodium* parasites. Phytother Res 2018; 32(8): 1617-30.
[http://dx.doi.org/10.1002/ptr.6093] [PMID: 29733118]

[185] Li J, Niu D, Zhang Y, Zeng XA. Physicochemical properties, antioxidant and antiproliferative activities of polysaccharides from *Morinda citrifolia* L. (Noni) based on different extraction methods. Int J Biol Macromol 2020; 150: 114-21.
[http://dx.doi.org/10.1016/j.ijbiomac.2019.12.157] [PMID: 32006573]

[186] Chan-Blanco Y, Vaillant F, Pérez AM, Belleville MP, Zúñiga C, Brat P. The ripening and aging of noni fruits (*Morinda citrifolia* L.): microbiological flora and antioxidant compounds. J Sci Food Agric 2007; 87(9): 1710-6.
[http://dx.doi.org/10.1002/jsfa.2894]

[187] Almeida-Souza F, Cardoso FO, Souza BVC, *et al. Morinda citrifolia* Linn. Reduces parasite load and modulates cytokines and extracellular matrix proteins in C57BL/6 mice infected with *Leishmania* (*Leishmania*) *Amazonensis*. PLoS Negl Trop Dis 2016; 10(8): e0004900.
[http://dx.doi.org/10.1371/journal.pntd.0004900] [PMID: 27579922]

[188] Landázuri AC, Gualle A, Castañeda V, Morales E, Caicedo A, Orejuela-Escobar LM. *Moringa oleifera* Lam. Leaf powder antioxidant activity and cytotoxicity in human primary fibroblasts. Nat Prod Res 2021; 35(24): 6194-9.
[http://dx.doi.org/10.1080/14786419.2020.1837804] [PMID: 33118387]

[189] Bauri RK, Tigga MN, Kullu SS. A review on use of medicinal plants to control *parasites.* Indian J Nat Prod Resour 2015; 6: 268-77.

[190] Nwodo N, Ibezim A, Ntie-Kang F, Adikwu M, Mbah C. Anti-trypanosomal activity of nigerian plants and their constituents. Molecules 2015; 20(5): 7750-71.
[http://dx.doi.org/10.3390/molecules20057750] [PMID: 25927903]

[191] Obediah GA, Christian Obi N. Anti-plasmodial effect of *Moringa oleifera* seeds in *Plasmodium berghei* infected albino rats. Biochem Pharmacol: Open Access 2020; 9(1)
[http://dx.doi.org/10.35248/2167-0501.20.9.268]

[192] Shrivastava M, Prasad A, Kumar D. Evaluation of anti plasmodium potential of *Moringa oleifera* (Lam) in *Plasmodium yoelii* infected mice. Indian J Pharm Sci 2021; 83(6).

[193] Wan Omar A, Ngah ZU, Zaridah MZ, Noor Rain A. *In vitro* and *in vivo* antiplasmodial properties of some Malaysian plants used in traditional medicine. Infect Dis J Pakistan 2007; 16(4): 97-101.

[194] Alenzi FQ, Altamimi A, Kujan O, Tarakji B, Tamimi W, Bagader O. Antioxidant properties of *Nigella sativa.* J Mol Genet Med 2013; 7(3).
[http://dx.doi.org/10.4172/1747-0862.1000077]

[195] Awan MA, Akhter S, Husna AU, *et al.* Antioxidant activity of *Nigella sativa* Seeds Aqueous Extract and its use for cryopreservation of buffalo spermatozoa. Andrologia 2018; 50(6): e13020.
[http://dx.doi.org/10.1111/and.13020] [PMID: 29700838]

[196] El-Sayed SAES, Rizk MA, Yokoyama N, Igarashi I. Evaluation of the *in vitro* and *in vivo* inhibitory effect of thymoquinone on piroplasm parasites. Parasit Vectors 2019; 12(1): 37.

[http://dx.doi.org/10.1186/s13071-019-3296-z] [PMID: 30651142]

[197] Al-Turkmani MO, Mokrani L, Soukkarieh C. Antileishmanial apoptotic activity of *Nigella sativa* L. essential oil and thymoquinone triggers on *Leishmania tropica*. Indian J Exp Biol 2020; 58: 699-705.

[198] Nassef NAE, El-Melegy MA, Beshay EV, Al-Sharaky DR, Al-Attar TM. Trypanocidal effects of cisplatin alone and in combination with *Nigella sativa* oil on experimentally infected mice with *Trypanosoma evansi*. Iran J Parasitol 2018; 13(1): 89-99.
[PMID: 29963090]

[199] Bhalla G, Kaur S, Kaur J, Kaur R, Raina P. Antileishmanial and immunomodulatory potential of *Ocimum sanctum* Linn. and *Cocos nucifera* Linn. In murine visceral leishmaniasis. J Parasit Dis 2017; 41(1): 76-85.
[http://dx.doi.org/10.1007/s12639-016-0753-x] [PMID: 28316391]

[200] Hasan Khan N, Zhi Xia K, Perveen N. Phytochemical analysis, antibacterial and antioxidant activity determination of *Ocimum sanctum*. Pharm pharmacol int 2018; 6(6).
[http://dx.doi.org/10.15406/ppij.2018.06.00223]

[201] Ramamurthy J. Evaluation of antioxidant activity of *Ocimum sanctum*-an *in vitro* study. Int J Oral Sci 2021; 5001-5.

[202] Jadid N, Hidayati D, Hartanti SR, Arraniry BA, Rachman RY, Wikanta W. Antioxidant activities of different solvent extracts of *Piper retrofractum* Vahl. Using DPPH assay. AIP Conference Proceedings. 2017.

[203] Ismail SM, Chua KH, Aminuddin A, Ugusman A. *Piper sarmentosum* as an antioxidant: A systematic review. Sains Malays 2018; 47(10): 2359-68.
[http://dx.doi.org/10.17576/jsm-2018-4710-12]

[204] Hafizah AH, Zaiton Z, Zulkhairi A, Mohd Ilham A, Nor Anita MMN, Zaleha AM. *Piper sarmentosum* as an antioxidant on oxidative stress in human umbilical vein endothelial cells induced by hydrogen peroxide. J Zhejiang Univ Sci B 2010; 11(5): 357-65.
[http://dx.doi.org/10.1631/jzus.B0900397] [PMID: 20443214]

[205] Najib Nik A Rahman N, Furuta T, kojima S, Takane K, Ali Mohd M. Antimalarial activity of extracts of Malaysian medicinal plants. J Ethnopharmacol 1999; 64(3): 249-54.
[http://dx.doi.org/10.1016/S0378-8741(98)00135-4] [PMID: 10363840]

[206] Alshahrani MY, Rafi Z, Alabdallah NM, *et al.* A comparative antibacterial, antioxidant, and antineoplastic potential of *Rauwolfia serpentina* (L.) leaf extract with its biologically synthesized gold nanoparticles (R-AuNPs). Plants 2021; 10(11): 2278.
[http://dx.doi.org/10.3390/plants10112278] [PMID: 34834641]

[207] Azmi MB, Qureshi SA. Methanolic root extract of *Rauwolfia serpentina* benth improves the glycemic, antiatherogenic, and cardioprotective indices in alloxan-induced diabetic mice. Adv Pharmacol Sci 2012; 1-11.
[http://dx.doi.org/10.1155/2012/376429] [PMID: 23365565]

[208] Da Costa Sarmento N, Worachartcheewan A, Pingaew R, Prachayasittikul S, Ruchirawat S, Prachayasittikul V. Antimicrobial, antioxidant and anticancer activities of *Strychnos lucida* R. Br. Afr J Tradit Complement Altern Med 2015; 12(4): 122.
[http://dx.doi.org/10.4314/ajtcam.v12i4.18]

[209] Masendra M, Aristo B, Purba V, Lukmandaru G, Verick Purba BA. Antioxidant activity of *Swietenia macrophylla* king bark extracts. Wood Res 2021; 66(1): 57-70.
[http://dx.doi.org/10.37763/wr.1336-4561/66.1.5770]

[210] Moghadamtousi S, Goh B, Chan C, Shabab T, Kadir H. Biological activities and phytochemicals of *Swietenia macrophylla* King. Molecules 2013; 18(9): 10465-83.
[http://dx.doi.org/10.3390/molecules180910465] [PMID: 23999722]

[211] Cavin A, Hostettmann K, Dyatmyko W, Potterat O. Antioxidant and lipophilic constituents of

Tinospora crispa. Planta Med 1998; 64(5): 393-6.
[http://dx.doi.org/10.1055/s-2006-957466] [PMID: 17253260]

[212]   Warsinah W, Baroroh HN, Harwoko H. Phytochemical analysis and antioxidant activity of brotowali (*Tinospora crispa* L. Mier) Stem. Molekul 2020; 15(2): 73.
[http://dx.doi.org/10.20884/1.jm.2020.15.2.533]

[213]   Puspitasari RN. Antioxidant activity of Tinospora crispa extracted with different ethanol solvents. Bali Med J 2022; 11(3): 1107-10. Available from: https://www.balimedicaljournal.org/index.php/bmj/article/view/3467

[214]   Melia S, Novia D, Juliyarsi I. Antioxidant and antimicrobial activities of gambir (*Uncaria gambir* Roxb) extracts and their application in rendang. Pak J Nutr 2015; 14(12): 938-41.
[http://dx.doi.org/10.3923/pjn.2015.938.941]

[215]   Rauf A, Rahmawaty , Siregar AZ. The condition of *Uncaria gambir* roxb. As one of important medicinal plants in north sumatra Indonesia. Procedia Chem 2015; 14: 3-10.
[http://dx.doi.org/10.1016/j.proche.2015.03.002]

[216]   Hidayati M, Rahmatulloh A. Antioxidant activity of *Uncaria gambir* (Hunter) Roxb extracts. Trop J Nat Prod Res 2022; 6(8): 1215-8.
[http://dx.doi.org/10.26538/tjnpr/v6i8.9]

[217]   Rahman M, Khatun A. SM R, Rashid M. Antioxidant, antimicrobial and cytotoxic activities of *Vitis trifolia* Linn. J Dhaka Int Univ 2010; 1: 181-4.

[218]   Rahman HS, Rasedee A, Yeap SK, *et al.* Biomedical properties of a natural dietary plant metabolite, zerumbone, in cancer therapy and chemoprevention trials. BioMed Res Int 2014; 1-20.
[http://dx.doi.org/10.1155/2014/920742] [PMID: 25025076]

CHAPTER 5

Natural Products as a Therapeutic Approach in Regulating Autophagy for the Management of Neurodegenerative Diseases

Mani Iyer Prasanth[1,2], **Dicson Sheeja Malar**[1,2] and **Tewin Tencomnao**[1,2,*]

[1] *Natural Products for Neuroprotection and Anti-ageing Research Unit, Chulalongkorn University, Bangkok-10330, Thailand*

[2] *Department of Clinical Chemistry, Faculty of Allied Health Sciences, Chulalongkorn University, Bangkok-10330, Thailand*

Abstract: Autophagy is a complex phenomenon that occurs constantly in cells for maintaining the well-being of individuals. However, any dysregulation in the mechanism or the proteins involved leads to detrimental effects on several diseases including cancer, diabetes, and neurodegenerative diseases (NDs). Autophagy dysfunction is involved in the progression of NDs including Alzheimer's disease (AD), Parkinson's disease (PD), and Huntington's disease (HD). With the involvement being identified, autophagy has become a prospective target in ameliorating NDs. Natural products in the form of extracts and bioactive compounds were repeatedly reported for targeting autophagy-related proteins and the mechanism making them promising drug candidates against NDs. The current chapter briefly outlines the role of autophagy in NDs and the effect of selected natural products in restoring pathological outcomes.

Keywords: Autophagy, mTOR, Neurodegenerative diseases, Oxidative stress, Polyphenols, Phytomedicine.

INTRODUCTION

Autophagy is a form of cellular survival during nutrient starvation, which helps to clear the damaged and degraded cell structures such as proteins, lipids, and other cellular organelles from the system, thereby providing nourishment and energy to the cells. These organelles are engulfed by membrane-bound vesicles termed autophagosomes, which fuse with the lysosomes and form autolysosomes further leading to the degradation of dysfunctional materials by lysosomal acid hydrolases [1, 2]. However, the process is age-dependent; in other words, the rate

---

* **Corresponding author Tewin Tencomnao:** Natural Products for Neuroprotection and Anti-ageing Research Unit & Department of Clinical Chemistry, Faculty of Allied Health Sciences, Chulalongkorn University, Bangkok-10330, Thailand; Tel.: +66-2-218-1533; E-mail: tewin.t@chula.ac.th

of autophagy decreases during aging [3]. There are different types of autophagy such as macroautophagy, microautophagy, chaperone-mediated autophagy, mitophagy, and lipophagy, depending on the activity involved.

Macroautophagy deals with the clearance of damaged cell organelles and proteins from the cells [4 - 6]. It is one of the most studied processes in autophagy and several genetic players have been identified. In case of microautophagy, the cell debris is directly taken to the lysosome, and the autophagosome is not essential for the process [4, 7]. The chaperone-mediated autophagy can function without autophagosome, as the cytosolic chaperons aid in the transportation of degraded proteins into the lysosome. This process is connected to the pathogenesis of neurodegenerative diseases and cancer; however, the complete mechanism is still unclear. The other processes such as mitophagy deal with the degradation of damaged mitochondria and lipophagy deals with the degradation of damaged lipids [4].

Different molecular pathways have been reported to mediate autophagy. It is already known that the disruption and dysfunction of autophagy can occur *via* mTOR mediated pathway and can also take place independently of the pathway [8]. In the mTOR-dependent regulation, phosphatase and tensin homolog (PTEN) induce autophagy by blocking mTOR, while the class I PI3 kinase, and AKT inhibit autophagy by activating mTOR [9]. In mTOR-independent regulation, autophagy can be modulated through cAMP-Epac-PLC-ε, phosphoinositol, and Ca^{2+}-calpain-GSα pathways [10]. In addition, oxidative stress can activate autophagy *via* an mTOR-mediated/independent pathway [11].

AUTOPHAGY IN NEURODEGENERATIVE DISEASES

In a normal healthy human brain, the proper functioning of cells depends on the periodic clearance of misfolded, unused, and damaged proteins. In contrast to most cell types, neurons are post-mitotic, and therefore their cell division process will not dilute any toxic materials. In this regard, autophagy is essential for the survival and functioning of neurons, and it must prolong until the organism's lifetime. It should be noted that autophagy occurs constitutively in neurons [12, 13]. Abnormal protein aggregation, which could eventually lead to neurodegeneration can occur by the suppression of this neuronal autophagy, which highlights the prominence of autophagy in maintaining neuronal homeostasis and survival [14, 15]. Disruption in autophagy has been reported to be involved in aging and age-associated degenerative diseases including Alzheimer's disease (AD), Parkinson's disease (PD), and Huntington's disease (HD) [16]. Autophagy plays a significant role in eliminating the build-up of amyloid-β, hyperphosphorylated tau protein, α-synuclein, and clearing malfunctioning organelles. However, autophagy has been reported to show both decreases [17 - 20] and increases in amyloid-β expression [21, 22], indicating the paradoxical relationship. For instance, autophagic vacuoles act as sites of abnormal APP cleavage leading to Aβ generation [23, 24]. More in-depth studies on the contradictory reports imply that during the initial phase of AD, the accumulating Aβ can activate autophagy, and thereby the autophagosome-lysosomal system. However, during the later stages, the continuous accumulation of Aβ leads to abnormal autophagy and neuronal dysfunction, which accelerates AD symptoms [25 - 28]. Similar to AD, compelling pieces of evidence point to the link between PD and autophagy dysfunction, as the α-synuclein inclusions have been reported to modulate autophagic function [29], leading to decreased lysosome - autophagosome fusion and reduced protein degradation, genetic mutations in phosphatase and tensin homolog-induced putative kinase 1 (PINK1) and E3 ubiquitin ligase (Parkin) [30 - 33].

Moreover, autophagy could also play a key role in the incidence and development of ischemic stroke through HiF-1α/BNIP3, PINK1/Parkin, PKC/JNK, PI3K/Akt-mTOR, AMPK/mTORC1, and other pathways [34 - 39]. Oxygen glucose deprivation/reoxygenation can activate PINK1-mediated mitochondrial autophagy and play a role in its pathophysiological process. Also, ROS can activate mitochondrial autophagy *via* the PINK1/Parkin pathway [40], and remove damaged mitochondria [41]. Under normal conditions, the optimum level of ROS developed in the body aids in cell growth, development, and immunity. Despite that, during brain ischemia, there would be a decrease in cerebral blood flow leading to oxygen and glucose deficiency, causing oxidative stress. During this stage, FOXO3A mediates autophagy by inducing LC3, BNIP3, Beclin1, and Atg12, which may result in cell lysis and promote cell death [42 - 45].

Targeting autophagy can play a role in mediating neurodegenerative diseases, as suggested by some recent shreds of evidence. Compounds that could block the mTOR-C1-kinase activity, and can further reduce Aβ and tau pathologies, such as rapamycin, CCI-779, Torin1, or PP242, can be used as an activator of autophagy [46 - 48]. However, blocking the mTOR pathway completely might have a negative impact, as it plays a role in normal growth and metabolism [6]. Therefore, mTOR-independent pathways that could modulate autophagy can be focused. Autophagy is a complex process involving different and diverse mechanisms, it would be ideal to aim multiple targets using a cocktail of drugs to induce autophagy in subjects with neurodegenerative diseases [48]. However, this could also lead to disastrous effects, as too much autophagy may lead to the accumulation of large chunks of autophagosomes and undigested autolysosomes, which too can hinder axonal activity [3].

AUTOPHAGY, NEUROPROTECTION, AND PHYTOMEDICINES

The absence/non-function or aberrant activation of the autophagy machinery may lead to neuronal injury *via* oxidative damage in connection with protein overload and neuroinflammation, while regulating autophagy may aid protection in cell survival [49]. Drugs for the treatment of neurodegenerative diseases are in high demand, and the currently available cholinesterase inhibitors are not effective in treating AD [50, 51]. Naturally available medicinal flora can be used as an alternative product as recent research has reported the abilities of different plants and plant-derived compounds (commonly known as secondary metabolites) to regulate autophagy and induce neuroprotection [52].

Polyphenols are secondary metabolites from plant sources and are classified into four main groups, including phenolic acids, flavonoids, stilbenes, and lignans [53, 54]. Phenolic acids can be further divided as hydroxybenzoic acids and hydroxycinnamic acids, and flavonoids, which are subsequently classified into flavonols, flavones, flavanones, isoflavones, anthocyanidins, and flavonols. More than several hundred polyphenols have been discovered in edible parts of plants including fruits, vegetables, nuts, and seeds, which also exert neuroprotective effects [52]. Polyphenols can either activate or inhibit autophagy during NDs depending on the cellular need to exhibit neuroprotective activity (Fig. **1**). Among these, several phytochemicals including baicalein, silibinin, berberine, and curcumin have been reported to modulate autophagy to exhibit protection in the respective model systems of neurodegenerative diseases (Table **1**).

The following section briefs some of the medicinal plants and their constituents that have potential implications against neurodegenerative diseases, where autophagy comes into play.

MODULATION OF AUTOPHAGY BY PLANT EXTRACTS/ COMPOUNDS TO AMELIORATE NEUROLOGICAL DYSFUNCTION

Herbal Teas' and Their Constituents

Habitual tea consumption can reduce the risk of neurocognitive disorders [79]. The extracts of green tea, oolong tea, hibiscus tea, safflower tea, and ginger tea were previously reported to exhibit neuroprotective effects. The extracts could reduce ROS accumulation, regulate antioxidant mechanisms, activate cell signaling pathways, induce neurite outgrowth, and protect neuronal cells against various toxic insults (Aβ, glutamate, α-synuclein) to offer neuroprotection [80 - 85]. One of the most studied polyphenols Epigallocatechin-3-gallate (EGCG), which is commonly seen in tea extracts was reported to modulate autophagy in several experimental studies. For instance, EGCG induced sirt-1 mediated autophagy against prion protein to inhibit mitochondrial apoptotic pathway in SH-SY5Y cells [86]. In mouse brains, EGCG attenuated autophagy *via* AKT/AMPK/mTOR pathway to protect against ischemia/reperfusion injury [87]. EGCG also attenuated impairment in learning and memory in rats upon stress through the restoration of hippocampal autophagic flux [88].

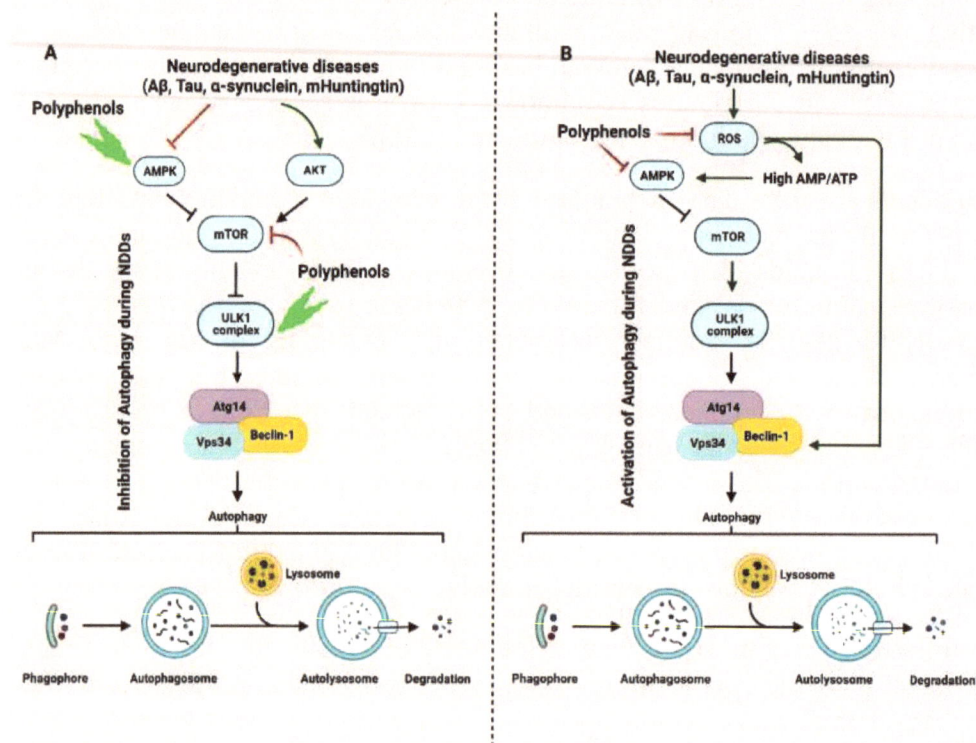

Fig. (1). Misfolded proteins play a dual role in influencing autophagy, either by inhibiting or activating the process, ultimately contributing to the progression of neurodegeneration. (**a**) Misfolded proteins hinder the activation of AMPK while promoting the AKT pathway, resulting in the activation of mTOR. This mTOR activation subsequently suppresses autophagy, leading to the accumulation of misfolded proteins within cells, thereby exacerbating the process of neurodegeneration. (**b**) Accumulation of misfolded proteins leads to the generation of ROS, causing a disruption in cellular energetics. This disturbance triggers an abnormal activation of AMPK, which induces autophagy as a compensatory mechanism to restore cellular homeostasis contributing to neurodegeneration. Depending on the cellular context, plant polyphenols exhibit a bidirectional influence on autophagy regulation. They can activate autophagy by mitigating the inhibitory effects of the AKT/mTOR pathway or inhibit autophagy by attenuating AMPK activation providing a therapeutic avenue for the management of NDs.

Table 1. Phytoconstituents against neurodegenerative diseases *via* modulating autophagy.

Compound	Plant source	Model system	Mechanism of action	Reference
Curcumin	*Curcuma longa*	SH-SY5Y transfected with A53T α-synuclein	Ameliorated PD pathology by downregulating mTOR/p70S6K signaling and inducing macroautophagy.	[55]
Berberine	*Berberis vulgaris*	APP/tau/PS1 mouse model	Decreased the extracellular and intracellular Aβ levels and activated autophagy.	[56]
		Neuro-2a cells expressing TDP-43	Activated autophagy and reversed the formation of insoluble TDP-43 aggregates.	[57]
		Transgenic N171-82Q mice	Enhanced autophagy-dependent degradation of mutant huntingtin and extended survival of HD mice.	[58]
α-Arbutin	*Arctostaphylos uva-ursi*	SH-SY5Y cells	AMPK and autophagy pathway-mediated neuroprotective effect.	[59]
Puerarin	*Pueraria lobata*	Rat	Protected against ischemia/reperfusion injury by suppressing autophagy.	[60]
Breviscapine	*Erigeron breviscapu*	Sprague-Dawley rats	Exhibited neuroprotective effect against cerebral ischemia by inhibiting astrocytic autophagy.	[61]
Orientin	*Passiflora* sp.	APP/PS1 mice	Decreased Aβ deposition by enhancing autophagosome clearance.	[62]
Oleuropein aglycone	*Olea europaea*	Transgenic TgCRND8 mice	Improved cognitive function and reduced Aβ plaques *via* autophagy induction.	[63]
Tomatidine	*Lycopersicon esculentum*	*C. elegans*	Enhanced mitochondrial biogenesis and showed PINK-1/DCT-1-related mitophagy-mediated healthspan improvement.	[64]
		Neuro-2a cells	Exhibited neuroprotection against ischemic injury by inducing lysosomal activity through TFEB-related pathways.	[65]
Schizandrin	*Schisandra chinensis*	PC12 cells	Protected against cerebral ischemia through autophagy attenuation mediated by AMPK/mTOR pathway.	[66]
Glycyrrhizic acid	*Glycyrrhiza glabra*	SHSY5Y cells	Upregulated LC3B II/I conversion, beclin 1 expression, and autophagy induction to protect the cells against 6-Hydroxydopamine-induced toxicity.	[67]

(Table 1) cont.....

Compound	Plant source	Model system	Mechanism of action	Reference
Cornel iridoid glycoside	*Cornus officinalis*	Rats	Facilitated the clearance of tau oligomers through autophagy induction and improved memory.	[68]
Genistein	*Glycine max*	Rats	Restored behavioral and biochemical functions through autophagy-mediated clearance of Aβ and tau against sporadic AD.	[69]
Euxanthone	*Polygala caudate*	PC12 cells and Sprague-Dawley rats	Protected against memory impairment, oxidative stress, and autophagy against Aβ$_{1-42}$-induced neurotoxicity.	[70]
Astragaloside IV	*Astragalus membranaceus*	Sprague-Dawley rats	Exhibited neuroprotective effect against ischemia/reperfusion injury through the induction of autophagy.	[71]
Capsaicin	*Capsicum annuum*	3xTg transgenic mice	Decreased Aβ, phosphorylated tau-mediated pathology by inducing microglia activation, and autophagy through TRPV1 activation.	[72]
Silibinin	*Silybum marianum*	Primary cultures of cortical neurons	Exhibited neuroprotective effect against H$_2$O$_2$-induced oxidative stress by inhibition of autophagy.	[73]
Silymarin	*Silybum marianum*	Swiss albino mice	Protected against MPTP-induced increase in α-synuclein and reduction in dopamine content through the modulation of autophagy.	[74]
Wogonin	*Scutellaria baicalensis*	SH-SY5Y-APP and BACE1 cells	Promoted Aβ clearance through mTOR-dependent autophagy.	[75]
Baicalein	*Scutellaria baicalensis*	SH-SY5Y cells and C57BL/6J mice	Protected against rotenone-induced neurotoxicity and mitochondrial dysfunction through induction of autophagy.	[76]
		Sprague-Dawley rats	Induced mitochondrial autophagy *via* miR-30b and SIRT1/AMPK/mTOR pathway against 6-hydroxydopamin--induced PD.	[77]
Hesperidin and hesperetin	Citrus fruits	Neuro-2a cells	Exhibited protective effect and improved Aβ-impaired glucose utilization by attenuating autophagy.	[78]

Ginger extract has been reported to exert a neuroprotective effect against monosodium glutamate toxicity in experimental rats through the suppression of Aβ accumulation and alteration of neurotransmitter levels [85]. *In vivo* studies also reported the beneficial effects of the extract against AD and PD by improving memory impairment induced by Aβ$_{1-42}$ plaque and alleviating cognitive dysfunctions [89 - 91]. Various studies highlighted that ginger tea's neuroprotective effect was activated by its bioactive components and in PC-12 cells, 6-gingerol attenuated hypoxia-induced autophagy through miR-10--mediated suppression of BNIP3 [92]. The compound also exerted a neuroprotective effect against cerebral ischemia/reperfusion injury through the regulation of autophagy by activating transient receptor potential vanilloid subfamily 1 (TRPV1) as well as inducing the dissociation between TRPV1 and Fas-associated factor 1 (FAF1) [93]. Hydroxysafflower yellow A, the pigment present in safflower tea, was identified to modulate PI3K/AKT/mTOR signaling pathway thereby regulating ROS levels and autophagy to aid neuroprotection [94]. *Thunbergia laurifolia*, a widely used herbal tea in Thailand has been reported for its neuroprotective effect. The extract could ameliorate cognitive and emotional deficits in olfactorectomized mice [95]. In addition, the extract has shown a neuroprotective effect against glutamate-induced toxicity in HT-22 cells through mitophagy signaling [96].

Hibiscus sabdariffa inhibited autophagy by attenuating ER stress and inhibiting the MAPK pathway (p-p38 and p-JNK). The extract also aided in the suppression of JNK-mediated apoptosis, thereby increasing the survival of cells [97]. In the *C. elegans* model of AD, *H. sabdariffa* extract was able to extend the lifespan and prevent Aβ-induced paralysis by regulating DAF-16 and SKN-1 mediated pathways [98]. In ovariectomized Wistar rats, the spatial memory was improved and BDNF expression was significantly induced by the extract [99]. Additionally, in streptozotocin-induced AD, the extract was able to inhibit the amyloidogenic pathway, suppressing the expression of pro-inflammatory cytokines and downregulating p-p38, thereby showing neuroprotective effects [100].

Epidemiological studies correlate coffee consumption and decreased risk of neurodegenerative diseases [101]. The active ingredients in coffee including, caffeic acid, caffeine, and chlorogenic acid have been reported for their neuroprotective effects. Caffeic acid was reported to activate JNK/Bcl-2-mediated autophagy, which reduces α-synuclein expression [102]. It also plays a role in the regulation of autophagic processes, thereby regulating neurological disease [103, 104]. Chlorogenic acid ameliorates the detrimental effects of $A\beta_{25-35}$ in both SH-SY5Y cells and rats by increasing autophagic flux and autophagosome production, thereby increasing cell metabolism and leading to neuronal cell death [105]. It also reduced the conversion of LC3-I to LC3-II, Atg-4, and Beclin-1 expression, suggesting the suppression of autophagosomes and an increase in lysosomal activity [106].

Vitis vinifera and Its Constituent Resveratrol

Vitis vinifera (seed, leaf extract) has shown a neuroprotective effect against dopamine-induced neurotoxicity in dopaminergic neurons, brain ischemia/reperfusion injury in rats, and glutamate toxicity in hippocampal cells [107 - 109]. The flavones of the plant could regulate hippocampal neurons in transgenic AD mice (APP/PS1) through the inhibition of excessive autophagy [110]. Resveratrol, the active constituent of grapes was identified to be responsible for most of the activities. In chronic cerebral hypoperfusion rats, resveratrol improved cognitive function by activating autophagy mediated by AKT/mTOR signaling pathway [111]. The protection against traumatic brain injury by resveratrol was associated with the upregulation of synaptophysin, and attenuation of autophagy [112]. AMPK, the protein kinase responsible for the activities of resveratrol, exerts its effect *via* proteins such as SIRT1, which inhibit mTOR and induce autophagy, thereby eliminating damaged mitochondria and α-synuclein aggregates in PD models [113]. Resveratrol induces autophagy, in dopaminergic SH-SY5Y cells challenged with rotenone *via* haem oxygenase [114] and AMPK/SIRT1 signaling [113]. Moreover, neurotoxicity caused by $A\beta_{25-35}$ in PC12 cells is attenuated by resveratrol, through autophagy induction, which is partially mediated *via* activation of the TyrRS -PARP1-SIRT1 signaling pathway [115].

Ginkgo biloba and Its Constituents

The Chinese medicinal herb *G. biloba* has been in use for a long term for the treatment of brain disorders. *G. biloba* leaf extract (EGb-761 and Ginaton) treatment promoted the autophagic activities and restored lysosomal dysfunction, which could be identified from the upregulation of the markers LC3-II, LAMP-1, AMPK, mTOR, and Parkin against cerebral ischemia/reperfusion injury in rats [116, 117]. In Tau-transgenic mice of AD and neuronal cells, EGb-761 administration reduced cerebral p-Tau levels and improved cognitive function through the activation of autophagy, which was attributed to the compounds ginkgolide A, bilobalide, and flavonoids. In addition, long-term EGb-761 treatment was found to facilitate phosphorylated Tau transport to the lysosomes resulting in the degradation of the protein [118]. Upon ischemic stroke, intraperitoneal administration of bilobalide protected against brain injury by inhibiting autophagy through the activation of Akt/eNOS [119]. Ginkgolic acid has been found to facilitate the clearance of intracellular alpha-synuclein aggregates through the activation of autophagy in neuronal cells [120].

Panax ginseng and Its Constituents

Panax ginseng with its bioactive compounds including ginsenosides, gintonin, and gypenoside has been well reported for its neuroprotective effects. Pioneering studies imply that *P. ginseng* and its phytoconstituents exert their effect through the modulation of antioxidant mechanisms, inhibition of inflammation, stress, and apoptosis, and activation of several signaling pathways [121, 122]. The secondary metabolite ginsenoside Rg2 delayed D-galactose-induced brain aging and restored memory functions by increasing mitochondrial autophagic flux [123]. Ginsenoside Rb1 exhibits a neuroprotective effect against spinal cord injury through the inhibition of excessive autophagy [124]. 20(S)-protopanaxadiol, the metabolite of ginsenoside promotes neural stem cell differentiation by inducing autophagy indicating its regenerative properties [125]. The phytoestrogen gypenoside XVII protects against $A\beta_{25-35}$-induced toxicity by attenuating autophagic cell death through estrogen receptor-dependent activation of the PI3K/Akt pathway [126]. However, in PC12 cells expressing APP695swe and APP/PS1 mice, gypenoside XVII induced autophagy by activating transcription factor EB (TFEB) resulting in the clearance of $A\beta$ [127].

CONCLUSION

Since autophagy plays a dual role, it is necessary to find the optimum level of autophagy to induce maximum health benefits. A chain of events occurs between oxidative and inflammatory events, accumulation of proteins, damage in mitochondria, and balance shift between autophagy and proteasome, leading to neurodegenerative proteinopathies [49]. The beneficial neuroprotective, antioxidant, and anti-inflammatory effects produced by several phytochemicals are mostly related to rescuing autophagy. On the other hand, counteracting behavioral alterations, such as mitochondrial damage intracellular accumulation, and release of potentially detrimental substrates [49]. The majority of these positive effects in modulating autophagy have been proved majorly *in vitro* and in some *in vivo* studies. More *in vivo* and clinical shreds of evidence are further required to confirm this claim. Moreover, modulation of autophagy during neurodegenerative diseases may also have a negative impact, as the pathway is cross-linked with several cellular mechanisms. In this regard, it is also important to focus on neurodegenerative diseases-associated biomarkers that will aid in the proper quantification of the activity of autophagy in the human brain [48] and based on the pathological outcomes, nutraceuticals, which can act as autophagy modulators can be prescribed in addition to standard drugs for individuals with neurodegenerative diseases.

ABBREVIATIONS

AD	Alzheimer's Disease
AMPK	AMP-activated Protein Kinase
APP	Amyloid Precursor Protein
Aβ	Amyloid Beta
BNIP3	Bcl-2 Interacting Protein 3
EGCG	Epigallocatechin Gallate
eNOS	Endothelial Nitric Oxide Synthase
FAF1	Fas-associated Factor 1
FOXO3A	Forkhead Box O3
HD	Huntington's Disease
JNK	c-Jun N-terminal kinases
LAMP1	Lysosomal-associated Membrane Protein 1
MAPK	Mitogen-activated Protein Kinase
MPTP	1-Methyl-4-Phenyl-1,2,3,6-Tetrahydropyridine
mTOR	Mammalian Target of Rapamycin
ND	Neurodegenerative Diseases
PARP1	Poly [ADP-ribose] Polymerase 1
PD	Parkinson's Disease
PI3K	Phosphoinositide 3-kinases
PINK1	Phosphatase and Tensin Homolog-induced Putative Kinase 1
PKC	Protein Kinase C
PTEN	Phosphatase and Tensin Homolog
SIRT1	Sirtuin 1
TRPV1	Transient Receptor Potential Vanilloid Subfamily 1

ACKNOWLEDGEMENTS

DSM wishes to thank the Second Century Fund (C2F) for Postdoctoral Fellowship, Chulalongkorn University, Thailand, for the support. MIP wishes to thank the Ratchadaphiseksomphot Endowment Fund for Postdoctoral Fellowship, Chulalongkorn University.

REFERENCES

[1]   Rahman MA, Rhim H. Therapeutic implication of autophagy in neurodegenerative diseases. BMB Rep 2017; 50(7): 345-54.
[http://dx.doi.org/10.5483/BMBRep.2017.50.7.069] [PMID: 28454606]

[2]   Rasheduzzaman M, Yin H, Park SY. Cardiac glycoside sensitized hepatocellular carcinoma cells to TRAIL *via* ROS generation, p38MAPK, mitochondrial transition, and autophagy mediation. Mol Carcinog 2019; 58(11): 2040-51.
[http://dx.doi.org/10.1002/mc.23096] [PMID: 31392779]

[3]   Hara Y, McKeehan N, Fillit HM. Translating the biology of aging into novel therapeutics for Alzheimer disease. Neurology 2019; 92(2): 84-93.
[http://dx.doi.org/10.1212/WNL.0000000000006745] [PMID: 30530798]

[4]   Kobayashi S. Choose delicately and reuse adequately: The newly revealed process of autophagy. Biol Pharm Bull 2015; 38(8): 1098-103.
[http://dx.doi.org/10.1248/bpb.b15-00096] [PMID: 26235572]

[5]   Nakamura S, Yoshimori T. New insights into autophagosome-lysosome fusion. J Cell Sci 2017; 130(7): 1209-16.
[PMID: 28302910]

[6]   Mputhia Z, Hone E, Tripathi T, Sargeant T, Martins R, Bharadwaj P. Autophagy modulation as a treatment of amyloid diseases. Molecules 2019; 24(18): 3372.
[http://dx.doi.org/10.3390/molecules24183372] [PMID: 31527516]

[7]   Hafner Česen M, Pegan K, Špes A, Turk B. Lysosomal pathways to cell death and their therapeutic applications. Exp Cell Res 2012; 318(11): 1245-51.
[http://dx.doi.org/10.1016/j.yexcr.2012.03.005] [PMID: 22465226]

[8]   Ghosh I, Sankhe R, Mudgal J, Arora D, Nampoothiri M. Spermidine, an autophagy inducer, as a therapeutic strategy in neurological disorders. Neuropeptides 2020; 83: 102083.
[http://dx.doi.org/10.1016/j.npep.2020.102083] [PMID: 32873420]

[9]   Azad MB, Gibson SB. Role of BNIP3 in proliferation and hypoxia-induced autophagy: Implications for personalized cancer therapies. Ann N Y Acad Sci 2010; 1210(1): 8-16.
[http://dx.doi.org/10.1111/j.1749-6632.2010.05778.x] [PMID: 20973794]

[10]   Jimenez-Sanchez M, Thomson F, Zavodszky E, Rubinsztein DC. Autophagy and polyglutamine diseases. Prog Neurobiol 2012; 97(2): 67-82.
[http://dx.doi.org/10.1016/j.pneurobio.2011.08.013] [PMID: 21930185]

[11]   Murphy MP. How mitochondria produce reactive oxygen species. Biochem J 2009; 417(1): 1-13.
[http://dx.doi.org/10.1042/BJ20081386] [PMID: 19061483]

[12]   Maday S, Holzbaur ELF. Autophagosome biogenesis in primary neurons follows an ordered and spatially regulated pathway. Dev Cell 2014; 30(1): 71-85.
[http://dx.doi.org/10.1016/j.devcel.2014.06.001] [PMID: 25026034]

[13]   Maday S, Wallace KE, Holzbaur ELF. Autophagosomes initiate distally and mature during transport toward the cell soma in primary neurons. J Cell Biol 2012; 196(4): 407-17.
[http://dx.doi.org/10.1083/jcb.201106120] [PMID: 22331844]

[14]   Hara T, Nakamura K, Matsui M, *et al.* Suppression of basal autophagy in neural cells causes neurodegenerative disease in mice. Nature 2006; 441(7095): 885-9.
[http://dx.doi.org/10.1038/nature04724] [PMID: 16625204]

[15]   Komatsu M, Waguri S, Chiba T, *et al.* Loss of autophagy in the central nervous system causes neurodegeneration in mice. Nature 2006; 441(7095): 880-4.
[http://dx.doi.org/10.1038/nature04723] [PMID: 16625205]

[16]   Kovacs GG, Adle-Biassette H, Milenkovic I, Cipriani S, van Scheppingen J, Aronica E. Linking pathways in the developing and aging brain with neurodegeneration. Neuroscience 2014; 269: 152-72.
[http://dx.doi.org/10.1016/j.neuroscience.2014.03.045] [PMID: 24699227]

[17]   Boland B, Kumar A, Lee S, *et al.* Autophagy induction and autophagosome clearance in neurons: Relationship to autophagic pathology in Alzheimer's disease. J Neurosci 2008; 28(27): 6926-37.

[http://dx.doi.org/10.1523/JNEUROSCI.0800-08.2008] [PMID: 18596167]

[18] Spilman P, Podlutskaya N, Hart MJ, *et al.* Inhibition of mTOR by rapamycin abolishes cognitive deficits and reduces amyloid-β levels in a mouse model of Alzheimer's disease. PLoS One 2010; 5(4): e9979.
[http://dx.doi.org/10.1371/journal.pone.0009979] [PMID: 20376313]

[19] Tian Y, Bustos V, Flajolet M, Greengard P. A small-molecule enhancer of autophagy decreases levels of Aβ and APP-CTF *via* Atg5-dependent autophagy pathway. FASEB J 2011; 25(6): 1934-42.
[http://dx.doi.org/10.1096/fj.10-175158] [PMID: 21368103]

[20] Vingtdeux V, Chandakkar P, Zhao H, d'Abramo C, Davies P, Marambsud P. Novel synthetic small-molecule activators of AMPK as enhancers of autophagy and amyloid-β peptide degradation. FASEB J 2011; 25(1): 219-31.
[http://dx.doi.org/10.1096/fj.10-167361] [PMID: 20852062]

[21] Nilsson P, Loganathan K, Sekiguchi M, *et al.* Aβ secretion and plaque formation depend on autophagy. Cell Rep 2013; 5(1): 61-9.
[http://dx.doi.org/10.1016/j.celrep.2013.08.042] [PMID: 24095740]

[22] Yu WH, Cuervo AM, Kumar A, *et al.* Macroautophagy—a novel β-amyloid peptide-generating pathway activated in Alzheimer's disease. J Cell Biol 2005; 171(1): 87-98.
[http://dx.doi.org/10.1083/jcb.200505082] [PMID: 16203860]

[23] Nixon RA. Autophagy, amyloidogenesis and Alzheimer disease. J Cell Sci 2007; 120(23): 4081-91.
[http://dx.doi.org/10.1242/jcs.019265] [PMID: 18032783]

[24] Rahman MA, Rahman MS, Rahman MDH, *et al.* Modulatory effects of autophagy on app processing as a potential treatment target for alzheimer's disease. Biomedicines 2020; 9(1): 5.
[http://dx.doi.org/10.3390/biomedicines9010005] [PMID: 33374126]

[25] Nilsson P, Saido TC. Dual roles for autophagy: Degradation and secretion of Alzheimer's disease Aβ peptide. BioEssays 2014; 36(6): 570-8.
[http://dx.doi.org/10.1002/bies.201400002] [PMID: 24711225]

[26] O'Keefe L, Denton D. Using *Drosophila* models of amyloid toxicity to study autophagy in the pathogenesis of alzheimer's disease. BioMed Res Int 2018; 2018: 5195416.
[PMID: 29888266]

[27] Wen J, Fang F, Guo SH, *et al.* Amyloid β-derived diffusible ligands (ADDLs) induce abnormal autophagy associated with Aβ aggregation degree. J Mol Neurosci 2018; 64(2): 162-74.
[http://dx.doi.org/10.1007/s12031-017-1015-9] [PMID: 29260451]

[28] Liu J, Li L. Targeting autophagy for the treatment of alzheimer's disease: Challenges and opportunities. Front Mol Neurosci 2019; 12: 203.
[http://dx.doi.org/10.3389/fnmol.2019.00203] [PMID: 31507373]

[29] Tanik SA, Schultheiss CE, Volpicelli-Daley LA, Brunden KR, Lee VMY. Lewy body-like α-synuclein aggregates resist degradation and impair macroautophagy. J Biol Chem 2013; 288(21): 15194-210.
[http://dx.doi.org/10.1074/jbc.M113.457408] [PMID: 23532841]

[30] Matsuda N, Sato S, Shiba K, *et al.* PINK1 stabilized by mitochondrial depolarization recruits Parkin to damaged mitochondria and activates latent Parkin for mitophagy. J Cell Biol 2010; 189(2): 211-21.
[http://dx.doi.org/10.1083/jcb.200910140] [PMID: 20404107]

[31] Narendra D, Tanaka A, Suen DF, Youle RJ. Parkin is recruited selectively to impaired mitochondria and promotes their autophagy. J Cell Biol 2008; 183(5): 795-803.
[http://dx.doi.org/10.1083/jcb.200809125] [PMID: 19029340]

[32] Pickrell AM, Youle RJ. The roles of PINK1, parkin, and mitochondrial fidelity in Parkinson's disease. Neuron 2015; 85(2): 257-73.
[http://dx.doi.org/10.1016/j.neuron.2014.12.007] [PMID: 25611507]

[33] Nguyen TN, Padman BS, Lazarou M. Deciphering the molecular signals of PINK1/Parkin mitophagy. Trends Cell Biol 2016; 26(10): 733-44.
[http://dx.doi.org/10.1016/j.tcb.2016.05.008] [PMID: 27291334]

[34] Wang P, Shao BZ, Deng Z, Chen S, Yue Z, Miao CY. Autophagy in ischemic stroke. Prog Neurobiol 2018; 163-164: 98-117.
[http://dx.doi.org/10.1016/j.pneurobio.2018.01.001] [PMID: 29331396]

[35] Xie W, Zhu T, Zhou P, *et al.* Notoginseng leaf Triterpenes Ameliorates OGD/R-induced neuronal injury *via* SIRT1/2/3-Foxo3a-MnSOD/PGC-1α signaling pathways mediated by the NAMPT-NAD pathway. Oxid Med Cell Longev 2020; 1-15.
[http://dx.doi.org/10.1155/2020/7308386] [PMID: 33149812]

[36] Ahsan A, Liu M, Zheng Y, *et al.* Natural compounds modulate the autophagy with potential implication of stroke. Acta Pharm Sin B 2021; 11(7): 1708-20.
[http://dx.doi.org/10.1016/j.apsb.2020.10.018] [PMID: 34386317]

[37] Rubinsztein DC, Mariño G, Kroemer G. Autophagy and aging. Cell 2011; 146(5): 682-95.
[http://dx.doi.org/10.1016/j.cell.2011.07.030] [PMID: 21884931]

[38] Guaragnella N, Antonacci L, Passarella S, Marra E, Giannattasio S. Achievements and perspectives in yeast acetic acid-induced programmed cell death pathways. Biochem Soc Trans 2011; 39(5): 1538-43.
[http://dx.doi.org/10.1042/BST0391538] [PMID: 21936848]

[39] Huang X, Ding H, Lu J, Tang Y, Deng B, Deng C. Autophagy in cerebral ischemia and the effects of traditional Chinese medicine. J Integr Med 2015; 13(5): 289-96.
[http://dx.doi.org/10.1016/S2095-4964(15)60187-X] [PMID: 26343099]

[40] Roberts RF, Tang MY, Fon EA, Durcan TM. Defending the mitochondria: The pathways of mitophagy and mitochondrial-derived vesicles. Int J Biochem Cell Biol 2016; 79: 427-36.
[http://dx.doi.org/10.1016/j.biocel.2016.07.020] [PMID: 27443527]

[41] Wen Y, Gu Y, Tang X, Hu Z. PINK1 overexpression protects against cerebral ischemia through Parkin regulation. Environ Toxicol 2020; 35(2): 188-93.
[http://dx.doi.org/10.1002/tox.22855] [PMID: 31654556]

[42] Huo L, Bai X, Wang Y, Wang M. Betulinic acid derivative B10 inhibits glioma cell proliferation through suppression of SIRT1, acetylation of FOXO3a and upregulation of Bim/PUMA. Biomed Pharmacother 2017; 92: 347-55.
[http://dx.doi.org/10.1016/j.biopha.2017.05.074] [PMID: 28554130]

[43] Kume S, Uzu T, Horiike K, *et al.* Calorie restriction enhances cell adaptation to hypoxia through Sirt1-dependent mitochondrial autophagy in mouse aged kidney. J Clin Invest 2010; 120(4): 1043-55.
[http://dx.doi.org/10.1172/JCI41376] [PMID: 20335657]

[44] Wang H, Quirion R, Little PJ, *et al.* Forkhead box O transcription factors as possible mediators in the development of major depression. Neuropharmacology 2015; 99: 527-37.
[http://dx.doi.org/10.1016/j.neuropharm.2015.08.020] [PMID: 26279492]

[45] Zhang C, Li C, Chen S, *et al.* Hormetic effect of panaxatriol saponins confers neuroprotection in PC12 cells and zebrafish through PI3K/AKT/mTOR and AMPK/SIRT1/FOXO3 pathways. Sci Rep 2017; 7(1): 41082.
[http://dx.doi.org/10.1038/srep41082] [PMID: 28112228]

[46] Rahman MA, Bishayee K, Habib K, Sadra A, Huh SO. 18α-Glycyrrhetinic acid lethality for neuroblastoma cells *via* de-regulating the Beclin-1/Bcl-2 complex and inducing apoptosis. Biochem Pharmacol 2016; 117: 97-112.
[http://dx.doi.org/10.1016/j.bcp.2016.08.006] [PMID: 27520483]

[47] Rahman MA, Bishayee K, Sadra A, Huh SO. Oxyresveratrol activates parallel apoptotic and autophagic cell death pathways in neuroblastoma cells. Biochim Biophys Acta, Gen Subj 2017; 1861(2): 23-36.

[http://dx.doi.org/10.1016/j.bbagen.2016.10.025] [PMID: 27815218]

[48]   Gruendler R, Hippe B, Sendula Jengic V, Peterlin B, Haslberger AG. Nutraceutical Approaches of autophagy and neuroinflammation in alzheimer's disease: A systematic review. Molecules 2020; 25(24): 6018.
[http://dx.doi.org/10.3390/molecules25246018] [PMID: 33353228]

[49]   Limanaqi F, Biagioni F, Mastroiacovo F, Polzella M, Lazzeri G, Fornai F. Merging the multi-target effects of phytochemicals in neurodegeneration: From oxidative stress to protein aggregation and inflammation. Antioxidants 2020; 9(10): 1022.
[http://dx.doi.org/10.3390/antiox9101022] [PMID: 33092300]

[50]   Ferreira-Vieira TH, Guimaraes IM, Silva FR, Ribeiro FM. Alzheimer's disease: Targeting the cholinergic system. Curr Neuropharmacol 2016; 14(1): 101-15.
[http://dx.doi.org/10.2174/1570159X13666150716165726] [PMID: 26813123]

[51]   Volpato D, Holzgrabe U. Designing hybrids targeting the cholinergic system by modulating the muscarinic and nicotinic receptors: A concept to treat alzheimer's disease. Molecules 2018; 23(12): 3230.
[http://dx.doi.org/10.3390/molecules23123230] [PMID: 30544533]

[52]   Brimson JM, Prasanth MI, Malar DS, *et al.* Plant polyphenols for aging health: Implication from their autophagy modulating properties in age-associated diseases. Pharmaceuticals 2021; 14(10): 982.
[http://dx.doi.org/10.3390/ph14100982] [PMID: 34681206]

[53]   Manach C, Scalbert A, Morand C, Rémésy C, Jiménez L. Polyphenols: Food sources and bioavailability. Am J Clin Nutr 2004; 79(5): 727-47.
[http://dx.doi.org/10.1093/ajcn/79.5.727] [PMID: 15113710]

[54]   Pandey KB, Rizvi SI. Plant polyphenols as dietary antioxidants in human health and disease. Oxid Med Cell Longev 2009; 2(5): 270-8.
[http://dx.doi.org/10.4161/oxim.2.5.9498] [PMID: 20716914]

[55]   Jiang TF, Zhang YJ, Zhou HY, *et al.* Curcumin ameliorates the neurodegenerative pathology in A53T α-synuclein cell model of Parkinson's disease through the downregulation of mTOR/p70S6K signaling and the recovery of macroautophagy. J Neuroimmune Pharmacol 2013; 8(1): 356-69.
[http://dx.doi.org/10.1007/s11481-012-9431-7] [PMID: 23325107]

[56]   Huang M, Jiang X, Liang Y, Liu Q, Chen S, Guo Y. Berberine improves cognitive impairment by promoting autophagic clearance and inhibiting production of β-amyloid in APP/tau/PS1 mouse model of Alzheimer's disease. Exp Gerontol 2017; 91: 25-33.
[http://dx.doi.org/10.1016/j.exger.2017.02.004] [PMID: 28223223]

[57]   Chang CF, Lee YC, Lee KH, *et al.* Therapeutic effect of berberine on TDP-43-related pathogenesis in FTLD and ALS. J Biomed Sci 2016; 23(1): 72.
[http://dx.doi.org/10.1186/s12929-016-0290-z] [PMID: 27769241]

[58]   Jiang W, Wei W, Gaertig MA, Li S, Li XJ. Therapeutic effect of berberine on huntington's disease transgenic mouse model. PLoS One 2015; 10(7): e0134142.
[http://dx.doi.org/10.1371/journal.pone.0134142] [PMID: 26225560]

[59]   Ding Y, Kong D, Zhou T, *et al.* α-Arbutin protects against parkinson's disease-associated mitochondrial dysfunction *in vitro* and *in vivo.* Neuromolecular Med 2020; 22(1): 56-67.
[http://dx.doi.org/10.1007/s12017-019-08562-6] [PMID: 31401719]

[60]   Mei Z-G, Feng Z-T, Wang J-F, *et al.* Puerarin protects rat brain against ischemia/reperfusion injury by suppressing autophagy *via* the AMPK-mTOR-ULK1 signaling pathway. Neural Regen Res 2018; 13(6): 989-98.
[http://dx.doi.org/10.4103/1673-5374.233441] [PMID: 29926825]

[61]   Pengyue Z, Tao G, Hongyun H, Liqiang Y, Yihao D. Breviscapine confers a neuroprotective efficacy against transient focal cerebral ischemia by attenuating neuronal and astrocytic autophagy in the

penumbra. Biomed Pharmacother 2017; 90: 69-76.
[http://dx.doi.org/10.1016/j.biopha.2017.03.039] [PMID: 28343073]

[62] Zhong Y, Zheng Q, Sun C, Zhang Z, Han K, Jia N. Orientin improves cognition by enhancing autophagosome clearance in an alzheimer's mouse model. J Mol Neurosci 2019; 69(2): 246-53.
[http://dx.doi.org/10.1007/s12031-019-01353-5] [PMID: 31243684]

[63] Pantano D, Luccarini I, Nardiello P, Servili M, Stefani M, Casamenti F. Oleuropein aglycone and polyphenols from olive mill waste water ameliorate cognitive deficits and neuropathology. Br J Clin Pharmacol 2017; 83(1): 54-62.
[http://dx.doi.org/10.1111/bcp.12993] [PMID: 27131215]

[64] Fang EF, Waltz TB, Kassahun H, *et al.* Tomatidine enhances lifespan and healthspan in C. Elegans through mitophagy induction *via* the SKN-1/Nrf2 pathway. Sci Rep 2017; 7(1): 46208.
[http://dx.doi.org/10.1038/srep46208] [PMID: 28397803]

[65] Ahsan A, Zheng Y, Ma S, *et al.* Tomatidine protects against ischemic neuronal injury by improving lysosomal function. Eur J Pharmacol 2020; 882: 173280.
[http://dx.doi.org/10.1016/j.ejphar.2020.173280] [PMID: 32580039]

[66] Wang G, Wang T, Zhang Y, Li F, Yu B, Kou J. Schizandrin protects against OGD/R-induced neuronal injury by suppressing autophagy: Involvement of the AMPK/mTOR pathway. Molecules 2019; 24(19): 3624.
[http://dx.doi.org/10.3390/molecules24193624] [PMID: 31597329]

[67] Yang G, Li J, Cai Y, Yang Z, Li R, Fu W. Glycyrrhizic acid alleviates 6-Hydroxydopamine and corticosterone-induced neurotoxicity in SH-SY5Y cells through modulating autophagy. Neurochem Res 2018; 43(10): 1914-26.
[http://dx.doi.org/10.1007/s11064-018-2609-5] [PMID: 30206804]

[68] Yang C, Li X, Zhang L, Li Y, Li L, Zhang L. Cornel iridoid glycoside induces autophagy to protect against tau oligomer neurotoxicity induced by the activation of glycogen synthase kinase-3β. J Nat Med 2019; 73(4): 717-26.
[http://dx.doi.org/10.1007/s11418-019-01318-3] [PMID: 31190266]

[69] Pierzynowska K, Gaffke L, Hać A, *et al.* Correction of huntington's disease phenotype by genistein-induced autophagy in the cellular model. Neuromolecular Med 2018; 20(1): 112-23.
[http://dx.doi.org/10.1007/s12017-018-8482-1] [PMID: 29435951]

[70] Yuan H, Jiang C, Zhao J, *et al.* Euxanthone attenuates $A\beta_{1-42}$-induced oxidative stress and apoptosis by triggering autophagy. J Mol Neurosci 2018; 66(4): 512-23.
[http://dx.doi.org/10.1007/s12031-018-1175-2] [PMID: 30345461]

[71] Zhang Y, Zhang Y, Jin X, *et al.* The role of astragaloside iv against cerebral ischemia/reperfusion injury: Suppression of apoptosis *via* promotion of P62-LC3-autophagy. Molecules 2019; 24(9): 1838.
[http://dx.doi.org/10.3390/molecules24091838] [PMID: 31086091]

[72] Wang C, Huang W, Lu J, Chen H, Yu Z. TRPV1-mediated microglial autophagy attenuates alzheimer's disease-associated pathology and cognitive decline. Front Pharmacol 2022; 12: 763866.
[http://dx.doi.org/10.3389/fphar.2021.763866] [PMID: 35115924]

[73] Wang M, Li YJ, Ding Y, *et al.* Silibinin prevents autophagic cell death upon oxidative stress in cortical neurons and cerebral ischemia-reperfusion injury. Mol Neurobiol 2016; 53(2): 932-43.
[http://dx.doi.org/10.1007/s12035-014-9062-5] [PMID: 25561437]

[74] Tripathi MK, Rasheed MSU, Mishra AK, Patel DK, Singh MP. Silymarin protects against impaired autophagy associated with 1-Methyl-4-phenyl-1,2,3,6-tetrahydropyridine-induced parkinsonism. J Mol Neurosci 2020; 70(2): 276-83.
[http://dx.doi.org/10.1007/s12031-019-01431-8] [PMID: 31732923]

[75] Zhu Y, Wang J. Wogonin increases β-amyloid clearance and inhibits tau phosphorylation *via* inhibition of mammalian target of rapamycin: Potential drug to treat Alzheimer's disease. Neurol Sci

2015; 36(7): 1181-8.
[http://dx.doi.org/10.1007/s10072-015-2070-z] [PMID: 25596147]

[76]   Kuang L, Cao X, Lu Z. Baicalein protects against rotenone-induced neurotoxicity through induction of autophagy. Biol Pharm Bull 2017; 40(9): 1537-43.
[http://dx.doi.org/10.1248/bpb.b17-00392] [PMID: 28659545]

[77]   Chen M, Peng L, Gong P, *et al.* Baicalein induces mitochondrial autophagy to prevent parkinson's disease in rats *via* miR-30b and the SIRT1/AMPK/mTOR pathway. Front Neurol 2022; 12: 646817.
[http://dx.doi.org/10.3389/fneur.2021.646817] [PMID: 35237220]

[78]   Huang SM, Tsai SY, Lin JA, Wu CH, Yen GC. Cytoprotective effects of hesperetin and hesperidin against amyloid β-induced impairment of glucose transport through downregulation of neuronal autophagy. Mol Nutr Food Res 2012; 56(4): 601-9.
[http://dx.doi.org/10.1002/mnfr.201100682] [PMID: 22383310]

[79]   Feng L, Chong MS, Lim WS, *et al.* Tea consumption reduces the incidence of neurocognitive disorders: Findings from the Singapore longitudinal aging study. J Nutr Health Aging 2016; 20(10): 1002-9.
[http://dx.doi.org/10.1007/s12603-016-0687-0] [PMID: 27925140]

[80]   Zhang S, Duangjan C, Tencomnao T, Liu J, Lin J, Wink M. Neuroprotective effects of oolong tea extracts against glutamate-induced toxicity in cultured neuronal cells and β-amyloid-induced toxicity in *Caenorhabditis elegans*. Food Funct 2020; 11(9): 8179-92.
[http://dx.doi.org/10.1039/D0FO01072C] [PMID: 32966472]

[81]   Snow AD, Cummings JA, Tanzi RE, Lake T. *In vitro* comparison of major memory-support dietary supplements for their effectiveness in reduction/inhibition of beta-amyloid protein fibrils and tau protein tangles: key primary targets for memory loss. Sci Rep 2021; 11(1): 3001.
[http://dx.doi.org/10.1038/s41598-020-79275-1] [PMID: 33589649]

[82]   Cai Z, Hu X, Tan R, *et al.* Neuroprotective effect of green tea extractives against oxidative stress by enhancing the survival and proliferation of PC12 cells. Mol Cell Toxicol 2019; 15(4): 391-7.
[http://dx.doi.org/10.1007/s13273-019-0042-8]

[83]   Waggas AM. Neuroprotective evaluation of extract of ginger (*Zingiber officinale*) root in monosodium glutamate-induced toxicity in different brain areas male albino rats. Pak J Biol Sci 2009; 12(3): 201-12.
[http://dx.doi.org/10.3923/pjbs.2009.201.212] [PMID: 19579948]

[84]   Hong JT, Ryu SR, Kim HJ, *et al.* Neuroprotective effect of green tea extract in experimental ischemia-reperfusion brain injury. Brain Res Bull 2000; 53(6): 743-9.
[http://dx.doi.org/10.1016/S0361-9230(00)00348-8] [PMID: 11179838]

[85]   Hussein U, Hassan N, Elhalwagy M, *et al.* Ginger and propolis exert neuroprotective effects against monosodium glutamate-induced neurotoxicity in rats. Molecules 2017; 22(11): 1928.
[http://dx.doi.org/10.3390/molecules22111928] [PMID: 29117134]

[86]   Lee JH, Moon JH, Kim SW, *et al.* EGCG-mediated autophagy flux has a neuroprotection effect *via* a class III histone deacetylase in primary neuron cells. Oncotarget 2015; 6(12): 9701-17.
[http://dx.doi.org/10.18632/oncotarget.3832] [PMID: 25991666]

[87]   Wang L, Dai M, Ge Y, *et al.* EGCG protects the mouse brain against cerebral ischemia/reperfusion injury by suppressing autophagy *via* the AKT/AMPK/mTOR phosphorylation pathway. Front Pharmacol 2022; 13: 921394.
[http://dx.doi.org/10.3389/fphar.2022.921394] [PMID: 36147330]

[88]   Gu HF, Nie YX, Tong QZ, *et al.* Epigallocatechin-3-gallate attenuates impairment of learning and memory in chronic unpredictable mild stress-treated rats by restoring hippocampal autophagic flux. PLoS One 2014; 9(11): e112683.
[http://dx.doi.org/10.1371/journal.pone.0112683] [PMID: 25393306]

[89]   Mao QQ, Xu XY, Cao SY, *et al.* Bioactive compounds and bioactivities of ginger (*Zingiber officinale* roscoe). Foods 2019; 8(6): 185.
[http://dx.doi.org/10.3390/foods8060185] [PMID: 31151279]

[90]   Zeng G, Zhang Z, Lu L, Xiao D, Zong S, He J. Protective effects of ginger root extract on Alzheimer disease-induced behavioral dysfunction in rats. Rejuvenation Res 2013; 16(2): 124-33.
[http://dx.doi.org/10.1089/rej.2012.1389] [PMID: 23374025]

[91]   Huh E, Lim S, Kim HG, *et al.* Ginger fermented with *Schizosaccharomyces pombe* alleviates memory impairment *via* protecting hippocampal neuronal cells in amyloid beta $_{1-42}$ plaque injected mice. Food Funct 2018; 9(1): 171-8.
[http://dx.doi.org/10.1039/C7FO01149K] [PMID: 29171599]

[92]   Kang C, Kang M, Han Y, Zhang T, Quan W, Gao J. 6-Gingerols (6G) reduces hypoxia-induced PC-12 cells apoptosis and autophagy through regulation of miR-103/BNIP3. Artif Cells Nanomed Biotechnol 2019; 47(1): 1653-61.
[http://dx.doi.org/10.1080/21691401.2019.1606010] [PMID: 31043087]

[93]   Luo J, Chen J, Yang C, *et al.* 6-Gingerol protects against cerebral ischemia/reperfusion injury by inhibiting NLRP3 inflammasome and apoptosis *via* TRPV1 / FAF1 complex dissociation-mediated autophagy. Int Immunopharmacol 2021; 100: 108146.
[http://dx.doi.org/10.1016/j.intimp.2021.108146] [PMID: 34537481]

[94]   Jiang Y, Kou J, Han X, *et al.* ROS-dependent activation of autophagy through the PI3K/Akt/mTOR pathway is induced by hydroxysafflor yellow A-sonodynamic therapy in THP-1 macrophages. Oxid Med Cell Longev 2017; 2017: 1-16.
[http://dx.doi.org/10.1155/2017/8519169] [PMID: 28191279]

[95]   Rojsanga P, Sithisarn P, Tanaka K, Mizuki D, Matsumoto K. *Thunbergia laurifolia* extract ameliorates cognitive and emotional deficits in olfactorectomized mice. Pharm Biol 2015; 53(8): 1141-8.
[http://dx.doi.org/10.3109/13880209.2014.962059] [PMID: 25609149]

[96]   Vongthip W, Sillapachaiyaporn C, Kim KW, Sukprasansap M, Tencomnao T. *Thunbergia laurifolia* leaf extract inhibits glutamate-induced neurotoxicity and cell death through mitophagy signaling. Antioxidants 2021; 10(11): 1678.
[http://dx.doi.org/10.3390/antiox10111678] [PMID: 34829549]

[97]   Malar DS, Prasanth MI, Brimson JM, Verma K, Prasansuklab A, Tencomnao T. *Hibiscus sabdariffa* extract protects HT-22 cells from glutamate-induced neurodegeneration by upregulating glutamate transporters and exerts lifespan extension in *C. elegans via* DAF-16 mediated pathway. Nutr Healthy Aging 2021; 6(3): 229-47.
[http://dx.doi.org/10.3233/NHA-210131]

[98]   Koch K, Weldle N, Baier S, Büchter C, Wätjen W. *Hibiscus sabdariffa* L. Extract prolongs lifespan and protects against amyloid-β toxicity in *Caenorhabditis elegans*: Involvement of the FoxO and Nrf2 orthologues DAF-16 and SKN-1. Eur J Nutr 2020; 59(1): 137-50.
[http://dx.doi.org/10.1007/s00394-019-01894-w] [PMID: 30710163]

[99]   Lorenzana-Martínez G, Santerre A, Andrade-González I, Bañuelos-Pineda J. Effects of *Hibiscus sabdariffa* calyces on spatial memory and hippocampal expression of BDNF in ovariectomized rats. Nutr Neurosci 2022; 25(4): 670-80.
[http://dx.doi.org/10.1080/1028415X.2020.1804095] [PMID: 32787648]

[100]   El-Shiekh RA, Ashour RM, Abd El-Haleim EA, Ahmed KA, Abdel-Sattar E. *Hibiscus sabdariffa* L.: A potent natural neuroprotective agent for the prevention of streptozotocin-induced Alzheimer's disease in mice. Biomed Pharmacother 2020; 128: 110303.
[http://dx.doi.org/10.1016/j.biopha.2020.110303] [PMID: 32480228]

[101]   Bae JM. History of coffee consumption and risk of Alzheimer's disease: A meta-epidemiological study of population-based cohort studies. Dement. Neurocogn. Dement Neurocognitive Disord 2020; 19(3): 108-13.

[http://dx.doi.org/10.12779/dnd.2020.19.3.108] [PMID: 32985150]

[102] Zhang Y, Wu Q, Zhang L, *et al.* Caffeic acid reduces A53T α-synuclein by activating JNK/Bcl-- -mediated autophagy *in vitro* and improves behaviour and protects dopaminergic neurons in a mouse model of Parkinson's disease. Pharmacol Res 2019; 150: 104538.
[http://dx.doi.org/10.1016/j.phrs.2019.104538] [PMID: 31707034]

[103] Tomiyama R, Takakura K, Takatou S, *et al.* 3,4-dihydroxybenzalacetone and caffeic acid phenethyl ester induce preconditioning ER stress and autophagy in SH-SY5Y cells. J Cell Physiol 2018; 233(2): 1671-84.
[http://dx.doi.org/10.1002/jcp.26080] [PMID: 28681934]

[104] Kim HM, Kim Y, Lee ES, Huh JH, Chung CH. Caffeic acid ameliorates hepatic steatosis and reduces ER stress in high fat diet–induced obese mice by regulating autophagy. Nutrition 2018; 55-56: 63-70.
[http://dx.doi.org/10.1016/j.nut.2018.03.010] [PMID: 29960159]

[105] Loos B, Engelbrecht AM, Lockshin RA, Klionsky DJ, Zakeri Z. The variability of autophagy and cell death susceptibility. Autophagy 2013; 9(9): 1270-85.
[http://dx.doi.org/10.4161/auto.25560] [PMID: 23846383]

[106] Gao L, Li X, Meng S, Ma T, Wan L, Xu S. Chlorogenic acid alleviates $A\beta_{25-35}$-induced autophagy and cognitive impairment *via* the mTOR/TFEB signaling pathway. Drug Des Devel Ther 2020; 14: 1705-16.
[http://dx.doi.org/10.2147/DDDT.S235969] [PMID: 32440096]

[107] Ben Youssef S, Brisson G, Doucet-Beaupré H, *et al.* Neuroprotective benefits of grape seed and skin extract in a mouse model of Parkinson's disease. Nutr Neurosci 2021; 24(3): 197-211.
[http://dx.doi.org/10.1080/1028415X.2019.1616435] [PMID: 31131731]

[108] Kadri S, El Ayed M, Cosette P, *et al.* Neuroprotective effect of grape seed extract on brain ischemia: A proteomic approach. Metab Brain Dis 2019; 34(3): 889-907.
[http://dx.doi.org/10.1007/s11011-019-00396-2] [PMID: 30796716]

[109] Duangjan C, Rangsinth P, Zhang S, Gu X, Wink M, Tencomnao T. *Vitis vinifera* leaf extract protects against glutamate-induced oxidative toxicity in HT22 hippocampal neuronal cells and increases stress resistance properties in *Caenorhabditis elegans.* Front Nutr 2021; 8: 634100.
[http://dx.doi.org/10.3389/fnut.2021.634100] [PMID: 34179052]

[110] Zhang P, Maimaiti Z, Aili G, Yuan F, Xiao H. *Vitis vinifera* L. Flavones regulate hippocampal neurons *via* autophagy in APP/PS1 alzheimer model mice. Evid Based Complement Alternat Med 2022; 2022: 1-7.
[http://dx.doi.org/10.1155/2022/8554184] [PMID: 36091589]

[111] Wang N, He J, Pan C, *et al.* Resveratrol activates autophagy *via* the AKT/mTOR signaling pathway to improve cognitive dysfunction in rats with chronic cerebral hypoperfusion. Front Neurosci 2019; 13: 859.
[http://dx.doi.org/10.3389/fnins.2019.00859] [PMID: 31481868]

[112] Feng Y, Cui Y, Gao JL, *et al.* Neuroprotective effects of resveratrol against traumatic brain injury in rats: Involvement of synaptic proteins and neuronal autophagy. Mol Med Rep 2016; 13(6): 5248-54.
[http://dx.doi.org/10.3892/mmr.2016.5201] [PMID: 27122047]

[113] Wu Y, Li X, Zhu JX, *et al.* Resveratrol-activated AMPK/SIRT1/autophagy in cellular models of Parkinson's disease. Neurosignals 2011; 19(3): 163-74.
[http://dx.doi.org/10.1159/000328516] [PMID: 21778691]

[114] Lin TK, Chen SD, Chuang YC, *et al.* Resveratrol partially prevents rotenone-induced neurotoxicity in dopaminergic SH-SY5Y cells through induction of heme oxygenase-1 dependent autophagy. Int J Mol Sci 2014; 15(1): 1625-46.
[http://dx.doi.org/10.3390/ijms15011625] [PMID: 24451142]

[115] Deng H, Mi M. Resveratrol attenuates Aβ25–35 caused neurotoxicity by inducing autophagy through

the TyrRS-PARP1-SIRT1 signaling pathway. Neurochem Res 2016; 41(9): 2367-79.
[http://dx.doi.org/10.1007/s11064-016-1950-9] [PMID: 27180189]

[116] Yihao D, Tao G, Zhiyuan W, Xiaoming Z, Lingling D, Hongyun H. *Ginkgo biloba* leaf extract (EGb-761) elicits neuroprotection against cerebral ischemia/reperfusion injury by enhancement of autophagy flux in neurons in the penumbra. Iran J Basic Med Sci 2021; 24(8): 1138-45.
[PMID: 34804431]

[117] Li X, Zhang D, Bai Y, Xiao J, Jiao H, He R. Ginaton improves neurological function in ischemic stroke rats *via* inducing autophagy and maintaining mitochondrial homeostasis. Neuropsychiatr Dis Treat 2019; 15: 1813-22.
[http://dx.doi.org/10.2147/NDT.S205612] [PMID: 31308674]

[118] Qin Y, Zhang Y, Tomic I, *et al. Ginkgo biloba* extract EGb 761 and its specific components elicit protective protein clearance through the autophagy-lysosomal pathway in tau-transgenic mice and cultured neurons. J Alzheimers Dis 2018; 65(1): 243-63.
[http://dx.doi.org/10.3233/JAD-180426] [PMID: 30010136]

[119] Zheng Y, Wu Z, Yi F, *et al.* By activating Akt/eNOS bilobalide B inhibits autophagy and promotes angiogenesis following focal cerebral ischemia reperfusion. Cell Physiol Biochem 2018; 47(2): 604-16.
[http://dx.doi.org/10.1159/000490016] [PMID: 29794436]

[120] Vijayakumaran S, Nakamura Y, Henley JM, Pountney DL. Ginkgolic acid promotes autophagy-dependent clearance of intracellular alpha-synuclein aggregates. Mol Cell Neurosci 2019; 101: 103416.
[http://dx.doi.org/10.1016/j.mcn.2019.103416] [PMID: 31654699]

[121] Tan X, Gu J, Zhao B, *et al.* Ginseng improves cognitive deficit *via* the RAGE/NF-κB pathway in advanced glycation end product-induced rats. J Ginseng Res 2015; 39(2): 116-24.
[http://dx.doi.org/10.1016/j.jgr.2014.09.002] [PMID: 26045684]

[122] Hu S, Han R, Mak S, Han Y. Protection against 1-methyl-4-phenylpyridinium ion (MPP+)-induced apoptosis by water extract of ginseng (Panax ginseng C.A. Meyer) in SH-SY5Y cells. J Ethnopharmacol 2011; 135(1): 34-42.
[http://dx.doi.org/10.1016/j.jep.2011.02.017] [PMID: 21349320]

[123] Zhang J, Chen K, Zhou Y, *et al.* Evaluating the effects of mitochondrial autophagy flux on ginsenoside Rg2 for delaying D-galactose induced brain aging in mice. Phytomedicine 2022; 104: 154341.
[http://dx.doi.org/10.1016/j.phymed.2022.154341] [PMID: 35870376]

[124] Wang P, Lin C, Wu S, *et al.* Inhibition of autophagy is involved in the protective effects of ginsenoside Rb1 on spinal cord injury. Cell Mol Neurobiol 2018; 38(3): 679-90.
[http://dx.doi.org/10.1007/s10571-017-0527-8] [PMID: 28762191]

[125] Chen S, He J, Qin X, *et al.* Ginsenoside metabolite 20(S)-protopanaxadiol promotes neural stem cell transition from a state of proliferation to differentiation by inducing autophagy and cell cycle arrest. Mol Med Rep 2020; 22(1): 353-61.
[http://dx.doi.org/10.3892/mmr.2020.11081] [PMID: 32319663]

[126] Meng X, Wang M, Sun G, *et al.* Attenuation of Aβ25–35-induced parallel autophagic and apoptotic cell death by gypenoside XVII through the estrogen receptor-dependent activation of Nrf2/ARE pathways. Toxicol Appl Pharmacol 2014; 279(1): 63-75.
[http://dx.doi.org/10.1016/j.taap.2014.03.026] [PMID: 24726523]

[127] Meng X, Luo Y, Liang T, *et al.* Gypenoside XVII enhances lysosome biogenesis and autophagy flux and accelerates autophagic clearance of Amyloid-β through TFEB activation. J Alzheimers Dis 2016; 52(3): 1135-50.
[http://dx.doi.org/10.3233/JAD-160096] [PMID: 27060963]

CHAPTER 6

Propitious Effects of Natural Bioactives for Osteoporosis: Special Emphasis From Marine Source

Shravya Shanbhag[1], Palak Parekh[1] and Maushmi S. Kumar[2,*]

[1] *Shobhaben Pratapbhai Patel School of Pharmacy and Technology Management, SVKM's NMIMS, V. L. Mehta Road, Vile Parle (West), Mumbai-400056, India*

[2] *Somaiya Institute for Research and Consultancy, Somaiya Vidyavihar University, Vidyavihar (East), Mumbai-400077, India*

Abstract: Osteoporosis is one of the most significant health issues on the globe. The activity of osteoclast cells is connected to altered hormone levels and other factors such as age. The condition is characterized by increased bone fragility and loss of bone tissue. Osteoporosis, osteopetrosis, and Paget's disease are frequently caused by an imbalance in the production and function of osteoclasts and osteoblasts. The disease's early signs are scarcely noticeable. It results in gradual bone loss, which eventually makes the patients more prone to fractures. Osteoporosis must be avoided since the fractures caused by it have substantial medical expenses and morbidity. Bisphosphonates are used in the treatment of osteoporosis, along with hormone therapy, selective estrogen receptor modulators (SERMs), calcitonin, strontium ranelate (SR), and other treatments. Marine Natural Products (MNPs) have also had a significant impact on bone metabolism by preventing osteoclastogenesis. These MNPs are generated from a variety of marine resources, including marine cyanobacteria, soft corals, mollusks, fish, dinoflagellates, algae, sponges, and mangroves. Numerous plant and herb species are also effective in the treatment of osteoporosis. We check if these plant-based bio-actives may replace hormonal and synthetic drug-based treatments. This chapter also throws light on any possible effect of COVID-19 that might be on the body, particularly the musculoskeletal system.

Keywords: Bisphosphonates, COVID-19, Hormone therapy, Marine natural bio-actives, Osteoporosis, Plant-based bio-actives.

INTRODUCTION

Osteoporosis is called a "silent" disease as its indications generally do not appear until a bone is broken with one or more vertebrae fractures. Systemic skeletal

---

[*] **Corresponding author Maushmi S. Kumar:** Somaiya Institute for Research and Consultancy, Somaiya Vidyavihar University, Vidyavihar (East), Mumbai-400077, India; E-mail: maushmiskumar@gmail.com

Pardeep Kaur, Tewin Tencomnao, Robin and Rajendra G. Mehta (Eds.)

osteoporosis is a disorder hallmarked by lower bone density, micro-architectural degradation of bone tissue, and greater fracture risk. It is one of the most frequent reasons for fractured bones in older people [1].

Our bones are living tissues that continuously repair themselves all our lives to help give shape, movement, and support to our bodies. During childhood and adolescence, the body replaces old bone faster, and after the age of 20, we may begin to lose bone faster than it is formed [2]. Exercise, Ca^{2+}, and vitamin D are essential for maintaining bone density and preventing bone loss. One should also avoid too much alcohol consumption and smoking. Bone diseases can make bones brittle, and the most common reason for fractures is osteoporosis. The onset of osteoporosis is one of the realities of aging. Other examples of bone problems include low bone density, Paget's disease, and osteogenesis imperfecta [2].

The most serious issue caused by osteoporosis is fracture, which may be the primary recognizable sign of the disease in patients. Annually, approximately 15 lakh people experience severe fractures because of bone disease. Fracture risk increases with age, and it occurs more in women. Commonly broken bones include vertebrae in the spine, forearm, and hip (Fig. **1**).

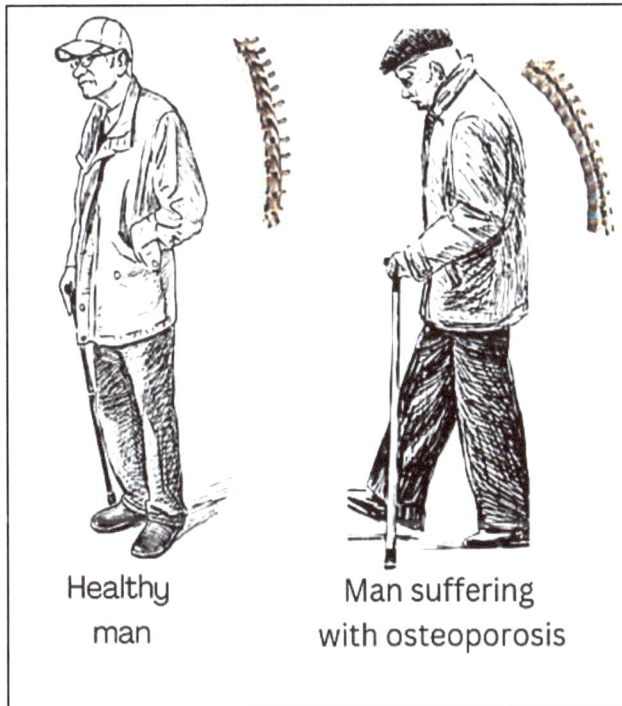

Fig. (1). Internal structure of a healthy bone and a bone affected with osteoporosis.

The global prevalence of osteoporosis is about 18.3% reported based on the incidences from 86 studies spanning five continents [3]. The latest studies from Africa indicate that osteoporosis and associated fractures are on the rise across the continent (Fig. **2**).

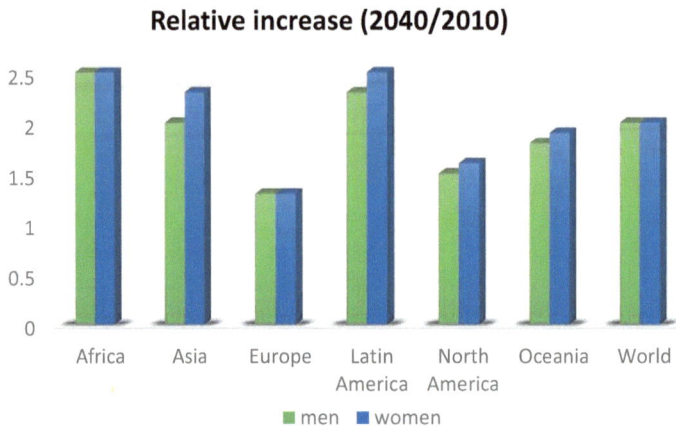

Fig. (2). High fracture risk in men and women in 2040 relative to 2010 by world region.

Other studies indicate strongly that the occurrence of osteoporosis and other bone diseases will continue to rise due to a sedentary lifestyle and lack of physical exercise. Earlier people used to work in agriculture farms and household chores were manual which involved a lot of physical work, however with the advent of the digital revolution, the job profile has changed over the last decade and more and more people are involved in the IT industry which involves sedentary lifestyle, which has resulted in a reduction of age with the onset of bone disease.

Their risk factors for osteoporosis have been categorized into modifiable and non-modifiable types. Modifiable risk factors can be controlled by bringing in some adjustments in our daily lifestyle whereas non-modifiable risk factors are beyond our control. Alcohol consumption, weight, smoking, dietary calcium deficiency and physical inactivity are modifiable osteoporosis risk factors. For non-modifiable osteoporosis, risk factors include sex, age, nationality, and genetic characteristics. These factors might be more common in terms of gender as well [3].

OSTEOPOROSIS- PATHOGENESIS AND MORPHOLOGIC FEATURES

Osteoporosis is traditionally categorized into two types. Primary osteoporosis is a result of osteopenia in the absence of an underlying disease or medication. It is further subdivided into two types a) idiopathic, which occurs in young and juveniles, and b) involutional, which occurs in postmenopausal women and the elderly. Secondary osteoporosis is caused due to some underlying diseases such as chronic anemia, hepatic disease, acromegaly, *etc.*, or as a side effect of medication [4]. Other forms of osteoporosis have a systemic skeletal distribution, except for disuse or immobilization osteoporosis, which is limited to the affected limb. The most common osteoporotic fractures are femoral neck fractures, vertebral crushes, and wrist fractures. The medullary cavity gets enlarged, and the cortex starts thinning [4]. Histologically, osteoporosis can be active or inactive. Active osteoporosis is distinguished by increased bone remodeling, resulting in accelerated turnover. There is a rise in the number of osteoclasts with an increase in the resorptive surface, as well as an increase in the quantity of osteoid with an increase in the osteoblastic surface. Osteoid seams are normal in width [4]. Inactive osteoporosis is distinguished by negligible bone formation and decreased resorptive activity, *i.e.*, decreased turnover. Inactive osteoporosis includes histological changes such as a decrease in the number of osteoclasts with decreased resorptive surfaces and a normal or less amount of osteoid with diminished osteoblastic surface. The width of osteoid seams is typically reduced or normal [4]. There are usually no symptoms in the initial stages of osteoporosis. However, after the bones have enfeebled due to osteoporosis, one may experience height loss over time, stooped posture, backache due to vertebral compression fractures (VCFs), and brittle bone [2].

TREATMENT FOR OSTEOPOROSIS

Bisphosphonates

Bisphosphonates are the most prescribed drugs for osteoporosis in both men and women, who are at high fracture risk. Alendronate, Ibandronate, Risedronate, and Zoledronic acid are some examples of bisphosphonates. If medications are not taken properly as recommended, side effects such as abdominal pain, nausea, and heartburn symptoms may occur. Among the side effects of bisphosphonates are flu or fever. They can also have low levels of calcium in one's blood. Another rare complication is the development of a crack in one's middle femur bone, which can lead to delayed healing of the jawbone [5, 6].

Denosumab Injections

Denosumab injections (Prolia, Xgeva) are RANK (Receptor activator of nuclear factor kappa-B) ligand inhibitors used for the treatment of osteoporosis in women who are predisposed to fractures after menopause, as well as osteoporosis in men. Denosumab produces comparable or improved bone density outcomes than bisphosphonates and lowers the risk of fractures of all kinds. Denosumab is administered every six months *via* a subcutaneous shot. Like bisphosphonates, denosumab can result in jaw osteonecrosis, thighbone fractures, or cracks. According to recent studies, there may be an increased risk of vertebral fractures if this medication is discontinued [7].

Selective Estrogen Receptor Modulator (SERM) Therapy

SERM is an estrogen-based therapy used for treating osteoporosis. It performs various functions, including reproduction in the body. The hormone estrogen also influences the brain. Estrogen is required for the proper closure of epiphyseal growth plates during osteogenesis in both males and females. Depending on the target organ, SERMs bind to the estrogen receptor with high affinity and have different estrogen agonists and antagonists' properties. Certain SERMs, like bazedoxifene and raloxifene, have estrogen activity in the bone and thus avoid bone loss, improve BMD, and reduce the risk of vertebral column fracture. For women who have not yet reached menopause, SERM's adverse effects include night sweats, vaginal discharge, hot flashes and leg cramps, and irregular menstrual cycles. Although, current drug treatments have been shown to improve BMD and reduce the risk of fracture; long-term use has been linked to a variety of side effects. As a result, the search for new effective drugs with minimum side effects is still ongoing. Furthermore, the only prophylactic agent available for osteoporosis is Ca^{2+} and vitamin D. Interest in employing herbal plants to treat osteoporosis has increased because of the result of recent developments in phytomedicine [8].

Antiosteoporotic Bioactives Extracted from Plants and Animals

Bioactive compounds from plants are used in herbal medicine to protect the human skeleton. Few intensively researched herbal plants have shown anti-osteoporotic effects in *in vitro* and *in vivo* studies. *Rhizoma alismatis, Rhizoma curculiginis,* and *Hemidesmus indicus* (L)R. Br, *Passiflora foetida, Cissus quadrangularis,* and *Dalbergia sissoo* are some of the herbal-based plants that have shown promise in combating osteoporosis [9]. We have attempted to understand the anti-osteoporotic characteristics of various medicinal plants, along with their effects on osteoclasts, osteoblasts, and bone remodeling of the medicinal herbs' families belonging to Berberidaceae, Fabaceae, Arecaceae, and Labiatae in Table **1**.

Table 1. Anti-osteoporotic effects of plant families.

Fabaceae	*Glycine max* L. (Fabaceae), scientifically known as soybean, is primarily indigenous to Southwest Asia. It contains a high concentration of flavonoids and proteins like, biochanin A, genistein, and daidzein. Isoflavones have been shown to preserve trabecular microstructure in animal models of bone loss. Soybean phytoestrogens have been shown to influence the metabolism of bones in postmenopausal women. Isoflavones might be utilized as a nutritional supplement for the prevention of postmenopausal osteoporosis by enhancing bone turnover indicators, BMD, and bone strength in postmenopausal women. Genistein is an estrogenic isoflavone that influences bone. It inhibits bone degradation and facilitates B-lymphopoiesis in the bone marrow without having an estrogenic effect in the uterus [10].
Beriberidaceae	Epimedium plants belong to the Berberidaceae family. They are deciduous perennials with a low growth rate. They are also referred to as bishop's hat, barrenwort, and fairy wings. Other species' leaves, such as *E. pubescens Maxim, E. brevicornum Maxim, E. koreanum Nakai, and E. sagittatum Maxim* have traditionally been used in China to treat menopause and osteoporosis-associated diseases. Icarin, epimedin C, and epimedin B are all found in the Epimedium crude extract. These compounds are antiosteoporotic components of Epimedium plants, preventing bone resorption and activating bone formation, & Ca^{2-} reabsorption in the urine. The flavonoids in Epimedium have estrogenic activity and promote osteoblast maturation by increasing the content of alkaline phosphatase (ALP), bone morphogenetic protein-2 (BMP-2), and core binding factor 1 (Cbf1). They increase osteoprotegerin (OPG) expression and decrease the expression of RANKL, which suppresses osteoclast formation. The most pharmacokinetically active flavonoid was discovered to be Icariin a glucoside derivative of the Epimedium plant [10].
Labiatae	*Salvia miltiorrhguiza* Bunge (also referred to as 'dan shen' or 'red sage root') is a Chinese herb from the Labiatae family that has traditionally been used to treat cardio-cerebral disorders. Pharmacologically, *S. miltiorrhiza* has been observed to have anticoagulant, improved blood flow, free radical scavenging, anti-inflammatory, and mitochondrial protective properties. Tanshinones (tanshinone I, tanshinone IIA, 16-dihydrotanshinone I, cryptotanshinone) and phenolics have been discovered through phytochemical studies *of S. miltiorrhiza* Bunge (salvianolic acid A, protocatechuic aldehyde, and salvianolic acid B). Treatment with *S. miltiorrhiza* significantly prevents the loss of trabecular bone mass and bone mineral density, as well as TRAP activity and oxidative stress parameters such as malondialdehyde (MDA) and nitric oxide (NO) in rodents caused by sex hormone deficiency. Salvianolic acid A, derived from *S. miltiorrhiza* Bunge, has been shown to reduce bone loss in rats given long-term prednisone. This is accomplished by controlling osteogenesis and inhibiting adipogenesis in bone marrow stromal cells. Salvianolic acid B, on the other hand, has been shown to inhibit glucocorticoid-induced cancellous bone loss and suppress adipogenesis. It influences bone marrow stromal cell (MSC) differentiation into osteoblasts and increases osteoblastic activity [11].

(Table 1) cont.....

Arecaceae	Oil palm, a member of the palm family (Arecaceae), is primarily grown for its oil. It is widely grown along the equator in its native West and Central Africa along with Asian countries such as Indonesia and Malaysia. *Elaeis guineensis* (African oil palm) is the most widely planted Arecaceae Family species, with *Attalea maripa* (Maripa palm) and *Elaeis oleifera* (American oil palm) being less well-known [12]. *Elaeis guineensis* palm oil is well known due to its rich vitamin E content. Vitamin E is a mutual term for the antioxidant and anti-inflammatory properties of tocopherol and tocotrienol isoforms, as well as other useful effects on the human body. Tocotrienol's anti-oxidative and anti-inflammatory properties are useful for its effective anti-osteoporotic agent. Both inflammation and oxidative stress are known to play roles in osteoporosis. Oxidative stress is also known to increase osteoclast signaling while also promoting differentiation. By affecting differentiation and survival rates, oxidative stress has been found to impair osteoblasts [13]. In nature, there are four distinct forms of each isoform of tocopherols and tocotrienols: α-, β-, γ-, and δ-. Tocotrienol is a suitable anti-osteoporotic drug due to its anti-inflammatory and anti-oxidative effects. Aktifanus *et al.* (2012) and Soelaiman *et al.* (2012) also found that tocotrienol supplementation decreased single-labeled surfaces while increasing double-labeled surfaces in ovariectomized rats. Additionally, as compared to the untreated control group, ovariectomized rats who received 30 and 60 mg/kg body weight of palm vitamin E had substantially better bone mineral density at the femur and vertebrae. Studies have also demonstrated that palm vitamin E can increase bone calcium levels in the femur and vertebra of orchidectomized and ovariectomized rats [14, 15].

The safety of herbal medication needs to be thoroughly investigated. Herbs are generally thought to be safe with minimum side effects. According to the studies, hepatotoxicity is the most reported toxic effect of herbal remedies. Before conducting definitive clinical trials, accurate research of bioactive compounds and scientific details concerning their safety and toxicity is required. Plant extracts influence bone metabolism by acting directly on bone cells, reducing oxidative stress and inflammation, and raising sex hormone levels [16]. However, proper human clinical trials will be required to confirm their bone-shielding effects.

MARINE NATURAL PRODUCTS (MNPS)

Seeking the right remedy for bone-linked diseases is a matter of major concern these days. Recent treatments, such as bisphosphonates, hormone therapy, SERM therapy, strontium ranelate, *etc.* are good at thwarting bone loss but have harmful aftereffects. Natural products from plants and marine plants and organisms are rapidly overtaking synthetic drugs because they have lesser aftereffects and are better suited for long-period use. Numerous marine-derived bioactive compounds or marine extracts have also been found to have a significant impact on bone metabolism regulation by lowering trabecular separation and increasing bone density, number, thickness, and cancellous bone volume. MNPs such as non-isoprenoids, quinones, terpenoids, brominated compounds, isoprenoids, nitrogen sulfur heterocyclics, nitrogen heterocyclics, and steroids may also promise to be useful in the therapy of bone-related disorders and in regulating bone metabolism

[16]. Marine microorganisms, plants, invertebrates such as sponges, cyanobacteria, fungi, dinoflagellates, algae, tunicates, bryozoans, mollusks, and fishes are known sources of biologically active compounds (Fig. **3**).

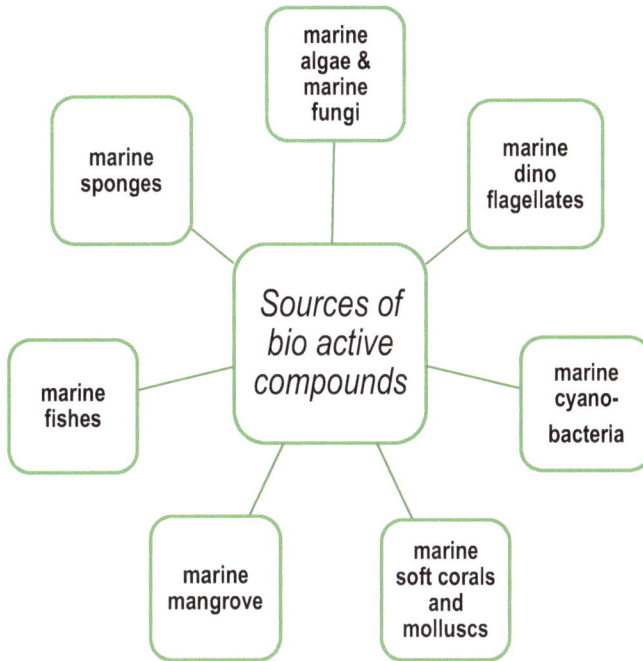

Fig. (3). Possible sources of bioactive compounds from marine source.

Sponges

Among marine organisms, sponges remain one of the most promising sources of pharmacologically active compounds. Their skeletons are used for scaffold development in tissue engineering and regeneration owing to their potential in cell conductive and inductive framework formation [16]. Nandi and colleagues investigated whether IGF-1 and BMP-2 impregnation of converted sponge scaffold aided in the excellent formation of osseous tissue. This means that the combination of marine sponges with these GFs and only marine sponges can be used to create a promising biomaterial for bone repair and augmentation [16 - 18]. To target cell components, salicylihalamides A is the first marine V-ATPase inhibitor suggested in drug development. V-ATPase is present on the plasma membrane of osteoclasts, where it activates osteoclast-secreted acid hydrolases and acidifies the bone surface. Therefore, the suppressive effect of salicylihalamides A for V-ATPase is beneficial in osteoporosis remedy [16].

Cyanobacteria

Biselyngbyaside is a glycosylated 18-membered macrolide compound that is obtained from the marine cyanobacterium *Lingpa* spp. It is conjugated with 1,3 diene, two olefins, and a side chain at C 17. At low concentrations, it inhibits macrophages in the bone marrow and RANKL-induced osteoclastogenesis in RAW 264.7 cells, and it even suppresses osteoblast-mediated osteoclast differentiation in co-cultures [19].

Fungi

Diaporthe sp. HLY-1 is a mangrove-associated fungal strain, which yielded the polyketide mycoepoxydiene (MED). By attempting to suppress RANKL-induced osteoclast differentiation, MED aided in the prevention of bone loss [20].

Dinoflagellates

Symbioimine is an amphoteric metabolite consisting of a distinctive 6,6,6-tricyclic iminium ring structure and an aryl sulfate moiety. It was produced from the symbiotic marine dinoflagellate *Symbiodinium* spp. It inhibited RAW 264.7 cell differentiation into osteoclasts, making it a potent anti-resorptive drug that shows its potential in the prevention and treatment of postmenopausal osteoporosis [21].

Algae

Padina pavonica extract is used as a nutrient supplement against osteoporosis. The extract enhances the uptake and fixation of Ca^{2+} by osteoblasts *in vitro*, it also works as an effective phytoestrogen, raising both bone collagen and bone mass. *Sargassum horneri* contains an anabolic agent with osteoblastic bone formation and bone resorption inhibitory characteristics. Alginate and fucoidan play an important role in bone tissue engineering. Alginate scaffolds incorporated with stem cells are widely checked for bone tissue regeneration [22].

Mangroves

In the past few decades, Halophytes have been a source of new bioactive chemicals. It is a known fact that halophytes live in hard environments, which causes them to produce healing substances that include polyphenols, flavonoids, and saponins. A potential source of a drug that inhibits adipogenesis while promoting osteoblastogenesis is the herbaceae family. Like this, *S. herbacea* extract improves bone formation in MC3T3-E1 pre-osteoblasts by increasing the expression of markers for osteoblastogenesis, including BMP-2, osteocalcin, collagen-I, and alkaline phosphatase activity [23].

Soft Corals

Marine soft corals are known to be a rich source of interesting, physiologically, and structurally active chemicals. A class of biologically active substances known as diterpenoids, which are derived from marine soft corals, have been confirmed to have anti-inflammatory, antioxidant, and anti-osteoporotic properties [22].

Molluscs

There are many different species of mollusks, an invertebrate group with a wide distribution, in estuarine and marine ecosystems occurring throughout the world. Molluscs are regarded as a significant group of organisms that can yield chemicals with possible medicinal uses. It is interesting to note that gastropods or bivalves account for 98% of bioactive chemicals. The organic matrix found in molluscan shells has the power to control calcium deposition and mineralization [24, 25].

Fishes

Fish oils and fish protein hydrolysates are the main sources of bioactive substances with medicinal uses. Waste products from the preparation of seafood such as skin, fins, fish bones, gills, and trimmed muscles, have been under study as potential sources of bioactive peptides, omega fatty acids, *etc.* Marine fish are a valuable resource for the nutraceutical, food, and pharmaceutical industries. One of the marine collagen items advertised as supplements to increase bone strength and density is gelatine, also known as collagen hydrolysate. Animal studies have demonstrated that fish collagen hydrolysates have a protective effect against osteoporosis. Studies have also shown that the gelatine present in cod bone may reduce bone resorption in rats that have had their ovary removed, hence preventing bone loss [26]. A diet high in collagen protein may boost and elongate the therapeutic value of calcitonin in osteoporosis patients, especially in postmenopausal women. Long-chain polyunsaturated fatty acids with the numbers n-6 and n-3 are thought to be mostly found in marine fish (PUFAs) [26]. Arachidonic acid stimulates bone production in low doses but inhibits it in large amounts. Prostaglandin E2 is important for bone metabolism and is synthesized by PUFAs [16].

FUTURE SCOPE OF MARINE BIOACTIVE FOR TREATMENT OF OSTEOPOROSIS

Based on extensive research, natural products have now emerged as a possible source for several medications during the past few decades. When compared to terrestrial, the marine ecosystem offers a wider variety of resources for human nutrition and health. MNPs and marine nutraceuticals have been extremely popular due to their impressive bioactivities. The clinical trial status for a few MNPs have been shown in Table **2**. However the potential of marine resources' anti-osteoporotic compounds—which are necessary for osteoporosis prevention and reversal—needs to be further studied. Therefore, it is essential to find bioactive compounds with anti-osteoporotic action in marine resources. The ability of these bioactive molecules to control immunological mediators including immune receptors, transcription factors, and important components like RANKL/OPG should also be examined. These new metabolites or chemicals could play an important role in the treatment of skeletal disorders in the future [16, 27, 28].

Table (2). Marine natural products status in preclinical and clinical trials [16].

Name	Source	Status
Phorbaketal A	Marine Sponge *Phorbas* spp.	Preclinical (Osteoporosis)
Largazole	Marine cyanobacteria *Symploca* spp.	Phase 1 Clinical (Cancer, Osteoporosis)
Biselyngbyaside	Marine cyanobacteria *Lyngbya* spp.	Preclinical (Osteoporosis)
Mycoepoxydiene	Mangrove-associated fungal strain. *Diaporthe* spp.	Preclinical (Osteoporosis)
Amphiricinin	Marine dinoflagellate *Amphiricinin* spp.	Preclinical (Osteoporosis)
Symbioimine	Marine dinoflagellate *Symbiodinium* spp.	Preclinical (Osteoporosis)
Fucoidan	Marine brown alga *Undaria pinnatifida*	Clinical (Osteoporosis)
Alginate	Marine algae	Preclinical and clinical (Osteoporosis)
Diterpenoids	Marine Soft Corals	Preclinical and clinical (Osteoporosis)
n-6 and n-3, long chain PUFAs	Marine Fish	Clinical (Osteoporosis)

Osteoporosis – Result of Novel Coronavirus

The SARS-CoV-2 (severe acute respiratory syndrome coronavirus 2) infection led to COVID-19 is now a global epidemic and a serious threat to people's lives and health. Through ACE2 (angiotensin-converting enzyme 2) receptors, SARS-Co-2 can impair several organs in the body. It might also affect osteoclasts and osteoblasts directly or indirectly, which could cause osteoporosis. A crucial hormone for bone health, vitamin D also possesses immunomodulatory effects that are relevant in the COVID-19 pandemic scenario. With COVID-19 infection, proinflammatory cytokine production rises, and immobility can lead to bone resorption and loss in very ill individuals, particularly the elderly and those having compromised immune systems [29, 30]. In most parts of the world, it is well-established that glucocorticoids are helpful in the treatment of COVID-19. Glucocorticoids may speed up bone loss in elderly patients receiving COVID-19 clinical treatment, thereby increasing the risk of developing osteoporosis in them. The effects of SARS-CoV-2 on the human body are influenced by various factors, but it has been determined that binding to the ACE2 receptor is mostly responsible for these effects. Many organs and tissues like adipose tissue, kidney, heart, and small intestine exhibit the highest levels of ACE2 expression. In a prior study, Saemi Obitsu *et al.* discovered that after SARS infection, various skeletal irregularities, including reduced bone mass and osteonecrosis, were seen in individuals after SARS recovery [31]. Through activation with RANKL, differentiation into osteoclast-like cells was reported to be increased by overexpressing SARS-CoV accessory protein 3a/X1 in the murine macrophage cell line RAW264.7. These findings suggest that the SARS-CoV accessory protein 3a/X1 accelerates osteoclastogenesis, which in turn lowers bone density and speeds up bone resorption [31].

During the COVID-19 lockdown, people did not step out of their homes. Hence, there was a lack of physical activities. Also, as people stayed indoors, they did not get enough vitamin D as they were not exposed to sunlight thus leading to vitamin D deficiency. Numerous studies have revealed that patients with vitamin D deficiency are more likely to be affected by COVID-19. Vitamin D is a critical hormone for bone health. Patients with vitamin D deficiency have a high risk of osteoporotic fractures, and numerous disorders are linked to it. In patients with vitamin D insufficiency, osteoporotic fractures, bone turnover, and bone loss are increased. Individuals with vitamin D deficit had approx. 4.59 times higher likelihood of testing positive for COVID-19 than patients who do not have a deficiency [32]. Fig. (**4**) depicts the factors connecting COVID-19 and osteoporosis.

To sum up, with the firming up of precaution measures, the development of vaccines, and the rise in vaccinated populations, there has been an effective control of COVID-19 in many countries and regions. The long-term impact of this pandemic on human health will require further investigation, specifically the effect on osteoporosis.

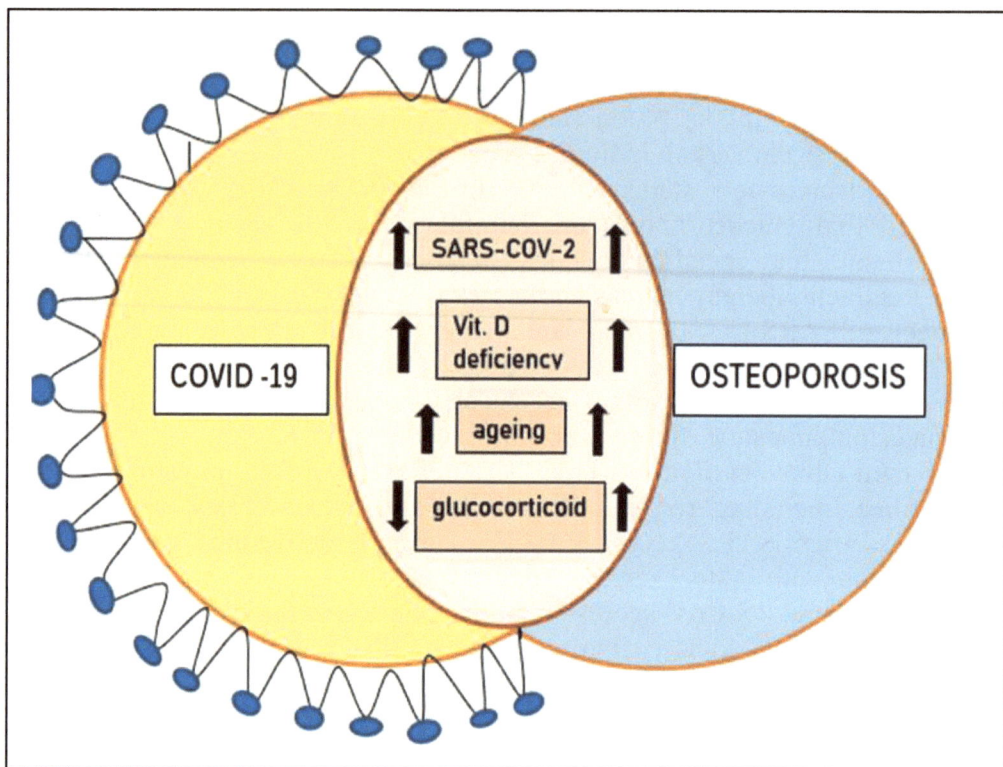

Fig. (4). COVID-19 and osteoporosis.

Since COVID-19 vaccines are new, their side effects are also a concern for everyone, the short-term effects were seen within a day after the vaccination and were also known through personal experiences, but the long-term effects are unknown. Even though scientists have studied the available evidence, the long-term ill effects of this vaccine if any need to be investigated. Elderly COVID-19 patients with vitamin D deficits treated with glucocorticoids are at increased risk of osteoporosis and need to be screened and diagnosed and be given immediate treatment to prevent fractures.

CONCLUSION

Medicinal constituents found in herbal and marine plants as well as marine organisms can aid in the prevention and cure of osteoporosis. These plant extracts and bioactive components have been shown to have anti-osteoporotic properties in numerous animal and cellular investigations. These biological extracts either directly affect bone cells or reduce oxidative stress, which both have an impact on bone remodeling. By promoting bone and reducing its reabsorption, these substances can enhance bone density and reduce the risk of bone fracture. Fracture prevention also requires improvements in cognitive, motor, and muscular coordination. To confirm their bone-protective properties, a full-fledged human clinical investigation is necessary. The usage of botanical compounds as a prevention for osteoporosis also faces problems of selectivity, standardization, and safety. To encourage its usage in osteoporosis prevention, these issues must be resolved. Going forward, we will be successful in developing plant-based and marine-based alternative treatments that can fight bone diseases with minimal side effects. The future looks promising indeed!

ABBREVIATIONS

SERMs	Selective Estrogen Receptor Modulators
SR	Strontium Ranelate
MNPs	Marine Natural Products
VCFs	Vertebral Compression Fractures
RANKL	Receptor Activator of Nuclear factor Kappa-B ligand
BMD	Bone Mineral Density
ALP	Alkaline Phosphatase
BMP-2	Bone Morphogenetic Protein-2
Cbf1	Core Binding Factor 1
OPG	Osteoprotegerin
MDA	Malondialdehyde
NO	Nitric Oxide
MSC	Marrow Stromal Cell
IGF-1	Insulin-like Growth Factor 1
V-ATPase	Vacuolar-type ATPase
MED	Mycoepoxydiene
PUFAs	Polyunsaturated Fatty Acids
SARS-CoV-2	Severe Acute Respiratory Syndrome Coronavirus 2
ACE2	Angiotensin-Converting Enzyme 2

ACKNOWLEDGEMENTS

We acknowledge SVKM's NMIMS and Somaiya Vidyavihar University for providing support while authoring the chapter.

REFERENCES

[1]   National Institutes of Health. Calcium-fact sheet for health professionals. Office of dietary supplements national institutes of health. 2020.

[2]   Osteoporosis overview National institute of arthritis and musculoskeletal and skin diseases Available from: https://www.bones.nih.gov/health-info/bone/osteoporosis/overview Accessed June 3, 2021.

[3]   Salari N, Ghasemi H, Mohammadi L, *et al.* The global prevalence of osteoporosis in the world: A comprehensive systematic review and meta-analysis. J Orthop Surg Res 2021; 16(1): 609.
[http://dx.doi.org/10.1186/s13018-021-02772-0] [PMID: 33397415]

[4]   Mohan H. Textbook of pathology. 7th edition: Jaypee brothers Medical Publishers, New Delhi 2015.
[http://dx.doi.org/10.5005/jp/books/12412]

[5]   Abrahamsen B, Eiken P, Brixen K. Atrial fibrillation in fracture patients treated with oral bisphosphonates. J Intern Med 2009; 265(5): 581-92.
[http://dx.doi.org/10.1111/j.1365-2796.2008.02065.x] [PMID: 19141097]

[6]   Caplan L, Pittman CB, Zeringue AL, *et al.* An observational study of musculoskeletal pain among patients receiving bisphosphonate therapy Mayo Clinic Proceedings 2010; 85(4): 341-8.
[http://dx.doi.org/10.4065/mcp.2009.0492]

[7]   Shen CL, Klein A, Chin KY, *et al.* Tocotrienols for bone health: A translational approach. Ann N Y Acad Sci 2017; 1401(1): 150-65.
[http://dx.doi.org/10.1111/nyas.13449] [PMID: 28891093]

[8]   Riggs BL, Hartmann LC. Selective estrogen-receptor modulators - mechanisms of action and application to clinical practice. N Engl J Med 2003; 348(7): 618-29.
[http://dx.doi.org/10.1056/NEJMra022219] [PMID: 12584371]

[9]   Jolly J, Chin KY, Alias E, Chua K, Soelaiman I. Protective effects of selected botanical agents on bone. Int J Environ Res Public Health 2018; 15(5): 963.
[http://dx.doi.org/10.3390/ijerph15050963] [PMID: 29751644]

[10]   Liu XL, Li JH, Yang YF, Zhu JY. Floral development of *Gymnospermium microrrhynchum* (Berberidaceae) and its systematic significance in the Nandinoideae. Flora 2017; 228: 10-6.
[http://dx.doi.org/10.1016/j.flora.2017.01.002]

[11]   Guo Y, Li Y, Xue L, *et al. Salvia miltiorrhiza*: An ancient Chinese herbal medicine as a source for anti-osteoporotic drugs. J Ethnopharmacol 2014; 155(3): 1401-16.
[http://dx.doi.org/10.1016/j.jep.2014.07.058] [PMID: 25109459]

[12]   Baricevic DE. BARTOL T V Pharmacology 11 The biological/pharmacological activity of the Salvia genus. The Genus Salvia 2000; p. 143.

[13]   Zhao L, Fang X, Marshall M, Chung S. Regulation of obesity and metabolic complications by gamma and delta tocotrienols. Molecules 2016; 21(3): 344.
[http://dx.doi.org/10.3390/molecules21030344] [PMID: 26978344]

[14]   Ha H, Bok Kwak H, Woong Lee S, *et al.* Reactive oxygen species mediate RANK signaling in osteoclasts. Exp Cell Res 2004; 301(2): 119-27.
[http://dx.doi.org/10.1016/j.yexcr.2004.07.035] [PMID: 15530848]

[15]   Soelaiman IN, Ming W, Abu Bakar R, *et al.* Palm tocotrienol supplementation enhanced bone formation in oestrogen-deficient rats. Int J Endocrinol 2012; 1-7.
[http://dx.doi.org/10.1155/2012/532862] [PMID: 23150728]

[16]   Chaugule SR, Indap MM, Chiplunkar SV. Marine natural products: New avenue in treatment of osteoporosis. Front Mar Sci 2017; 4: 384.
[http://dx.doi.org/10.3389/fmars.2017.00384]

[17]   Lin Z, Solomon KL, Zhang X, *et al. In vitro* evaluation of natural marine sponge collagen as a scaffold for bone tissue engineering. Int J Biol Sci 2011, 7(7). 968-77.

[http://dx.doi.org/10.7150/ijbs.7.968] [PMID: 21850206]

[18]   Nandi SK, Kundu B, Mahato A, Thakur NL, Joardar SN, Mandal BB. *In vitro* and *in vivo* evaluation of the marine sponge skeleton as a bone mimicking biomaterial. Integr Biol 2015; 7(2): 250-62.
[http://dx.doi.org/10.1039/C4IB00289J] [PMID: 25578396]

[19]   Yonezawa T, Mase N, Sasaki H, *et al.* Biselyngbyaside, isolated from marine cyanobacteria, inhibits osteoclastogenesis and induces apoptosis in mature osteoclasts. J Cell Biochem 2012; 113(2): 440-8.
[http://dx.doi.org/10.1002/jcb.23213] [PMID: 21678460]

[20]   Asagiri M, Takayanagi H. The molecular understanding of osteoclast differentiation. Bone 2007; 40(2): 251-64.
[http://dx.doi.org/10.1016/j.bone.2006.09.023] [PMID: 17098490]

[21]   Kim HK, Woo ER, Lee HW, *et al.* The correlation of *Salvia miltiorrhiza* extract-induced regulation of osteoclastogenesis with the amount of components tanshinone I, tanshinone IIA, cryptotanshinone, and dihydrotanshinone. Immunopharmacol Immunotoxicol 2008; 30(2): 347-64.
[http://dx.doi.org/10.1080/08923970801949133] [PMID: 18569089]

[22]   Morgan AMA, Lee HW, Lee SH, Lim CH, Jang HD, Kim YH. Anti-osteoporotic and antioxidant activities of chemical constituents of the aerial parts of *Ducrosia ismaelis*. Bioorg Med Chem Lett 2014; 24(15): 3434-9.
[http://dx.doi.org/10.1016/j.bmcl.2014.05.077] [PMID: 24953601]

[23]   Karadeniz F, Kim JA, Ahn BN, Kwon M, Kong CS. Effect of *Salicornia herbacea* on osteoblastogenesis and adipogenesis *in vitro*. Mar Drugs 2014; 12(10): 5132-47.
[http://dx.doi.org/10.3390/md12105132] [PMID: 25310765]

[24]   Anand TP, Rajaganapathi J, Edward JK. Antibacterial activity of marine molluscs from Portonovo region. Indian J Mar Sci 1997; 26: 206-8.

[25]   Benkendorff K. Molluscan biological and chemical diversity: Secondary metabolites and medicinal resources produced by marine molluscs. Biol Rev Camb Philos Soc 2010; 85(4): 757-75.
[http://dx.doi.org/10.1111/j.1469-185X.2010.00124.x] [PMID: 20105155]

[26]   Han X, Xu Y, Wang J, *et al.* Effects of cod bone gelatin on bone metabolism and bone microarchitecture in ovariectomized rats. Bone 2009; 44(5): 942-7.
[http://dx.doi.org/10.1016/j.bone.2008.12.005] [PMID: 19124090]

[27]   Folmer F, Jaspars M, Solano G, *et al.* The inhibition of TNF-α-induced NF-κB activation by marine natural products. Biochem Pharmacol 2009; 78(6): 592-606.
[http://dx.doi.org/10.1016/j.bcp.2009.05.009] [PMID: 19445900]

[28]   Rosen HN, Drezner MK, Rosen CJ, Schmader KE, Mulder JE. Overview of the management of osteoporosis in postmenopausal women. Monografiaen 2017.

[29]   Sundram K, Sambanthamurthi R, Tan YA. Palm fruit chemistry and nutrition. Asia Pac J Clin Nutr 2003; 12(3): 355-62.
[PMID: 14506001]

[30]   Kellerman RD, Bope ET. Conn's current therapy Elsevier Health Sciences 2017.

[31]   Obitsu S, Ahmed N, Nishitsuji H, *et al.* Potential enhancement of osteoclastogenesis by severe acute respiratory syndrome coronavirus 3a/X1 protein. Arch Virol 2009; 154(9): 1457-64.
[http://dx.doi.org/10.1007/s00705-009-0472-z] [PMID: 19685004]

[32]   Katz J, Yue S, Xue W. Increased risk for COVID-19 in patients with vitamin D deficiency. Nutrition 2021; 84: 111106.
[http://dx.doi.org/10.1016/j.nut.2020.111106] [PMID: 33418230]

CHAPTER 7

Pathogenesis of Atherosclerosis and Coronary Heart Disease: Epidemiology, Diagnostic Biomarkers and Prevention by Nutraceuticals, Functional Foods, and Plant-Derived Therapies

Prabhnain Kaur[1,*], Ritu Dahiya[1], Ginpreet Kaur[2], Harpal S. Buttar[3,*], Douglas W. Wilson[4] and Istvan G. Telessy[5]

[1] *Department of Pharmacology, Delhi Pharmaceutical Sciences and Research University, Pushp Vihar, New Delhi, India*

[2] *Shobhaben Pratapbhai Patel School of Pharmacy and Technology Management, SVKM's NMIMS, Mumbai-56, Maharashtra, India*

[3] *Department of Pathology and Laboratory Medicine, Faculty of Medicine, University of Ottawa, Ottawa, Ontario, Canada*

[4] *Formerly, School of Medicine Pharmacy and Health, Durham University, Thornaby TS17 6BH, UK; and Centre for Ageing and Dementia Research, Swansea University, SA2 8PP, U.K.*

[5] *Department of Pharmaceutics, Faculty of Pharmacy, University of Pécs, Hungary, and MedBioFit Lpc. Fácán sor 25. Gödöllö, Hungary*

Abstract: Atherosclerosis is characterized by hardening/narrowing of arteries and reduction of blood flow to vital organs. Animal models and human research show that endothelial dysfunction and plaque development precede the pathogenesis of atherosclerosis, and related coronary heart disease, neurological, and renal disorders. Cardiac CT-scans are used to detect atherosclerosis. Early diagnosis of atherosclerosis reduces mortality, morbidity, and healthcare expenditures. Biomarkers like C-reactive protein, IL-6, IL-8, phospholipase A2, cardiac troponin, MicroRNA, miR-21, and other endothelial inflammation biomarkers are novel targets for monitoring atherosclerosis-related cardiovascular disorders. Anti-platelet and anti-cholesterol drugs are used in the treatment of atherogenesis and blood vessel clots. However, cholesterol-lowering drugs may cause serious adverse effects. Thus, safe and cost-effective non-pharmacological anti-atherogenic and anticoagulant therapies are urgently needed. Nutraceuticals, functional foods, plant-derived therapies, antioxidant/anti-inflammation, foods/fruits/vegetables, and lifestyle changes (*e.g.*, physical activity, less alcohol, smoking cessation) reduce atherogenesis, diabetes mellitus, obesity, hypertension,

* Corresponding authors Prabhnain Kaur and Harpal S. Buttar: Department of Pharmacology, Delhi Pharmaceutical Sciences and Research University, Pushp Vihar, New Delhi, India and Department of Pathology and Laboratory Medicine, Faculty of Medicine, University of Ottawa, Ottawa, Ontario, Canada; E-mails: prabhnain.kaur91@gmail.com, hsbuttar@bell.net

LDL, and C-reactive protein in all age groups, especially younger people. Overwhelming evidence suggests that regular physical activity (30 min/day), cessation of cigarette smoking, and consumption of antioxidant nutraceuticals rich in flavonoids and retinoids, fresh vegetables and fruits, omega-3 PUFA, culinary spices, probiotics, Mediterranean-type diet, and "DASH DIET" lower the risk of atherogenesis and cardiovascular diseases. This review summarizes current advances in the diagnosis and management of atherosclerosis and related cardiovascular illnesses with plant-based and wholesome diets, including the Mediterranean diet, DASH DIET, and lifestyle changes. New preventative measures and alternative therapies, including dietary interventions and plant-based foods may be the most cost-effective ways to manage atherosclerosis and cardiovascular illnesses.

Keywords: Coronary heart disease, Culinary spices, DASH diet, Diagnostic biomarkers, Healthful foods, Mediterranean diet, Nutraceuticals, Pathophysiology of atherosclerosis, Stroke.

INTRODUCTION

Cardiovascular diseases (CVDs) are among the most prevalent chronic illnesses that affect the people worldwide. In both developed and developing nations, CVDs continue to be the main cause of morbidity and mortality [1]. CVDs include atherosclerosis, hypertension, myocardial infarction, heart failure, arrhythmias, valvular heart disease, coagulopathies, and stroke. According to the Registrar General of India (2001–2003), CVDs are the main cause of mortality and morbidity in India, with the highest percentage (25%) recorded in Southern India. Additionally, it was mentioned that CVDs contributed nearly 26% of adult fatalities all across India in the years 2001 to 2003, and that number is predicted to rise to 32% in the years 2010 to 2013 [2]. Globally, the incidence of CVD-related fatalities increased by 41% between 1990 and 2013, and about 17.6 million deaths were attributed to CVDs in 2016. The CVDs not only place a very high financial and emotional strain on families but also escalate the economic healthcare burden on society [3].

Atherosclerosis has been identified by several researchers as the primary underlying cause of many CVDs. The word *athero* means hardening and *sclerosis* means gruel in the Greek language which gave us the phrase atherosclerosis, *i.e.*, accumulation of lipids in the endothelium. In 1904, Marchand originally identified atherosclerosis as the fatty degeneration and stiffness of the blood vessels [4]. It was further characterized as a progressive degenerative process with cholesterol buildup in the small and medium arterial walls and intimal plaque formation in the endothelium [5, 6]. The slow arterial inflammation leads to the buildup of macrophages and white blood cells, which triggers a chronic inflammatory response in the arterial walls (Fig. **1**). Low-density lipoproteins (LDL), which carry triglycerides and cholesterol, further encourage this pathological process without providing enough high-density lipoprotein (HDL) to remove triglycerides and cholesterol from the macrophages [6].

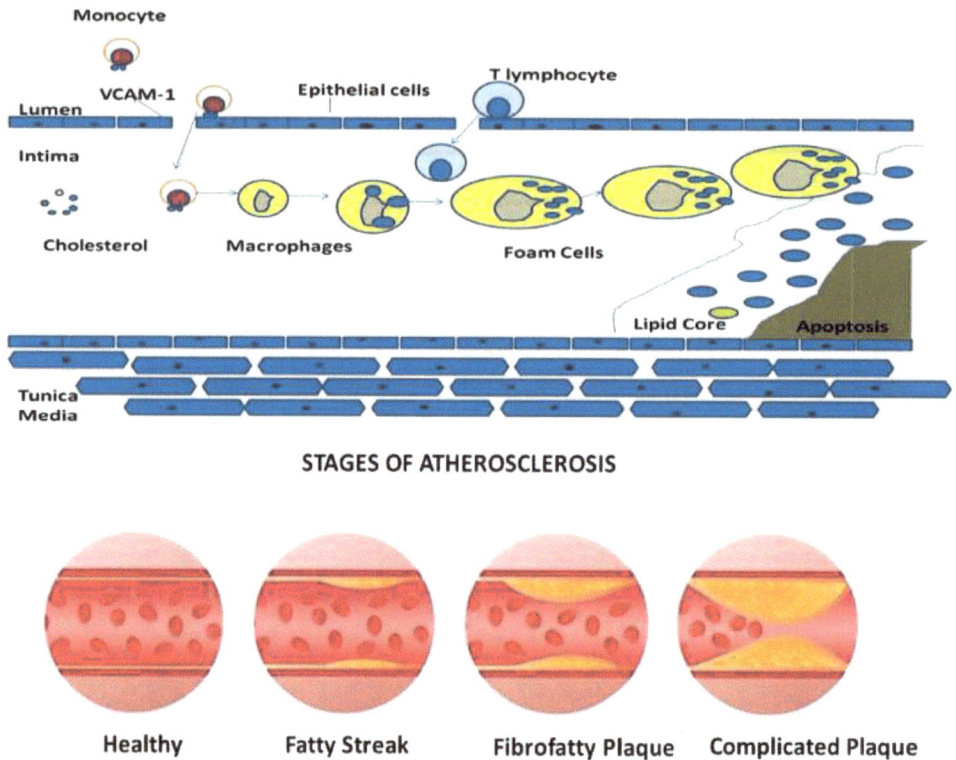

Fig. (1). Schematic illustration of the development of atherosclerosis, including stages of arterial plaque formation.

Atherosclerosis, hypertension, hyperlipidemia, and hyperglycemia are typical CVD risk factors. Tobacco smoking, poor nutrition, lack of exercise, and low socioeconomic level lead to obesity, diabetes mellitus, and CVD in children and adults. Particularly hazardous risk factors are sugary drinks and salty foods. Atherosclerosis, plaque formation, obesity, and diabetes are the main cardiovascular risk factors linked to poor diets and lifestyles. Heart-healthy meals and exercise are the most cost-effective ways to preserve cardiovascular health. Diet and cardiovascular health are strongly linked [7]. This study emphasizes on early atherosclerosis diagnosis with blood-based biomarkers and CVD prevention with dietary treatments, plant-derived medicines, probiotics, exercise, and smoking cessation.

PATHOGENESIS OF ATHEROSCLEROSIS

Atherosclerosis, also known as arteriosclerosis, is a slowly developing multi factorial arterial disease whose exact aetiology remains unknown as yet. Age-related oxidative stress in the endothelium of blood vessels, chronic inflammatory response to leukocyte infiltration in artery walls, obesity, diabetes mellitus, smoking, and deposition of LDL and triglycerides in the arterial lining without adequate removal by HDL are the main potential causes of endothelial damage in arteries. The oxidative stress-induced chronic inflammation in the arterial vessels' endothelium is considered the major initiating cause that encourages the cellular growth as well as the infiltration and retention of lipoproteins in the arterial walls. Various researchers have shown that atherosclerosis is positively correlated with a marked increase in the plasma concentration of LDL and a significant reduction in the plasma level of HDL. Hypercholesterolemia and biochemical oxidation of LDL are considered to be the main culprits causing harm to the endothelial cells of the arteries. The macrophages can quickly identify the oxidised LDL, which encourages the growth of foam cell formation in the endothelium. On the other hand, HDL encourages the reuptake of cholesterol through a mechanism called the cholesterol reverse transport process, which lowers the incidence of atherosclerosis. Additionally, HDL is a strong antioxidant that prevents foam cells formation and the oxidation of LDL.

Atherogenesis triggers endothelial dysfunction, which is set off by oxidative stress and the generation of free radicals (ROS). Fig. (**2**) represents the atherosclerosis-induced plaque formation in the arterial blood vessel. The two important physiological functions of the endothelial cell are the secretion of nitric oxide (NO), and the production of the antioxidant enzyme superoxide dismutase (SOD), which prevent the development of atherogenic plaques. NO has potent vasodilator properties and also exerts anti-inflammatory effects by preventing platelet aggregation. SOD, on the other hand, is a potent antioxidant agent that works to protect cell membranes by scavenging reactive oxygen species. Any type of smoking causes oxidative stress in the arterial endothelium and promotes atherosclerosis and hypertension. Diabetes-induced hyperglycemia also contributes to endothelial dysfunction by increasing the generation of ROS, which sets off an inflammatory cascade [8]. Once the endothelium is damaged, LDL and other macromolecules are transported in caveolae into the vascular intima. The interaction of this transferred LDL with the matrix proteoglycans allows for its retention. The smooth muscle cells (SMC) boost the synthesis of proteoglycans in the intima and consequently produce lipid buildup within the intima that elevates vessel wall stress and further increases LDL binding. The reactive oxygen species further enhance this process and cause LDL to oxidize into superoxide anion, hydrogen peroxide, and lipid peroxide. Dietary antioxidants and enzymes like glutathione peroxidase can counteract the effects of ROS. Atherosclerosis is enhanced by low levels of this enzyme and intracellular glutathione. In addition, the oxidized LDL molecule can promote angiogenesis, or the formation of new blood vessels in the plaque by stimulating leukocyte recruitment and foam cell generation in the fatty streak [9].

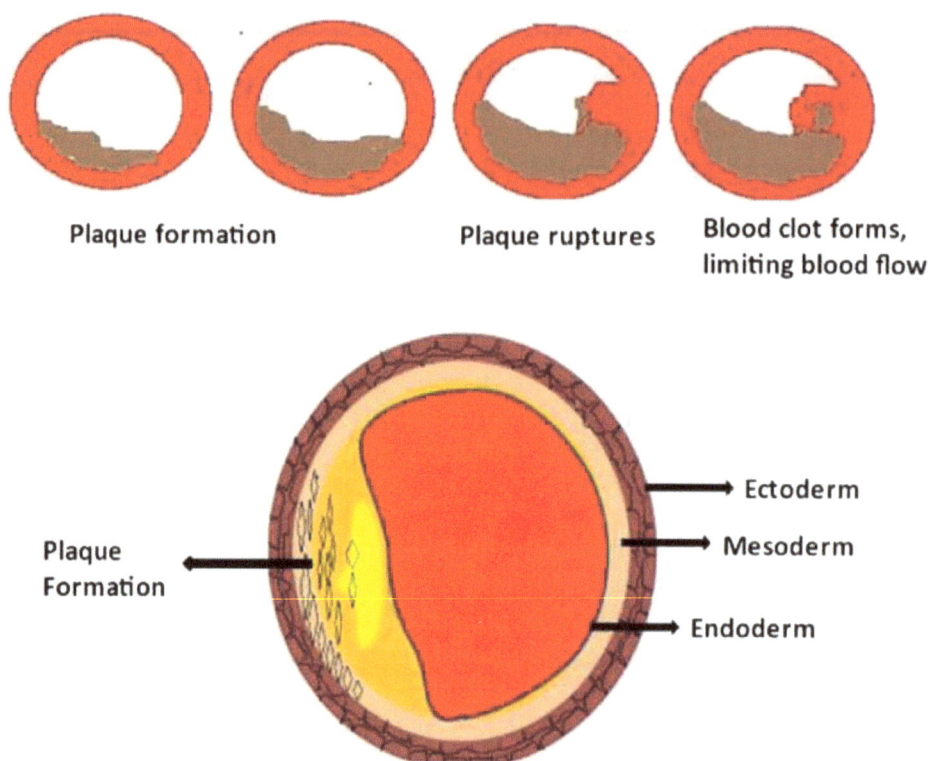

| Plaque formation | | Plaque ruptures | Blood clot forms, limiting blood flow |

Fig. (2). Diagrammatic representation of atherosclerosis-induced plaque formation in the arterial blood vessel.

Biochemically modified LDL is formed and gets deposited in the vascular intima by promoting leukocyte adhesion molecule (LAM) and chemokine production, and maintaining leukocyte recruitment. Furthermore, this vicious cycle encourages endothelial and smooth muscle cells to produce more pro-inflammatory cytokines. Through a positive feedback loop, these pro-inflammatory cytokines cause the production of LAM and chemo-attractive cytokines [10].

The macrophages that attack the oxidized LDL cause the oxidized LDL to appear foamy when examined histopathologically. Chronic endothelial inflammation results from foam cell activation [11]. Since these foam cells are difficult to move around, they build up locally and serve as a source of pro-inflammatory cytokines like IL-1, TNF-α, and chemokines like IL-1, which in turn boost the expression of cell adhesion molecules and draw immune and inflammatory cells, thereby promoting the progression of plaques [12].

The two main distinguishing characteristics of the necrotic core of the atherosclerotic plaque are lipids and a fibrous cap, which surrounds it and contains dead foam cells, macrophages, SMC, lymphocytes, and extracellular matrix (ECM). The plaque wall can be externally remodeled to compensate for the luminal constriction and restricted blood flow [13]. This lumen-narrowing condition can lead to ischemia, which manifests as angina pectoris-like symptoms. Continuous atheromatous plaque growth may cause fibrous cap disruption or hemorrhage with or without calcification.

NO has been shown to suppress the expression of pro-inflammatory molecules including nuclear factor-κB (NF-κB) and adhesion molecules like monocyte chemoattractant protein-1 (MCP-1), selectins (E & P), intracellular cell adhesion molecule-1 (ICAM-1), and vascular cell adhesion molecule-1 (VCAM-1) in experimental studies. Additionally, numerous studies have demonstrated that too many ROS decrease cellular antioxidant defenses and promote the activity of superoxide dismutase, which in turn causes lipid peroxidation, DNA damage, atherosclerosis, and vascular endothelial dysfunction [14, 15].

Epidemiology

As stated earlier, atherosclerosis is a major cause of CVDs, however, the incidence varies depending on the population's ethnicity. According to reports, about 610,000 people per year in the United States alone die from CVDs. The biggest cause of death in the world, coronary heart disease claims over 370,000 lives annually. Men are more likely than women to have atherosclerosis because estrogens have a cardio-protective effect [16].

In people aged 30 to 79 years, or 1.5% of the population, 58 million cases of carotid stenosis were reported globally, according to Song *et al.* [17]. It has been noted that despite controlled plasma LDL-cholesterol levels, atherogenic dyslipidemia is relatively common throughout the world, particularly in individuals on statins. It has been noted that Middle Eastern populations exhibit a different profile of plasma lipid abnormalities than communities in other regions of the world [18]. In contrast to prior research conducted in 1992-1993, the prevalence of low plasma HDL cholesterol and high plasma triglyceride levels increased by 41.8% in 2006, bolstering the idea that atherogenesis is extremely common in Latin America.

Diagnostic Biomarkers

As it is apparent from the foregoing, a complex multifactorial pathophysiology underlies the etiology of atherosclerosis. After accounting for the conventional CVD risk factors, some blood-based biomarkers have been linked with elevated cardiovascular risk (Table **1**). Several of these biomarkers have been added to the risk prediction models, either individually or in combination to determine if they would improve the model's capacity for atherogenic prediction and related CVD (Fig. **3**). Here we discuss the recently published research on blood-based biomarkers, and consider if adding these biomarkers would be beneficial in clinical decision-making. Age, blood pressure, cholesterol levels, gender, diabetes mellitus, and smoking frequency are all included in the commonly used risk prediction models to categorize those subjects at risk for known or suspected CVD. Their measurements may sometimes underestimate the risk of long-term cardiovascular disease, however, vigorous research is going on for finding robust biomarkers that when combined with conventional risk variables, can precisely predict the risk of CVD. For example, CRP, IL-6, IL-18, BNP, and cardiac troponin 1, to name a few of them.

Table 1. Novel blood-based diagnostic biomarkers and their indications.

S. No.	Biomarker	Indication
1.	C Reactive protein	Peripheral artery disease in cardiovascular adverse events is associated with elevated plasma hs-CRP.
2.	IL-6	AMI risk increases with plasma IL-6.
3.	IL-18	High baseline IL-18 levels are independently associated with CV death.
4.	Cardiac troponin	Even without ACS, troponin increases below the MI threshold may indicate CAD and increased cardiovascular risk.
5.	Brain natriuretic peptide	High NT-proBNP levels increase mortality in stable CAD & ACS patients.
6.	Cystatin C	Enhanced coronary artery calcium deposition progression.
7.	Lipoprotein-associated phospholipid A2	Plasma Lp-PLA2 levels suggest vascular inflammation and atherosclerotic susceptibility, predicting future cardiovascular events.
8.	Micro RNAs	CAD patients had greater miR-223 levels and higher mortality and AMI risk.
9.	Osteocalcin	OC levels raise the risk of atherosclerosis due to vascular calcification.
10.	Angiogenin	ANG elevation precedes CHF.
11.	Monocyte chemoattractant protein-1	Upregulated MCP-1 precede CHD events

(Table 1) cont.....

S. No.	Biomarker	Indication
12.	Placental growth factor	Elevated PlGF concentrations were substantially related to adverse outcomes (death or nonfatal MI).
13.	Pregnancy-associated plasma protein-A (PAPP-A)	Elevated in unstable angina and MI patients.
14.	Soluble CD40 ligand	Carotid atheroma patients with high intraplaque lipid content have sCD40L, indicating high-risk lesions.

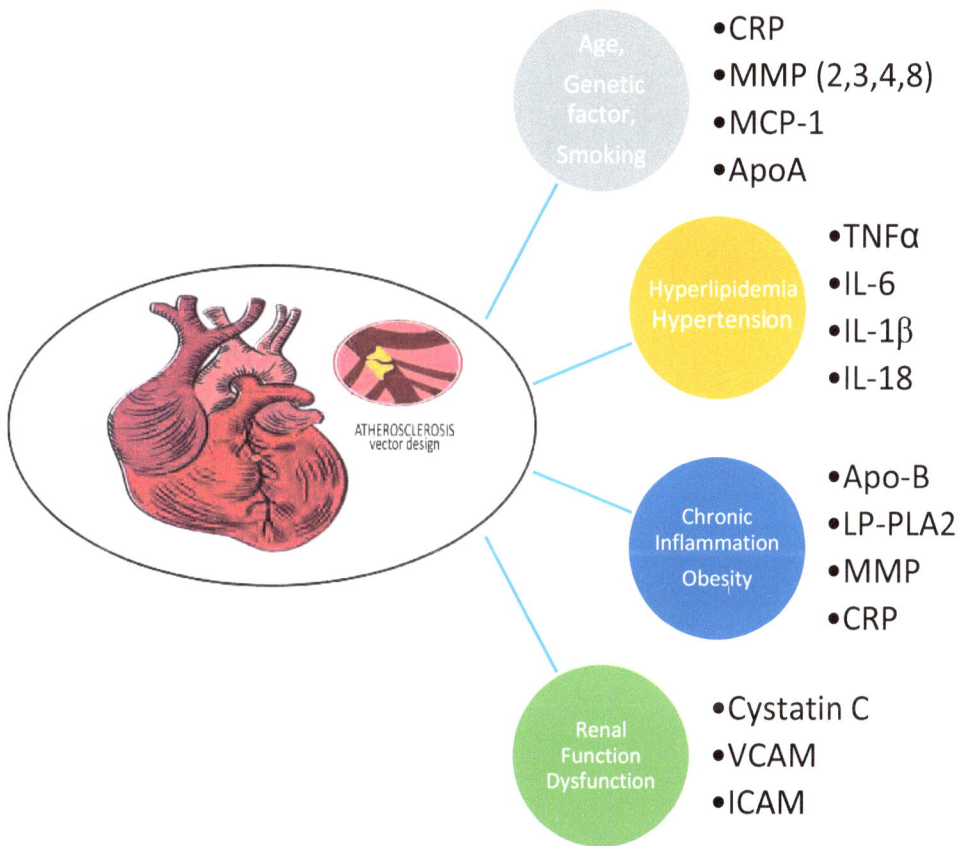

Fig. (3). Different risk factors and diagnostic biomarkers associated with atherosclerosis and CVD diagnosis and disease progression

C Reactive Protein (CRP)

CRP is a pentraxin family member that is produced by liver hepatocytes in response to certain cytokines. For acute inflammatory diseases, this proinflammatory molecule has undergone the most comprehensive research.

Within 48 hours, it can reach a peak value of 300 mg/L of blood. CRP is regarded as a trustworthy clinical diagnostic biomarker due to its analytical stability, repeatable results, and commercial availability of highly-sensitive tests with good precision.

Atherosclerotic plaque cells may also locally produce CRP in addition to hepatocytes [19]. Ridker *et al.* have provided data in support of the use of hsCRP to predict cardiovascular events [20]. Higher levels of hs-CRP are associated with onset diabetes, incident hypertension, myocardial infarction (MI), ischemic stroke, and cardiovascular mortality [21, 22].

Based on hs-CRP levels, Sabatine *et al.* divided PEACE study participants into 3 risk categories: 1, 1-3, and >3 mg/L blood [19, 21]. Patients with peripheral arterial disease (PAD) were studied by Vidula *et al.* for CRP. Each 50% increase in CRP was associated with a higher chance of dying from any cause or a CVD after 4 years of follow-up [23].

Future risk estimation is increased by adding hsCRP to standard Framingham risk variables. In this sizable cohort of women without baseline CVD, adding hsCRP to a risk prediction model using only Framingham risk factors had no effect. The model including hsCRP better predicted subsequent events. 20% of women were categorized as having a 10-year CVD risk >5% after adding hsCRP [24].

The Reynolds Risk Score was developed by Ridker *et al.* [20] based on the data obtained from a cohort of 24,558 women participating in the Health Study who did not have cardiovascular disease (CVD). In order to enhance the accuracy of cardiovascular risk prediction, the ultimate model that was selected incorporated eight characteristics that hold clinical significance. These factors encompass age, cigarette usage, systolic blood pressure, lipid profile, parental history of myocardial infarction, and high-sensitivity C-reactive protein (hsCRP). The utilisation of the Reynolds Risk Score did not yield a significant enhancement in the c-statistic in comparison to the Framingham risk factors. Nevertheless, it resulted in the reclassification of 40-50% of women who were initially categorised as having intermediate risk. The Reynolds Risk Score demonstrated clinically significant risk prediction in women, with the conventional Framingham risk markers, for the majority of individuals who were classified [25].

Interleukin-6 (IL-6)

Through the oxidant and antioxidant balance, IL-6 maintains chronic inflammation in CVD. The pro-inflammatory cytokine with anti-inflammatory myokine properties is IL-6. In humans, the IL-6 gene produces this protein. The expression of IL-6 is essential for host defense mechanisms. It is tightly regulated by intracellular pathways, the deregulation of which can lead to aberrant IL-6 expression and both short-term and long-term inflammatory disorders.

A single-chain glycoprotein with a molecular weight of 26 kDa, IL-6 is produced by activated macrophages, endothelial cells, monocytes, and adipose tissue. The principal procoagulant cytokine, IL-6, stimulates the growth of SMCs and the release of the MCP-1 from macrophages, which promotes the process of amplifying the inflammatory cascade. Endothelial cells express ICAM-1 in response to IL-6 [26, 27]. Infusions of recombinant IL-6 encouraged the growth of fatty lesions in the animal atherosclerosis model [28]. Elevated levels of interleukin-6 (IL-6) were detected in atherosclerotic plaque in humans, particularly in the regions of stable and unstable plaque known as the shoulders [29, 30]. Furthermore, IL-6 was observed to co-localize with the angiotensin II type 1 receptor (AT-1 receptor) in these areas [31]. The stimulation of the AT-1 receptor by the action of IL-6 leads to the occurrence of angiotensin II-induced vasoconstriction, the production of free radicals, and impairment of endothelial function [32]. In a recent study conducted by Maier *et al.*, it was found that individuals with Acute Coronary Syndrome (ACS) exhibited elevated levels of IL-6 specifically at the site of coronary plaque rupture, as compared to the levels observed in the systemic circulation [33].

The COVID-19 pandemic has drawn further attention to IL-6 signaling in CADs. This pro-atherogenic cytokine was enhanced by smoking, cardiovascular risk factors that lead to lung inflammation, obesity, and stress from obesity during the SARS-CoV-2 cytokine storm. High IL-6 levels have been linked to adverse health outcomes, including dyslipidemia, hypertension, glucose deregulation, acute myocardial infarction (AMI), or unstable angina.

IL-6 is released as a result of atherosclerosis, and there exists evidence of IL-6 along with cardiovascular risk in people with elevated hs-CRP. Numerous studies have correlated poor IL-6 signaling to endothelial dysfunction and atherothrombosis. Furthermore, higher plasma IL-6 levels have been linked to a higher risk of AMI in healthy males [34].

Increased CVD episodes have been correlated to greater plasma IL-6 concentrations, according to reports. In the first 48 hours following hospital admission, Biasucci *et al.* reported noticeably higher IL-6 levels in patients, which increased morbidity and mortality in those with unstable angina [34]. The Fast Revascularization during Instability in Coronary Artery Disease II (FRISC II) study's 24 experiments' findings validated the prognostic value of IL-6 and suggested that individuals with high IL-6 levels may benefit from an early invasive operation [35]. Additionally, numerous prospective studies have shown that baseline IL-6 levels are a highly accurate predictor of the development of CVDs in people who appear to be in good health and are asymptomatic [36 - 39].

A meta-analysis of IL-6 as a biomarker of CVD was performed by Zhang *et al.* Their analysis included information from 288,738 healthy individuals, who represented 14,607 non-CVD controls, and 5,400 CVD patients. It was found that over 7 years, cardiovascular events were linked with higher IL-6 levels in unhealthy adults. Thus, the symptoms of cardiovascular disease are brought to light by chronic inflammation. IL-6 levels were found to be related to hypertension and hypercholesterolemia, in contrast to triglycerides. Due to the genetic polymorphism and diversity of IL-6 genes, it was hypothesized that IL-6 may not be a robust biomarker for all studied populations.

Interleukin-18 (IL-18)

IL-18 is a cytokine that promotes inflammation and is strongly expressed in a wide range of cell types [40]. The expression of matrix metalloproteases (MMPs) is stimulated by IL-18 in addition to interferon (IFN) production and the subsequent activation of the Th1 immune response [41 - 43]. The multiple functions of IL-18 make it an essential and potent mediator for the development of atherosclerotic plaque as well as for the instability of the plaque and stroke susceptibility. It has been discovered that human atherosclerotic plaques express IL-18 more often, particularly in lesions that are more likely to rupture, where it is mostly present in plaque macrophages [41, 44]. In double-knockout animals, IL-18 and apo-E displayed decreased lesion diameters, further supporting IL-18's proatherogenic activity, but in apoE-deficient mice, the control of IL-18 by IL-1--binding protein inhibited the formation and progression of atherosclerotic plaques [45, 46]. The administration of interleukin-18 (IL-18), even in the absence of T cells, was found to expedite the development of atherosclerosis in a manner dependent on interferon (IFN) [47]. Furthermore, IL-18 not only initiated but also promoted a transition to a susceptible plaque phenotype by reducing the amount of collagen in the arterial wall and altering the ratio of the cap to the core of the plaque [48, 49]. Subsequent investigations have indicated that elevated baseline levels of IL-18 were autonomously linked to subsequent mortality related to cardiovascular events throughout a 3.9-year follow-up period [42]. However, after 5.9 years, the predictive value of IL-18 concentrations for such outcomes diminished, hence raising scepticism over the use of this particular biomarker [50 - 54]. The research encompassed a total of 1,229 individuals who were diagnosed with CHD through angiographic examination.

An increased risk for eventual CHD events was linked to elevated baseline IL-18 concentrations in a cohort trial (PRIME) carried out in France and the Northern

Islands [55, 56]. However, no apparent correlation was found when the data from the two populations were evaluated simultaneously. No statistically significant association between men and women was established in these trials since there were numerous confounding variables present. This extensive population-based case-cohort analysis suggests that IL-18 may only be a reliable indicator of future CVD incidents in males living in regions with a high absolute risk of CHD. The therapeutic usefulness of IL-18 as a CVD biomarker must therefore be determined by additional well-designed research.

Cardiac Troponin

Cardiovascular troponins T and I control the calcium-mediated interaction of actin and myosin. These regulatory proteins may be unique to the myocardium and are encoded by different genes. Cardiovascular troponins are used to diagnose MI, evaluate the prognosis of ACS patients, and identify people who might benefit from early invasive therapy [57 - 59]. Elevation of troponins above the MI threshold may indicate the incidence of CAD and an increased risk of CVD even in patients without ACS. Troponin-I levels did not rise over baseline levels during stress testing the detection of a 70% coronary stenosis using a diagnostic cut-off value of 0.02 ng/mL troponin-I. This cut-off value was considerably lower than the troponin-I value for this assay (0.07 ng/mL), which corresponded to the 99th percentile of a reference population [60].

Agewall *et al.* employed an alternative troponin-I assay in their examination of 468 consecutive patients who were admitted to the coronary care unit due to suspected myocardial infarction. Following a median duration of 40 months of observation, the unadjusted mortality rates were found to be 5.9% among individuals with undetectable levels of troponin-I, and 23.2% among those with detectable troponin-I values that fell below the diagnostic threshold for myocardial infarction (MI). It is worth noting that the diagnostic cutoff for MI in this particular assay was approximately equivalent to the 99th percentile of a reference population (P < 0.01) [61]. Based on the findings of these investigations, it has been shown that troponin-I elevations of a relatively mild nature, namely those that do not exceed the 99th percentile of a reference sample, have the ability to serve as a predictive indicator for angiographic coronary artery disease (CAD) and subsequent cardiovascular events.

Participants in the aforementioned studies with suspected CAD were hospitalized in the coronary care unit for suspected MI or referred for coronary angiography. Zethelius and colleagues evaluated the prognostic value of mildly elevated troponins in 1,203 males with a mean age of 71. Following the traditional risk variables, all individuals had a greater chance of dying from any cause for those with a troponin-I level of 0.04 mcg/L, or the 99th percentile of a reference group, following a median follow-up of 7.9 years. A troponin-I cut-off of 0.04 mcg/L accurately predicted death and the occurrence of CHD events in persons without CVD at baseline in 80% and 85% of cases, respectively [62].

Brain Natriuretic Peptide (BNP)

BNP is produced and released by the ventricular myocardium in response to myocardial stretch, while pro-inflammatory cytokines and neurohormones can also trigger BNP release [63, 64]. In both persons with and without CVD, BNP and NT-proBNP have been studied as CVD risk predictors. Omland *et al.* discovered that stable coronary artery disease in ACS patients had higher long- and short-term mortality when NT-proBNP levels were greater [64]. The use of NT-prognostic proBNPs has also been investigated in other ACS investigations. For instance, Khan *et al.* examined the effects of NT-proBNP in 473 patients with successive ST-segment elevation myocardial infarction (STEMI) 24 hours following the onset of unfavorable symptoms. The authors concluded that STEMI and elevated NT-proBNP levels may offer more prognostic data beyond clinical criteria [65]. Vascular risk can be predicted in ACS patients with normal troponin levels utilizing NT-proBNP. In the Bad Nauheim ACS and Prognosis in ACS (PACS) registries, it was found that NT-proBNP levels > 474 pg/mL were linked to increased death after 173 days in 213 patients [66]. In the ICTUS study, Windhausen and associates investigated whether NT-proBNP forecasts the value of routine invasive therapy in ACS patients with positive troponins. Increased NT-proBNP levels did not independently predict recurrent MI throughout the follow-up period or identify patients who would benefit from routine invasive therapy, but they did strongly predict death at 1 year (HR 5.0, 95% CI 2.1-11.6 for the highest quartile compared to the lowest 3 quartiles) [67].

Multiple researchers have suggested that NT-proBNP may serve as a potential predictor for stable coronary artery disease. The combination of the NT-proBNP parameter with clinical risk indicators, including echocardiographic parameters, CRP, treadmill exercise capacity, and New York Heart Association Classification of increased cardiovascular event, resulted in a statistically significant increase in the area under the ROC curve from 0.76 to 0.80 (P = 0.006) [68]. An elevated risk of cardiovascular death (hazard ratio [HR] 1.69, 95% confidence interval [CI] 1.38-2.07), fatal or non-fatal congestive heart failure (HR 2.35, 95% CI 1.86-2.98), and fatal or non-fatal stroke (HR 1.63, 95% CI 1.26-2.12) was observed with each standard deviation increase in log-transformed NT-proBNP levels. However, no significant association was found between log-transformed NT-proBNP levels and fatal or non-fatal myocardial infarction (HR 1.02, 95% CI 0.87 I). The inclusion of NT-proBNP in a conventional risk factor model resulted in a statistically significant increase in the area under the receiver operating characteristic (ROC) curve for cardiovascular mortality, from 0.74 to 0.77 (p < 0.05) [69]. Following multivariable adjustment, the Heart Protection Study observed a significant association between elevated NT-proBNP levels (highest quintile compared to lowest quintile) and a 2.3-fold higher risk of cardiovascular death, myocardial infarction, stroke, or revascularization. This study included a cohort of 20,536 patients who were followed for an average duration of 5 years [70].

Olsen *et al.* examined the prognostic value of NT-proBNP in a sizable population sample of 2,656 randomly chosen Danes, only 5% of whom had experienced an MI or stroke in the past. Only one standard deviation increase in log (NT-proBNP) was discovered to be a significant predictor of the composite end-point of cardiovascular death, non-fatal MI, or non-fatal stroke after 4.9 years of follow-up (HR 1.56, 95% CI 1.33-1.83) [71].

Cystatin C

The CST3 gene encodes cystatin C, which is a clinical indicator of kidney function. Its ability to predict new or worsening cardiovascular disease has been reported by several investigators. Cystatin C may also predict amyloid-related brain illnesses like Alzheimer's disease. This new clinical biomarker of kidney malfunction and moderate glomerular filtration rate reduction are considered a better indicator than serum creatinine measure and elevated CVD risk. Ix *et al.* diagnosed 990 stable CAD patients using Cystatin C [72]. The authors found that after correcting for established cardiovascular risk factors, those in the highest quartile of cystatin C levels had a higher risk of all-cause mortality, cardiovascular events, and acute heart failure. In another study of 509 subjects with type I diabetes and no cardiovascular disease, Maahs and co-workers examined the role of cystatin C and coronary artery calcium score development. Cystatin C outperformed blood creatinine or glomerular filtration rate as a superior predictor of coronary artery calcium development during a follow-up of 2.5 years [73].

Lipoprotein-Associated Phospholipase A2 (Lp-PLA2)

Lp-PLA2, a calcium-independent enzyme belonging to the phospholipase A2 family, serves as an additional biomarker for atherosclerosis. Atherosclerotic lesions, specifically complicated plaques, and thin cap coronary lesions that rupture or detach inside the arterial bloodstream, exhibit a higher prevalence. The production of the substance is attributed to monocytes, macrophages, T-lymphocytes, and mast cells. The plasma isoform of Lp-PLA2 is conveyed with LDL, HDL, and very low-density lipoprotein (VLDL) [74, 75].

LDL serves as a reservoir for Lp-PLA2 until it undergoes oxidation. Following the process of LDL oxidation within the artery wall, Lp-PLA2 enzymatically cleaves an oxidised phosphatidylcholine component of the lipoprotein particle. This cleavage occurs by the hydrolysis of a short acyl group at the sn-2 position of phospholipids. As a result, two very influential mediators, namely LysoPC and oxFA, are generated. These mediators possess significant pro-inflammatory and pro-atherogenic properties [76]. LysoPC has been observed to promote apoptosis in macrophages, as well as stimulate macrophage proliferation, SMC dysfunction, and endothelial dysfunction. Lp-PLA2 has been proposed as a potential mediator connecting plaque inflammation and LDL oxidation within the arterial intima [74, 77 - 80]. Multiple studies have yielded findings suggesting that the early assessment of ACS Lp-PLA2 may not serve as a reliable predictor for the recurrence of CVD [81 - 83]. Hence, further investigations are necessary to ascertain the clinical use of this biomarker.

MicroRNAs

MicroRNAs are endogenous gene expression regulators and are involved in the pathophysiology of inflammation-induced chronic diseases. Stable circulating miRNAs are novel biomarkers for CVDs. Modulation of miR-21 is regarded as a robust clinical biomarker of atherosclerosis and regulator of plaque formation. MicroRNAs (miRNAs or miRs) are 17-25 nucleotide non-coding RNAs that interfere with messenger RNA's 3' untranslated region (UTR) to regulate gene expression at the translational level [84]. The miRNAs and mRNAs affect protein synthesis, producing diseases like atherogenesis [85]. It was observed that miRNAs activate, proliferate, and senescence atherosclerosis. AMI and severe vascular disease increase PBMC miR-21 expression [86, 87]. A higher level of miR-21 macrophages makes foam cells in the endothelium. Berkan *et al.* have shown the miR-486-5p downregulation to atherosclerotic plaque formation [88 - 90].

Hypothyroidism patients with high thyroxine stimulating hormone (TSH) and MiR-146a may be inflicted with severe atherosclerosis. TSH promotes endothelial dysfunction, which in turn stimulates smooth muscle cell proliferation [91, 92]. OBS patients with elevated carotid IMT exhibited higher miR-664a-3p levels [93]. Post-stent MiR-195 may indicate ischemia. miR-195 inhibits SMC proliferation and neointima. Reduced stenting promotes adverse ischemia events two years later [94]. Hyperhomocysteinemia-induced inflammation and VSMC proliferation increase atherosclerosis risk [95]. Hyperhomocysteinemia and atherosclerosis patients expressed more miR-217 than controls [96]. Silent information regulator 1 modulates endothelial function by suppressing miR-217 [97].

The downregulation of miR-126, which inhibits the proliferation of SMC and the Notch1 inhibitor delta-like 1 homolog, may indicate cerebral atherosclerosis [98]. According to research, miR-126 and miR-143 had an impact on the severity of cerebral atherosclerosis in aged people [99]. In antiphospholipid syndrome, antiphospholipid antibodies change the protein expression and microRNAs, which helps to cause atherosclerosis. A biomarker of early atherogenesis may be miR-19b/miR-124, which has been linked to inflammation and thrombosis [100, 101] and maybe one. Apoe -/-mice exhibit an increase in the fibrous cap of atherosclerotic carotid lesions due to SMC survival and proliferation brought on by miRNA-210 overexpression [102]. In CAD patients, higher miR-146a/146b expression was linked to atherosclerosis [103]. miR-221 and miR-222 are regarded as diagnostic, theranostic, and prognostic indicators in atherosclerosis and inflammatory diseases [104]. In a demographic and ethnic subgroup analysis, Liu *et al.* found significant associations between microRNA-146a rs2910164 polymorphism and CVD risk. MicroRNA-196a2, rs11614913, microRNA-499, and its SNP (Single Nucleotide Polymorphism) rs3746444 have all been found to increase the risk of CVD [105].

Four miRNAs, including miR-1, miR-208a/b, miR-133a, and miR-499 are increased and move through the bloodstream after AMI [106 - 109]: (1) miR-1 (vital for early cardiogenesis and present in cardiac and skeletal muscles; increases apoptosis and worsens oxidative stress in injured cardiomyocytes; produced in AMI implies cardiac myocyte necrosis as its cause; downregulated in hypertrophic hearts); (2) miR-133a (encourages cardiogenesis, heart function, and pathology; collaborates with miR-1 to regulate the early stages of cardiogenesis and regulates cardiac conductance); (3) MiR-208a According to a research by Liu *et al.* [110], miR-208a and miR-370 may help with CAD patient diagnosis, and combining the two miRNAs may enhance CAD diagnosis.

Eight CAD biomarkers were found by Chen *et al.*, including miR1, miR-21, miR-126, miR-133, miR-145, miR-208, miR-223, and miR-499. Patients with coronary artery stenosis displayed elevated miR-21 [111] after experiencing cardiac stress for 24 hours. After the beginning of symptoms, miR-126 levels and hsCRP were decreased in AMI patients. The administration of aspirin decreased miR-126. MiR-145 lower levels indicated CAD severity [112, 113]. MiR-223 is a promising cardiovascular death biomarker since, in contrast to other miRNAs, its levels were higher in CAD patients and were linked to an elevated risk of mortality and AMI [114, 115].

Despite the improvements in assessing the diagnostic value of miRNAs as potential CVD biomarkers [115], there are still many difficulties and unanswered problems. First, more research needs to be done on the therapeutic relevance of miRNA-based CVD phenotypic regulation. Secondly, How do mRNAs and miRNAs affect gene expression? Thirdly, the detection and management of atherosclerosis-related CVD may be aided by circulating or tissue-resident miRNAs. Fourthly, it is unknown how co-morbidities affect the levels of miRNA. Fifth, more research is necessary to understand how statins alter miRNA expression.

Osteocalcin (OC)

Bone osteoblasts release non-collagenous synthetic protein osteocalcin (OC). The complex of OC and calcium ions governs hydroxyapatite crystals in the bone extracellular matrix [116, 117]. Osteoblasts, chondrocytes, and osteoblast-like VSMCs produce pro-protein OC. Uncarboxylated OC (uOC) pro-protein lacks signal peptide. 1,25(OH)2D3 increases OC expression in humans and rats, whereas it decreases OC expression in mice [118]. However, clinical observational trial results are inconsistent regarding OC expression [119]. About 20% of cOC enters the bloodstream and the rest binds to bone calcium. cOC reduces osteoclast resorption in bone, and active bone resorption can decarboxylate cOC into uOC. Vitamin K reduces ucOC's bone mineral binding affinity and prevents its release into blood [120, 121]. How cOCs enter into the bloodstream and subsequently into the blood vessels to produce calcification remains unknown [118]. It has been suggested that dietary supplements and vitamin K may alter OC isoforms, energy metabolism, and atherosclerosis [122]. Low-ucOC can cause abdominal aortic calcification [123, 124].

OC is not only connected to bone functions; it can also affect some other physiological processes, including brain growth and function, which helps explain how cognitive ability declines with age [125]. In addition to improving glucose tolerance and promoting male fertility by raising testosterone production, OC can stimulate the expression of cyclin D1, insulin, and adiponectin (an insulin-sensitizing adipokine) in adipocytes and pancreatic cells [126 - 129].

OC increases CVD-related morbidity, mortality, and vascular calcification. Endochondral or membranous bones, like cartilage, are likewise biomineralized by OC. To create VSMC osteoblast-like, it decreases markers of smooth muscle cells and enhances osteogenic markers such as alkaline phosphatase [130]. Rached *et al.* claim that FoxO1 controls the physiology of osteoblasts, oxidative stress, atherosclerosis, and bone remodeling [131].

OC causes endothelial necrosis and dysfunction that promotes arteriosclerosis. Also, FFA overload impairs endothelial function [132, 133]. OC stimulates PI3-kinase/Akt and protects endothelial cells from FFA [134]. Endothelial progenitor cells (EPCs), which form vascular endothelium in atherosclerosis patients, are promoted by OC [135]. EPCs exacerbate atherosclerotic changes and distinguish stable from unstable patients [136]. Diabetes and peripheral vascular disease lower EPCs. The EPC reduction may cause diabetic peripheral vascular issues [137].

Pancreatic beta cells and adipocytes regulate OC-mediated glucose and lipid metabolism [138]. OC boosts pancreatic beta cell insulin production and glucose tolerance [139, 140]. Low OC levels predicted T2DM in Japanese postmenopausal women [139]. Carotid atherosclerosis and low OC levels were found in T2DM and Chinese postmenopausal women [141, 142]. Patients with carotid artery dysfunction had a lesser concentration of OC [143]. In 1077 male Chang Feng study participants with normal glucose tolerance, OC independently predicted carotid atherosclerosis [144].

Subclinical vitamin K deficiency in Chronic Kidney Disease (CKD) patients produced c-OC. CKD worsened in heart disease patients, elevating dp-ucOC [145, 146]. According to a study by Jia *et al.*, OC increases the risk of vascular calcification. However, this study did not differentiate between cOC and unOC. More investigation is required on the connection between UnOC and vascular calcification [147]. HD patients showed lower c-OC and higher unOC than healthy ones [128]. Rapid bone turnover HD and pre-dialysis CKD patients had serum ucOC/intact OC ratios > 1.0 [148]. Kidney transplant recipients with greater serum OC exhibited lower VRI and poorer endothelial dysfunction [149 - 151]. It has been suggested that vascular reactivity reduces ESRD survival rates [149].

In a study, Yeap *et al.* revealed that total serum OC predicted all-cause and CVD-related mortality in 3,542 community-dwelling men aged 70-89 in a U-shaped distribution [151]. Whereas, Hwang *et al.* observed the opposite results [152]. After controlling for other CVD risk factors, total OC blood levels were not associated with CVD in 1,290 males aged 40–78 frequently followed at the Health Promotion Center as outpatients and hospitalized for 8.7 years. These inconsistencies require more investigations to determine if the altered bone turnover rate or OC's biological activities are responsible for causing atherosclerosis [152].

While a higher amount of serum OC has been linked to adverse cardiovascular events, atherosclerotic-induced CVD may be curable. Arguably, total OC may not indicate arterial calcification and atherosclerosis risk, but the physiologically active isoform of OC should be determined. Although a few ucOC/cOC tests are available, the clinical relevance of the test system accuracy is unclear due to OC comparability and heterogeneity [147], and ethnicity [153]. Furthermore, OC has a circadian cycle that peaks at night; therefore, blood sampling time may affect the results obtained [154]. In addition, vitamin K [155], vitamin D, and bone metabolism impact OC. In conclusion, the current research relating OC to atherosclerosis and vascular calcification may not predict the incidence of atherosclerosis and CVD with precision.

Angiogenin (ANG)

ANG is a 14-kDa protein ribonuclease (RNase) enzyme found in human tissues and bodily fluids including plasma, amniotic fluid, the tumor microenvironment, and cerebrospinal fluid. Additionally, it is discovered in cancer cells, nuclear, and stress-related cytoplasmic compartments. ANG plays a role in tissue regeneration, reproduction, innate immunity, neuro-protection, and anti-inflammation processes [156 - 159].

Angiogenesis and atherosclerosis are complicated phenomena [160, 161]. ANG may promote atherosclerotic plaque formation and the production of microvessels. Fragile and discontinuous endothelium-lined thin-walled vasculature lack VSMC support. The plaque-induced hemorrhage causes ACS and blood vessel occlusion [162]. Tissue plasminogen activator (tPA) and wound-healing proteases like metalloproteinases enhance plasmin generation [163, 164]. Since proteases weaken atherosclerotic plaque, the angiogenic factors may predict ACS [162].

Plasma ANG was identified by Krciki *et al.* as a biochemical risk factor in 107 patients with three-vessel CAD and 15 controls. The control group had coronary stenosis, an abnormal stress test result, aberrant segmental contractility, and ACS. Resistin, adiponectin, IL-8, and TNF-α were present in both groups. Gensini scores are employed to gauge the severity of CAD. It is a frequently used method of angiographic atherosclerosis quantification, where a score of 0 indicates the absence of atherosclerotic disease. Patients with CAD (414 ng/mL *vs.* 275, p = 0.02) and a higher Gensini score (0.06) were shown to have higher ANG levels [165].

In another study, Tello-Montoliu *et al.* assessed ANG in 396 ACS patients (63.4% men, mean age 67), 44 stable CAD, and 76 healthy controls (gensini score was p < 0.001). Death, recurrent ACS, revascularization, and heart failure were followed up to six months. At six months, elevated troponin T, electrocardiographic abnormalities, and ANG predicted worse outcomes (p = 0.008) [162].

Jiang *et al.* examined NT-proBNP in addition to evaluating ANG as a diagnostic marker for heart failure (HF). They discovered that in HF patients, ANG values were positively correlated (p 0.001). In individuals with heart failure (HFPEF),

ANG (426 ng/mL) and an intact ejection fraction predicted all-cause death. Patients with advanced troponin T exhibited ANG levels between 290 and 450 ng/mL [166]. 109 CHF patients (85 men, mean age 60) and 112 healthy controls were studied by Patel *et al.* They measured the plasma levels of ANG and BNP and discovered that CHF had statistically significantly higher levels of ANG than controls (p 0.001). Age, plasma glucose, insulin, and BNP were all favorably connected with ANG (p 0.001), although diastolic blood pressure was inversely correlated (p = 0.04) [167].

Angiogenesis, neovascularization, stress adaptation and survival, cell signaling processes, and stem cell homeostasis are all physiologically regulated by ANG. More research is needed on the function of ANG in cancer, microbial infection, and rare disorders including amyotrophic lateral sclerosis [168]. The biological tool ANG—Ribonuclease inhibitor 1 (RNH1), which protects RNA against RNAse [169], can be used to measure angiogenesis and to diagnose CVD, ACS, CAD, and CHF.

Monocyte Chemoattractant Protein-1 (MCP-1)

CC chemokine receptor 2 (CCR2) is primarily activated by MCP-1 and CCL-2 (Monocyte Chemotactic Protein -1), which regulate monocyte/macrophage movement and penetration into the arterial wall. MCP-1 is expressed by ECs, monocytes, and/or SMCs in response to cytokines, growth factors, oxLDL, and CD40L [170]. MCP-1 is also expressed in atherosclerotic lesions, particularly those with macrophage-rich areas [171]. MCP-1 induces thrombosis, oxidative stress, plaque neovascularization, endothelial cell migration, and smooth muscle cell proliferation [172]. The MCP-1/CCR2 pathway also results in MMPs103, indicating a role in plaque destabilization.

According to reports, apolipoprotein E-deficient animals treated with anti-monocyte MCP-1 gene therapy had their atherosclerosis stabilized. The degree of atherosclerosis and the presence of macrophages were both linked with MCP-1 expression. These findings suggest that MCP-1 may be a viable therapeutic target for atherosclerosis [173 - 175].

MCP-1 levels preceded CHD in a sizable case-cohort analysis from the MONICA/KORA Augsburg database, but other risk variables also predicted CHD risk [176, 177]. Therefore, additional clinical trials in a variety of populations are required before MCP-1 may be used as a therapeutic and diagnostic biomarker.

Placental Growth Factor (PLGF)

PLGF, a 50-kDa angiogenic protein containing a cysteine knot, and VEGF have 40% of the same amino acid sequence. The effects of VEGF may be exacerbated by PLGF hetero dimerization. The placenta is where PLGF is largely produced, while it is also expressed in the thyroid, heart, and lungs [178]. Only the early and advanced stages of atherosclerosis increase its expression [179]. PLGF has powerful proatherogenic properties in addition to its physiological roles during pregnancy. These consist of the development and movement of EC and SMC, the chemotactic attraction of circulating monocytes and macrophages to atherosclerotic lesions, and the overexpression of numerous cytokines, such as TNF-α [179, 180]. In apoE-deficient mice, PLGF decreases early atherosclerotic plaques and macrophages, increasing atherosclerosis. Periadventitial PLGF adenoviral gene transfer increased intimal thickness, neointimal macrophage accumulation, and adventitial neovascularization in hypercholesterolemic rabbit carotid arteries [181].

The prognostic potential of PLGF in ACS has only been studied in a small number of clinical trials. PLGF levels were assessed in 626 chest pain patients in emergency department and 547 CAPTURE placebo participants over 30 hospital days. In these two populations, elevated PLGF levels were linked to major negative outcomes (death or non-fatal MI) independently of troponin, sCD40L, and CRP [182]. Increased PLGF concentrations continued to be an important and independent predictor of mortality or MI during the follow-up period of the CAPTURE research, which was prolonged from 1 to 48 months [183]. The database, however, did not support the clinical utility of PLGF as a risk biomarker.

Pregnancy-Associated Plasma Protein-A (PAPP-A)

PAPP-A is a high-molecular-weight zinc-binding metalloproteinase that can release cells into the extracellular matrix and activate cells in unstable plaques. PAPP-A was abundantly expressed in both eroded and ruptured coronary and carotid plaques, particularly in cap and shoulder monocyte/macrophages, according to studies utilizing monoclonal antibodies [184, 185], while it was weakly expressed in a stable plaque. After PAPP-A eliminates IGF-binding proteins-4 and -5, insulin-like growth factor (IGF-1) can attach to cell-surface type-1 IGF receptors [186]. In addition to inhibiting plaque growth and destabilization, PAPP-A can degrade extracellular matrix, cell proliferation, differentiation, migration, inflammatory cell activation, LDL-cholesterol absorption, and cytokine release by IGF-1 [184].

In individuals with stable CHD and ACS, PAPP-A has been investigated as a clinical biomarker. In a brief trial, patients with unstable angina and MI had greater PAPP-A levels than the controls [184]. In 200 patients with ACS who lacked troponin, PAPP-A levels predicted ischemic heart episodes and revascularization over six months [187]. In the CAPTURE study, the estimation of PAPP-A levels predicted death and MI in patients with positive and negative troponin levels. In a multivariable analysis, PAPP-A, sCD40L, IL-10, and VEGF each independently predicted the result [188]. In STEMI patients, elevated PAPP-A levels predicted 12-month death and recurrent non-fatal MI [189]. In stable CHD patients, PAPP-A and its endogenous inhibitor, proMBP, were linked to complex angiographic stenosis morphology, impending death, and ACS [190, 191]. PAPP-A may prevent inflammation and tissue damage even if it produced unfavorable inflammatory results in some studies [192]. Recent research showed that a PAPP-A variation associated with ACS does not interact with proeosinophil major basic protein (proMBP), enabling more targeted testing [193]. Therefore, more clinical and mechanistic research is needed to fully explore PAPP-A's potential for ACS risk classification.

Soluble CD40 Ligand (CD40L)

CD40 and CD40L are co-expressed by all cells involved in atherosclerosis, activated T lymphocytes, vascular endothelial cells, smooth muscle cells, and monocytes/macrophages. Proatherogenic adhesion molecules, chemokines (including MCP-1), cytokines, growth factors, and MMPs are increased by CD40/CD40L interactions. Prothrombotic tissue factor and thrombomodulin are increased by CD40L [194]. OxLDL may upregulate CD40/CD40L [195]. CD40 signaling caused atherosclerosis in LDL receptor-deficient mice. Interrupting CD40 signaling dramatically slowed lesion growth. Mouse atheroma collagen lesions increased rapidly, changing plaque phenotype [196 - 198]. Plaque rupture cleaves CD40L. Soluble CD40L may activate ECs and other CD40-expressing cells in atherosclerotic plaques and produce a vessel wall proinflammatory cascade. High-risk carotid atheroma lesions cause an increase in intraplaque lipid content and sCD40L [199].

Some studies have connected sCD40L to fatal or non-fatal MI. Statins and abciximab elevated the levels of sCD40L in MI patients. Thus, sCD40L may predict ACS thrombotic risk and may be used as a potential biomarker in CVD.

COST-EFFECTIVE STRATEGIES TO PREVENT ATHEROSCLEROSIS AND CARDIOVASCULAR DISEASES

Particularly in low- and middle-income countries, urbanization, industrialization, and globalization have changed people's eating and lifestyle habits, which has raised the risk of non-communicable diseases (NCDs) like diabetes mellitus, obesity, atherosclerosis, hypertension, and cardiometabolic disorders (CMDs). The prevalence of NCDs has increased as a result of diets heavy in processed carbohydrates, saturated fats, high sugar, and salt content, and low in fresh produce. Numerous studies have established a connection between poor dietary practices, a sedentary lifestyle, excessive cigarette and alcohol use, and coronary heart disease, stroke, obesity, and diabetes. According to a study by Micha *et al.*, 1 in 2 CVD deaths in the US were caused by CMDs, and the majority of these deaths were linked to a diet low in fruits, vegetables, fiber, nuts and seeds, and seafood and high in red meat, saturated fat, processed foods, and high sodium levels [8]. It is now widely accepted that adopting healthy eating practices and consuming anti-inflammatory and antioxidant foods lower the incidence of NCDs.

The following sections discuss probiotics, fruits, vegetables, and anti-inflammatory diets that are thought to lower the incidence of NCDs and CMDs as well as morbidity and mortality from heart disease, stroke, and type 2 diabetes globally:

Berries: Rubus (Family: Rosaceae)

Berries are rich in fiber, vitamins, and antioxidant and anti-inflammation flavonoids. Berries help to lower LDL levels, blood pressure, and serum blood sugar [200, 201], whereas serum triglycerides and total cholesterol remain unaffected. Clinically recognized effects include cholesterol transferase inhibition and LDL-cholesterol peroxidation. Berries inhibit foam cell formation and plaque progression in the vascular intima, thus lowering atherosclerosis risk [200].

Beans: *Phaseolus vulgaris* (Family: Fabaceae)

Beans contain a high amount of soluble dietary fiber and have shown several health benefits, including heart health. Eating beans and pulses reduce the risk of atherosclerosis [202]. They can also minimize the dose and dose-related adverse effects of statin monotherapy, enhancing medication tolerance. One meta-analysis of 26 high-quality randomized control studies found that diets with roughly 1 serving (130 g) of beans daily had significantly lower LDL (bad) cholesterol than control diets [203, 204]. Another 2001 US epidemiological study found that eating legumes or beans three times a week compared to once a week reduced CVD risk by 11% and CHD risk by 22% [205]. In the large intestine, soluble dietary fibers ferment to short-chain fatty acids without intestinal enzyme hydrolysis. Short-chain fatty acids promote intestinal microbiota, decreasing hepatic absorption and increasing bile and fecal lipid excretion. Beans reduce LDL-cholesterol but not triglycerides.

Depending on the age and gender, the 2015–2020 Dietary Guidelines for Americans (DGA) recommend 1000–3200 calories per day in 12 different diet groups. To meet the weekly requirements for dark-green, red/orange, starchy, legumes, and other vegetables, a typical 2000-calorie diet is advised to consume 2.5 cups of equivalent (c-eq) of vegetables daily [205]. Fig. (**4**) shows various health benefits of consuming beans and legumes.

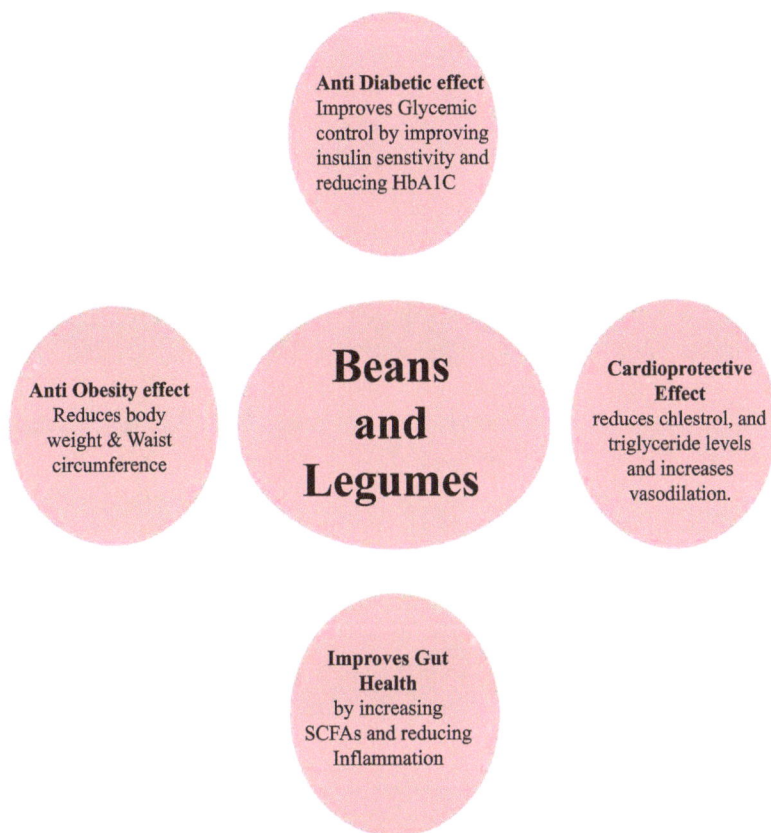

Anti Diabetic effect
Improves Glycemic control by improving insulin senstivity and reducing HbA1C

Anti Obesity effect
Reduces body weight & Waist circumference

Beans and Legumes

Cardioprotective Effect
reduces chlestrol, and triglyceride levels and increases vasodilation.

Improves Gut Health
by increasing SCFAs and reducing Inflammation

Fig. (4). Various health benefits of consuming beans and legumes.

Sea Food

High concentrations of omega-3 fatty acids (O-3 PUFA) found in seafood and fish meals lower the risk of atherosclerosis. Numerous studies have shown that omega-3 PUFA suppresses VCAM-1 and ICAM-1, cell membrane adhesion molecules that allow cells to interact and initiate an inflammatory response. ICAM-1 levels are decreased by fish flesh, whereas VCAM-1 levels are unaffected [206 - 208]. Carotid atherosclerosis risk is decreased by fish consumption. 3-n PUFA inhibits platelet and macrophage, cyclooxygenase, and lipoxygenase, as well as reducing endothelial inflammation and plaque progression. They also suppress hepatic triglyceride and apoprotein synthesis. They replace arachidonic acid (ERA) with EPA and DHA [209, 210].

Tomatoes and tomato products (Family: Solanaceae)

Lycopene, a carotenoid with anti-inflammatory and antioxidant properties, is abundant in tomatoes. Inflammation and CVD risk are reduced by retinoid-rich foods such as tomatoes and tomato products [211, 112]. Tomatoes cooked in olive oil express the most adhesion molecules and inflammatory proteins [213]. It has been reported that lycopene inhibits endothelial damage, LDL-cholesterol oxidation, foam cell production, and the proinflammatory cascade that causes plaque progression [214].

Onions (*Allium sativum, A. cepa* - Family: Amaryllidaceae)

One of the most widely used spices globally; onions are often used in their raw or processed forms. The high sulfate content of onions and the antioxidant polyphenolic flavonoid quercetin are primarily responsible for their health benefits. Onions also contain several vitamins (B1, B2, C), potassium, and selenium. Many studies have reported that onions' high sulfur content and quercetin reduce cellular inflammation and platelet agglutination, cause vasodilation, and increase NO levels in the endothelium. Onions protect against coronary heart disease and stroke by slowing plaque formation in the vascular intima [215, 216]. A 15-year cohort research found that allium and cruciferous vegetables, which are high in organic sulfur, help in scavenging ROS and decreasing the incidence of atherosclerotic vascular disorders [216].

Citrus Fruits

Lemons, oranges, and grapefruit are high in vitamins A and C, fiber, minerals, and antioxidant flavonoids. These exogenous antioxidants scavenge ROS in the arterial walls, thereby reducing atherosclerosis-related inflammation and LDL-cholesterol peroxidation [217]. According to Gorinstein *et al.*, citrus fruits protect against atherosclerosis by lowering plasma triglycerides in CVD patients [218]. Miwa *et al.* observed that the bioactive citrus fruit ingredient, hesperidin (500 mg/day), can lower plasma triglycerides in hyperlipidaemic and hypertriglyceridemia patients [219].

Culinary Spices

Culinary spices such as black pepper, ginger, cinnamon, chili, onion, garlic, and turmeric reduce atherosclerosis and CVD risk [220]. These spices contain natural antioxidants and anti-inflammatory agents that can scavenge ROS, lower blood lipid levels, and prevent platelet clumping. Black pepper contains a strong antioxidant, piperine, that reduces platelet aggregation and prevents the inflammatory cascade that causes arterial plaque development and progression [221]. Rosemary, a key Mediterranean spice, also has cardioprotection. It reduces headache, dizziness, hair loss, and bloating effects. Rosmanol and epirosmanol present in rosemary extract inhibit LDL-cholesterol peroxidation and prevent foam cell formation in the endothelium [222]. Traditional Ayurvedic remedies have frequently used turmeric to treat swellings, chronic inflammation, and gastrointestinal disorders. Curcumin and curcuminoids are the bioactive ingredients of turmeric, with antioxidant, anti-apoptotic and anti-cancer properties. Curcumin can inhibit NF-kB activity, making it an effective anti-inflammatory and anticancer agent. Curcumin helps to prevent cardiovascular and neurodegenerative diseases. Curcuminoids reduce plasma triglycerides and LDL-cholesterol and increase high-density lipoprotein (HDL) [223, 224]. However, curcumin's therapeutic usage is limited due to its poor solubility, less absorption from the intestine, and low systemic bioavailability. Novel methods (microencapsulation, nanocarrier, nanoformulation) are being developed to enhance the absorption, bioavailability, and biological activity of curcumin.

Flaxseeds (Family: Linaceae)

Flaxseeds are rich in fiber, vitamins, minerals, and unsaturated fats. Due to their high fiber content, flaxseeds have laxative properties and also help to increase HDL-cholesterol. Administration of flaxseeds supplemented diet for 14 weeks caused atherosclerosis plaque regression in rabbits fed a 40% high-cholesterol diet [225]. The bioactive ingredient of flax seeds is secoisolariciresinol diglucoside (SDG), which is a powerful anti-inflammatory and cholesterol-lowering lignan [226].

Beetroot (*Beta vulgaris*)- Family: Chenopodiaceae

Redbeet and sugarbeet are other names for beetroot. The biological effects of beetroot fruit and juice are attributed to the components betanin, beta-cyanin, and betalain, which have potent anti-inflammatory and antioxidant properties. Inorganic nitrate (NO), fiber, vitamins, minerals, and fiber are all abundant in beetroot juice. A kilogram of fresh beet juice contains roughly 250 mg of NO. Beetroot nitrates have potent antithrombotic and vasodilator effects on the body. Pro-inflammatory cytokines and platelet aggregation are decreased as a result of NO's reduction of platelet adhesion to the endothelium. Atherosclerosis and CVD risk are reduced by beetroot-rich diets [227, 228].

Whole grains (Families: Poaceae and Gramineae*)*

Whole grain cereals (bran, endosperm, and germ) consist of carbohydrates, fiber, and bioactive peptides, which possess anticancer, antioxidant, and antithrombotic properties. Several investigators have explored the CVD-reducing actions of whole grains. For instance, Jacobs and Gallaher found that frequent consumption of whole grain cereals reduced CHD risk by 20% to 40% in 17 prospective cohort studies [229]. In a meta-analysis of 12 prospective cohort studies, Anderson *et al.* found that whole grain eaters had a 26% lower risk of CHD [230].

Oats (Poaceae Grass, *Avena sativa*)

Oats contain beta-glucan and avenanthramides. These antioxidants suppress cytokines and adhesion molecules [4]. A study in mice showed that oats and oat bran diet lowered pro-inflammatory markers, enhanced endothelial nitric oxide synthesis (eNOS), and minimized plaque development in LDL receptor-deficient mice [231]. Oats also mitigated the risk of atherosclerosis and high LDL-cholesterol levels in humans [232 - 234]. Wu *et al.* observed that oats containing diet reduced LDL levels and inflammatory markers, including CRP and TNF-α in 716 Chinese CAD patients. It was concluded that oats fiber decreases plasma LDL levels and controls the inflammatory cascade that causes plaque development and revascularization [235].

Cocoa and Dark Chocolate

Theobroma cacao, a tropical plant seed, is the source of cocoa and dark chocolate products. Flavor-rich and pleasant taste chocolates are consumed all over the world. Their health advantages result from the antioxidant polyphenolics they absorb. Increased consumption of cocoa and dark chocolate, as reported by Djoussé *et al.*, resulted in decreased calcification of atherosclerotic plaques in the coronary arteries of 2,217 individuals [236]. Because cocoa and dark chocolate contain significant levels of polyphenols and NO, they have been shown to have anti-atherogenic properties. By lowering NOX2-mediated oxidative stress and increasing peripheral oxygenation in the hypoxic regions of the body, Lofferedo *et al.* discovered that a short-term intervention with dark chocolate, as opposed to milk chocolate, reduced atherosclerosis and improved physical function in people. Dark chocolate can therefore be a healthy addition to the diet of people who have a higher risk of developing atherosclerosis [237].

Olive Oil (Family: Oleaceae)

Olive oil is a liquid fat extracted from the fruit of *Olea europea*. Mediterranean cuisine traditionally uses olive oil as an essential fat product for frying and salad dressing. Olive oil has multiple therapeutic applications in addition to its cooking utilities. Due to its high concentration of antioxidant/anti-inflammation polyphenols, reduction of total cholesterol, increase in HDL cholesterol, and normalization of blood triglyceride lipids, numerous clinical trials have demonstrated that olive oil has cardioprotective and neuroprotective properties. Both extra virgin and extra refined olive oils are widely used in the Mediterranean diet and throughout the world. Extra virgin olive oil contains a larger level of antioxidant and anti-inflammation polyphenols than refined olive oil.

Widmer *et al.* discovered that the daily use of one ounce (30 ml) of extra virgin olive oil for four months dramatically improved participants' blood vessel function and lowered inflammatory markers in a randomized trial of 82 individuals with early atherosclerosis [238]. Polyphenols in olive oil offer a wide range of health-protective qualities, including anti-inflammatory, anti-allergic, anti-atherogenic, anti-thrombotic, and anti-mutagenic actions, according to an excellent review by Gorzynik-Debicka *et al.* According to certain theories, polyphenols can prevent or delay the onset of cancer, and cardiovascular, and neurological illnesses [239].

Nuts and Seeds

Humans consume a vast range of dry seeds and nuts. A nut is a fruit with a large amount of endosperm and a hard seed shell that gets harder with time, according to botany. The dry drupe form of some well-known nuts, including pecans (*Carya illinoensis*), almonds (*Prunus amygdalus*), macadamias (*Macadamia integrifolia*), candlenuts (*Aleurites moluccanus*), water caltrops (*Trapa bicornis*), and walnuts (*Juglans regia*), is known as drupes. Nuts and seeds are a great source of omega-3 fatty acids and amino acids. Nuts and seeds also contain phytosterols, bioactive phytochemicals, protein, fiber, vitamins, and non-sodium minerals. Regular nut and seed consumption has been associated with a reduced risk of CHD, and CVD, as well as other diseases like cancer, diabetes mellitus, obesity, and conditions of the brain (dementia, Alzheimer's, and Parkinson's disease). According to a cohort study's meta-analysis, people who said they ate nuts had a 37% (95% CI: 0.51 to 0.83) lower risk of CHD. The risk of CHD-related fatalities was almost 8.3% reduced for each weekly serving (or 30 g) of nuts [240]. The benefits of walnuts and walnut oil for cardiovascular health are linked to improved endothelial function, decreased levels of oxidative stress and pro-inflammatory cytokines, and increased cholesterol efflux from peripheral organs [241].

ANTIOXIDANT/ANTI-INFLAMMATORY DIETS AND THEIR POTENTIAL ROLE IN THE PREVENTION OF ATHEROSCLEROSIS AND CARDIOVASCULAR DISEASES

The anti-atherosclerogenic effects of dietary treatments in humans are a subject of disagreement among cardiovascular researchers. Some researchers think dietary adjustments can postpone the initiation of atherosclerosis and prevent the development of CHD, whereas others do not think there is a substantial difference when it comes to these outcomes [6]. In general, dietary adjustments advise cutting less on saturated fats and red meat because they both raise levels of LDH-cholesterol, or bad cholesterol, in the blood. Conversely, eating foods high in unsaturated fats such as avocados, walnuts, fatty fish, nuts, and seeds helps to lower the level of harmful cholesterol in the blood vessels. The consumption of omega-3 and omega-6 polyunsaturated fatty acids (PUFAs) found in marine foods and olive oil is recommended by several Dietary Guidelines as part of a heart-healthy diet [242]. Higher amounts of fruits, green vegetables, legumes, whole grains, dairy products, chicken, and PUFAs are included in the Mediterranean and DASH diets (Dietary Approaches to Stop Hypertension). Numerous carefully planned clinical studies using the Mediterranean and DASH diets have demonstrated that these diets lower the risk of atherosclerosis and CVD-related mortality and morbidity by containing antioxidant and anti-inflammatory ingredients, fewer carbohydrates, and more fiber, as well as probiotics that support healthy microbiota in the gut [243].

Mediterranean-Diet

The Mediterranean diet is acknowledged as a sustainable and beneficial dietary pattern for the prevention of CVDs by the World Health Organization and the United Nations Educational, Scientific, and Cultural Organization [244]. Vegetables, fruits, legumes, nuts, beans, whole grains, fish, poultry, eggs, dairy products, and a small amount of red wine make up the majority of the Mediterranean diet. To balance the diet's overall nutritional value, less red meat is introduced.

The primary source of unsaturated fat in the Mediterranean diet is olive oil. As previously mentioned, olive oil is the primary ingredient in all cooking and salad dressings, and regular use lowers both LDL and total cholesterol levels. Nuts and seeds featured in the Mediterranean diet also contain monounsaturated fat. Fatty fish including mackerel, herring, sardines, albacore tuna, salmon, and lake trout are also a part of the Mediterranean diet. Fatty fish are rich in omega-3 PUFA, which lowers inflammation in the body, stops blood clotting, enhances lipid profiles, and thus lessens the risk of stroke and heart failure.

A population-based study performed in Manhattan in 2014 with 1,374 participants (mean age 66 9 years, 60% female, 60% Hispanic, 18% White, and 19% Black) found that following the Mediterranean diet helped prevent the development of carotid atherosclerotic plaques, which in turn helped prevent cardiac vascular events [245].

Another study's results showed that Med-diet usage regularly reduced the indicators of systemic vascular inflammation and improved endothelial function (Fig. 5). Although the precise mechanism underpinning cardioprotective activity is unknown, it is believed that the high fiber, olive oil, and dietary antioxidant content of the Mediterranean-style diet reduced the temporary endothelial dysfunction that occurs in healthy persons after consuming a high-fat diet [246].

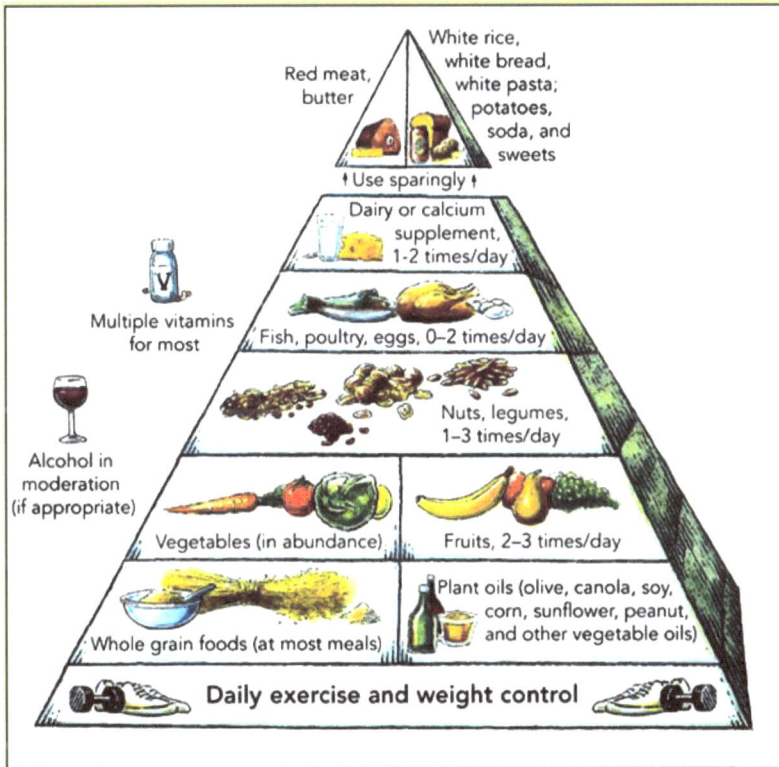

Fig. (5). Mediterranean-style dietary chart depicting portion sizes of various food products.

There is a wealth of data showing that Mediterranean-style diets, which are high in fiber, low in saturated fat, and low in glycemic load, reduce the risk of CVD, metabolic syndrome, and type 2 diabetes. Numerous research carried out in various nations discovered the ecological link between nutrition and the risk of coronary heart disease. Ancel Keys (1904–2004) and his colleagues created one long-term investigation, The Seven Countries investigation, in the 1950s with the primary goal of confirming a potential association between nutrition, lifestyle, and ischemic heart disease [247]. The Mediterranean diet, along with extra virgin olive oil or nuts, considerably lowers the incidence of CVD than the reduced fat diet alone, according to a multicentral trial conducted in Spain with 7,447 individuals who were at high risk for developing CVD [248].

Free Radical Scavenging Actions of Antioxidant and Anti-inflammatory Diets

Oxidative stress is characterized by an imbalance between the body's ability to detoxify ROS and reactive nitrogen species (NOS) and their production and accumulation. It is now widely acknowledged that excessive cellular death in the myocardium during myocardial infarction in humans is predominantly caused by unchecked oxidative stress [249]. Additionally, a great deal of research has shown that oxidative stress is a significant factor in the pathophysiology of atherosclerosis, CHD, and stroke [250]. The peroxidation of LDL cholesterol, which is followed by the activation of macrophages and production of cytokines/interleukins that result in foam cells and plaque deposits in the vascular intima, is a significant stage in the development of atherogenesis, as was previously indicated. Numerous studies' findings have shown that the creation and spread of intimal plaques in arterial blood arteries are mostly caused by the triggered cascade of LDL-cholesterol, macrophage activation, and smooth muscle cell inflammation by cytokines [251]. Exogenous antioxidants (such as vitamin C, E, Zn, and selenium) and endogenous glutathione scavenge ROS/NOS and subsequently prevent atherosclerosis and CVDs, whereas unchecked oxidative stress is the major contributory factor in the pathophysiology of atherosclerosis, CHD, heart attack, and stroke.

Vitamin C

This water-soluble vitamin or ascorbic acid plays an important physiological role in treating scurvy and repair of body organs and tissues. Its antioxidant properties assist in scavenging hydroxyl, superoxide, and ROS [4, 252]. Vitamin C's antioxidant effects are also linked to the prevention of atherosclerosis, and cardiovascular and neurological disorders. The antiatherogenic process appears to involve the prevention of LDL-cholesterol peroxidation, scavenging of oxidized LDL-cholesterol, and consequently the retardation of plaque formation.

One important component in the initiation of atherosclerosis and plaque formation is the adhesion of circulating monocytes to inflamed endothelial lining. It has been demonstrated that vitamin C decreases pro-inflammation cytokines and thereby prevents monocyte adherence to the endothelium. Vitamin C also increases the endothelium's capacity to produce NO, which encourages vasodilation and decreases blood pressure. Vitamin C helps to keep the cardiovascular system healthy and prevents plaque buildup in the coronary blood vessels when consumed regularly [253].

Vitamin E

Due to its strong anti-inflammatory and antioxidant properties, vitamin E has been linked to a range of health advantages, including improved skin, reduced risk of cancer, immune system modulation, and cardioprotective effects. However in multicenter clinical trials, vitamin E supplementation in the diet had no appreciable cardioprotective effects [254]. 40,000 men (4 years of follow-up) and nearly 80,000 women (8 years of follow-up) were enrolled in large-scale prospective research that discovered a significant reduction in the incidence of coronary heart disease with high doses of vitamin E supplements (>100 IU/d) [255]. The most biologically effective form of vitamin E for humans is D-alpha tocopherol, but other chemical forms of vitamin E's fat-soluble components are less helpful to the body. Table **2** shows different cellular and molecular targets of vitamin E against atherosclerosis

Table 2. Different cellular and molecular targets of vitamin E against atherosclerosis.

Target	Biological Function	References
LDL	Suppresses oxidation.	[256]
Lipoproteins	Thrombin generation assembly is suppressed.	[257]
Endothelial cells	Increases prostacyclin synthesis. Cytosolic phospholipase A_2 (cPLA2) and cyclooxygenase (COX) expression are increased. Agonist-induced monocyte adhesion suppressed cell-mediated LDL oxidation. Endothelial expression of adhesion molecules induced by oxidized LDL decreased.	[258 - 262]
SMC	SMC proliferation is reduced.	[263]
Platelets	Attenuated platelet adhesion, aggregation, and release reaction.	[264]
Neutrophils	Leukotriene (LT) synthesis suppressed.	[265]
Monocytes	Monocyte adhesion suppressed.	[266]

PUFAS

PUFAs consist of long chains comprising two or more double bonds between carbon atoms. Nuts, seeds, eggs, and seafood are exceptional sources of polyunsaturated fatty acids (PUFAs). Omega-3 and omega-6 fatty acids are the two primary classes of PUFAs. The chain length of the first double bond in the chemical structure of omega-3 PUFAs ranges from 18 to 22 carbon atoms [267]. Numerous *in vitro* and *in vivo* studies support omega-3 fatty acids' antiatherogenic properties. In addition, omega-3 fatty acids have been shown to influence lipid metabolism, plaque stability, and innate and adaptive immune function. To investigate the modulatory effects of omega-3 fatty acids on atherogenesis, apolipoprotein-E (apoE) deficient mice and LDL-receptor (LDLr) deficient mice were utilized. The development of atherosclerosis was accelerated in rodents fed a high-fat, Western-style diet [268 - 271].

Numerous researchers have investigated the fundamental mechanisms of omega-3 PUFA's protective role, including the protective changes in the structural integrity, fluidity, and morphology of cell membrane lipid rafts. Omega-3 PUFA not only reduced cellular inflammation but also improved cell signal transduction pathways leading to the modulatory action of key transcription factors, such as the inhibition of NF-κB and the activation of peroxisome proliferator-activated receptor [269, 272].

DASH-Diet (Dietary Approaches to Stop Hypertension)

Regular consumption of a flexible and balanced DASH diet is intended to reduce hypertension or elevated blood pressure. The DASH diet consists of foods that are rich in potassium, calcium, magnesium, fiber, and protein while being low in saturated fat, total fat, cholesterol, and sodium. The DASH diet promotes the consumption of whole grains, fat-free or low-fat dairy products, fruits, green vegetables, poultry, salmon, and nuts [273]. Reiterating, extreme care must always be taken to avoid unhealthy diets composed of saturated fatty acids, red meat, full-fat dairy products, tropical oils (coconut, palm, and palm kernel oils), sweet desserts, and sugar-loaded beverages, as these diets promote obesity, diabetes, and cardiometabolic syndrome.

Adherence to the DASH diet has been associated with improved cardiovascular health in adult humans, including a lower incidence of hypertension, type 2 diabetes, heart failure, coronary heart disease, stroke, and total mortality. High adherence to the DASH diet reduced the incidence of CVD in patients with cardiometabolic syndrome, according to a 2001-2005 study conducted by Liese *et al.* on 2,130 young people with diabetes mellitus (10 to 22 years old).

Probiotics and Prebiotics

Probiotics and fiber-rich prebiotics contain live bacteria such as Lactobacillus and Bifidobacterium that enhance the host's immune system and decrease the incidence of pathogenic bacterial and viral infections in the gastrointestinal tract. In humans, they also prevent inflammatory bowel disease (IBD), diabetes, obesity, and colorectal cancer. Consumption of probiotics produces an acidic environment in the gastrointestinal tract and modulates intestinal mucosa homeostasis, increases epithelial cell tolerance through cytoprotective action, binds the exo- and endotoxins produced by pathogenic bacteria, and prevents the invasion of pathogenic bacteria and viruses in the gastrointestinal tract. In contrast, dysbiosis in the intestine can result in acute and chronic inflammation due to an increase in pro-inflammatory cytokines production. Athletes can also develop leaky gut syndrome and respiratory ailments due to dysbiosis. Recent evidence suggests that gut microbiota generate endothelial lining-damaging metabolites such as trimethylamine (TMA) and secondary bile acids. This metabolite promotes atherosclerosis, increases monocyte adhesion to arterial walls, and consequently contributes to CHDand stroke. Prebiotics contain oligosaccharides that are indigestible and promote the development of beneficial bacteria in the gut. Live bacteria such as Lactobacillus, Bifidobacterium, and Streptococcus are well-studied and esteemed probiotics/prebiotics constituents. Fuentes *et al.* observed that *Lactobacillus plantarum* isolates (CECT 7527, 7528, and 7529) reduced circulating cholesterol and plaque formation in the vascular intima of hypercholesteremia patients in a randomized, double-blind clinical trial [274]. Compared to placebo, *Lactobacillus reuteri* (NCIMB 30242) significantly decreased LDL-C and total cholesterol [275].

L. bacillus and *L. plantarum* probiotics have been reported to be well tolerated and able to reduce cardiovascular risk [276]. Ingestion of bioactive compounds derived from plants, such as berberine, can modulate intestinal microflora and reduce the incidence of CVDs. Berberine stimulated Akkermansia in ApoE-/- rodents and decreased atherosclerosis in a mouse study [277]. Resveratrol protects against the cardiovascular risk of TMAO by modifying the expression of gastrointestinal microbiota and barrier genes [278]. Resveratrol decreased TMAO-induced atherosclerosis [279] by increasing hepatic bile acid (BA) metabolism and reducing gastrointestinal microbiota-mediated TMAO production.

As food supplements, probiotics are not regulated by the US FDA or other food and drug regulatory agencies. When purchasing probiotics, the consumer must therefore exercise due diligence and read the label attentively. If lactose intolerance prevents someone from consuming probiotics, they should search for lactobacillus and bifidobacterium in another food's ingredient list. Since probiotics are living organisms, they should be refrigerated, as heat and improper storage conditions would destroy the microorganisms they contain. In addition, effective manufacturing practices and quality control must be implemented during probiotics' production.

DISCUSSION

CVDs include atherosclerosis, hypertension, MI, arrhythmias, valvular heart disease, coagulopathies, and stroke, and they continue to be among the most prevalent chronic conditions affecting humans worldwide. These diseases significantly contribute to mortality, morbidity, and the economic burden of illness in Canada and elsewhere. Atherosclerosis is a progressive pathological condition in which the arterial blood vessels thicken and stiffen, thereby restricting blood flow to vital organs and tissues. Any form of smoking promotes atherosclerosis and hypertension by causing oxidative stress in the arterial endothelium. There is a significant increase in the search for cost-effective measures to prevent CVDs and CMDs associated with T2DM and obesity. Overwhelming evidence suggests that the consumption of the Mediterranean diet and DASH DIET reduces the risk of atherosclerosis, hypertension, and stroke, as they enhance lipid profile and blood sugar level, thereby lowering the incidence of non-genetic CVDs. The consumption of a Mediterranean diet rich in fresh fruits, vegetables, whole cereals, omega-3 fatty acids, dairy products, poultry, nuts and seeds, olive oil, and moderate amounts of red wine is associated with a reduction in mortality and morbidity due to CVDs and CMDs. Further, lifestyle modifications such as quitting smoking, consuming less alcohol, and exercising regularly (30 minutes per day) reduce the incidence of CVDs. Emerging evidence suggests that nutraceuticals (vitamins, minerals, and amino acids) contribute to overall health improvement beyond their fundamental nutritional functions. Nutraceuticals modulate gene and protein expression and alter endogenous metabolic pathways and homeostasis, thereby decreasing the risk of chronic diseases with multiple etiologies. The beneficial effects of bioactive flavonoids derived from plants are a result of their antioxidant and anti-inflammatory properties.

In addition to the traditional biomarkers used for the diagnosis of CHD and CMD, new biomarkers (C-reactive protein, IL-6, IL-8, phospholipase A2, cardiac troponin, MicroRNA, and miR-21) may provide sophisticated tools for the early diagnosis of atherosclerosis and CVDs, according to published evidence. For instance, elevated levels of C-reactive protein and hsCRP can predict peripheral arterial disease; cystatin C, which was once considered a biomarker for renal disease, is now used to assess the risk of CHD and CMD diseases. As previously indicated, lifestyle changes, quitting smoking, and heart-healthy diets play a significant role in reducing the risk of atherosclerosis, heart attack, and stroke. Increased consumption of fresh fruits, leafy vegetables, and PUFA, as well as citrus fruits, berries, and dark chocolate, which are high in antioxidants, has been associated with a reduction in the onset and progression of atherogenesis.

The increasing interest in the CVD-healing properties of nutraceuticals, functional foods, and plant-derived bioactive constituents, particularly natural compounds, is due to their therapeutic properties, cost-effectiveness, and lack of adverse effects. Various dietary patterns, such as the Mediterranean diet and the DASH DIET, have demonstrated beneficial effects in the prevention of atherogenesis by improving lipid concentrations and lowering blood sugar levels, as observed in preclinical and clinical studies. In addition to reducing the risk of atherosclerosis, these diets help obese patients maintain a decent control over weight gain and sugar levels.

In a randomized, double-blind, placebo-controlled clinical trial, Khatir *et al.* evaluated the antiatherogenic effects of saffron supplementation in 63 male and female patients (30-60 years old). The treatment group received 100.0 mg saffron-filled capsules once daily for six weeks, while the other group received placebo capsules. Using quantitative PCR, the expression levels of circulating miR-21 were determined in the blood of patients. Participants' fasting glucose, lipid profile, and anthropometric index were also measured before and after treatment. miR-21 expression levels in atherosclerosis patients treated with saffron decreased significantly compared to the placebo group (P= 0.04). The hip circumflex also diminished significantly following saffron supplementation (P values ranged from 0.049 to 0.006). In patients exposed to saffron, the expression of circulating miR-21 was found to be downregulated. The authors suggested that saffron supplementation could be a novel target therapy for the treatment of atherosclerosis, plaque formation, cardiovascular disease, and obesity [280]. To evaluate the efficacy, optimal dose schedules, and long-term safety of saffron supplementation for the treatment of atherosclerosis, CVDs, and obesity, however, further well-designed, randomized, multicenter, and place-controlled studies with large numbers of patients are required.

The human GI tract is inhabited by billions of microbiomes that participate in numerous physiological processes. Changes in the composition of gastrointestinal microbiota and their metabolites, such as trimethylamine-N-oxide, play a crucial role in the development of NCDs such as atherosclerosis, inflammatory bowel disease, autoimmune disorders, autism, obesity, and type 2 diabetes. To reduce TMA production by microbiota, novel therapies are being developed. Probiotics and prebiotics confer health benefits to the host by promoting healthy microbiota in the intestine, enhancing the integrity of the gut endothelium, and boosting the immune system.

Probiotics and fiber-rich prebiotics contain beneficial live bacteria (Lactobacillus, Bifidobacteria) that keep the intestine healthy, boost immune function, preserve endothelial integrity, and combat toxins and pathogens in the gastrointestinal tract. Accumulating scientific evidence suggests that the prevention of non-communicable diseases (such as obesity, diabetes, cardiovascular disease, Crohn's disease, rheumatoid arthritis, and colorectal cancer, to name a few) with probiotics and prebiotics represents a new frontier in biomedicine and biopharmacotherapy.

CONCLUSION

In this review, novel clinical biomarkers for the diagnosis and evaluation of cardiovascular functions and thrombogenicity for earlier risk estimation in high-risk patients with CAD and stroke are discussed. The clinical biomarkers would aid in evaluating and predicting adverse cardiovascular events related to atherosclerosis and CVDs. The consumption of antioxidant and anti-inflammatory diets, such as the Mediterranean diet, the DASH diet, functional foods, and nutraceuticals, as well as lifestyle modifications and quitting smoking, would aid in the prevention of atherosclerosis, CHD, and stroke.

Consumption of foods rich in omega-3 fatty acids, olive oil, and probiotics is associated with health promotion in humans and a reduced risk of cardiovascular diseases, brain-related diseases (depression, dementia, Alzheimer's disease, and Parkinson's disease), and certain types of cancer. Antioxidant and anti-inflammatory nutraceuticals and phytochemicals such as phenolics, flavonoids, retinoids, anthocyanins, and lycopene contribute to these health benefits by removing excessive free radicals from the body. However, it should be noted that megadoses of antioxidants and anti-inflammatory dietary supplements should be avoided. Large doses of nutraceuticals could be detrimental because they would interfere with the cell signals required for cell-to-cell communication.

Lactobacillus and bifidobacterium-containing probiotics promote healthy microflora in the gut, enhance the host's immune system and increase endothelial integrity, reduce the levels of pathogenic bacteria in the gastrointestinal tract, and prevent colorectal cancer in humans.

At the level of primary health promotion, holistic approaches are required for the prevention of cardiovascular diseases (CVDs) before some of the key underlying causes of these diseases severely affect an individual or a population. These holistic approaches will not only reduce the global economic burden of health care but also decrease hospital stays and increase workers' productivity by decreasing employee absenteeism.

ABBREVIATIONS

CVD	Cardiovascular Diseases
CHD	Coronary Heart Disease
LDL	Low-density Lipoproteins
HDL	High-density Lipoprotein
ROS	Reactive Oxygen Species
NO	Nitric Oxide
SOD	Superoxide Dismutase
LAM	Leukocyte Adhesion Molecule
CRP	C Reactive Protein
hsCRP	High-sensitivity C-reactive Protein
MI	Myocardial Infraction
PAD	Peripheral Artery Disease
IL-6	Interleukin-6
AT-1	Angiotensin 1 Receptor
ACS	Acute Coronary Syndrome
AMI	Acute Myocardial Infraction
FRISC II	Fragmingham and Fast Revascularization during Instability in Coronary Artery Disease II
IL-18	Interleukin-18
IFN	Interferon
MMP	Matrix Metalloproteases
CAD	Coronary Artery Disease
BNP	Brain Natriuretic Peptide
NT-proBNP	N-terminal pro-B-type Natriuretic Peptide
STEMI	ST-segment Elevation Myocardial Infarction
ROC	Receiver Operating Characteristic
CI	Confidence Interval
Lp-PLA2	Lipoprotein-associated Phospholipase A2
VLDL	Very Low Density Lipoprotein
LysoPC	Lysophosphatidylcholine
TSH	Thyroid Stimulating Hormone
CK-MB	Creatine Kinase-MB
SMC	Smooth Muscle Cells
OC	Osteocalcin

VSMC	Vascular Smooth Muscle Cells
GGCX	γ -Glutamyl Carboxylase
1,25(OH)2D3	1,25-dihydroxycholecalciferol
FFA	Free Fatty Acid
FoxO1	Forkhead box O-class (FoxO)
EPC	Endothelial Progenitor Cells
T2DM	Type 2 Diabetes Mellitus
CKD	Chronic Kidney Disease
ANG	Angiogenin
tPA	Tissue Plasminogen Activator
HFPEF	Heart Failure with Preserved Ejection Fraction
CHF	Chronic Heart Failure
ANG-RNH1	Angiogenin (ANG)-ribonuclease Inhibitor
MCP-1	Monocyte Chemoattractant Protein-1
CCR2	CC Chemokine Receptors 2
PlGF	Placental Growth Factor
apoE	Apolipoprotein E
VEGF	Vascular Endothelial Growth Factor
PAPP-A	Pregnancy-associated Plasma Protein-A
IGF-1	Insulin like Growth Factor -1
proMBP	Proform of the Eosinophil Major Basic Protein
EC	Endothelial Cells
NCD	Non Communicable Disease
CMD	Cardiometabolic Disease
DGA	Dietary Guidelines for Americans
3-nPUFA	Omega-3 Polyunsaturated Fatty Acids
DHA	Docosahexaenoic Acid
ERA	Arachidonic Acid
EPA	Eicosapentaenoic Acid
NOX-2	NADPH Oxidase 2
DASH	Dietary Approaches to Stop Hypertension
LDLr	Low Density Lipoprotein Receptor
SCFA	Short Chain Fatty Acid
TMAO	Trimethylamine N-oxide
VCAM	Vascular Cell Adhesion Molecule

ICAM	Intercellular Cell Adhesion Molecule
ApoA	Apolipoprotein A
HbA1C	Glycated Haemoglobin

REFERENCES

[1]   Bowry ADK, Lewey J, Dugani SB, Choudhry NK. The burden of cardiovascular disease in low- and middle-income countries: Epidemiology and management. Can J Cardiol 2015; 31(9): 1151-9.
[http://dx.doi.org/10.1016/j.cjca.2015.06.028] [PMID: 26321437]

[2]   India RG. Center for Global Health research. Causes Death India. 2003; p. 2001.

[3]   Global status report on noncommunicable diseases 2014. World Health Organization 2014.

[4]   Marchand F. Ueber atherosclerosis. Verhandlung Congresses Inn Med 1904; pp. 21-59.

[5]   Malekmohammad K, Sewell RDE, Rafieian-Kopaei M. Antioxidants and atherosclerosis: Mechanistic aspects. Biomolecules 2019; 9(8): 301-20.
[http://dx.doi.org/10.3390/biom9080301] [PMID: 31349600]

[6]   Visen PK, Visen AS, Visen SS, Buttar HS, Singh RB. Management of Type 2 diabetes and atherosclerosis with alternative therapies. World Heart J 2015; 7(1): 63-82.

[7]   Aziz M, Yadav KS. Pathogenesis of atherosclerosis a review. Med Clin Rev 2016; 2(3): 1-6.

[8]   Meier T, Gräfe K, Senn F, *et al.* Cardiovascular mortality attributable to dietary risk factors in 51 countries in the WHO european region from 1990 to 2016: A systematic analysis of the global burden of disease study. Eur J Epidemiol 2019; 34(1): 37-55.
[http://dx.doi.org/10.1007/s10654-018-0473-x] [PMID: 30547256]

[9]   Afshin A, Sur PJ, Fay KA, *et al.* Health effects of dietary risks in 195 countries, 1990–2017: A systematic analysis for the global burden of disease study 2017. Lancet 2019; 393(10184): 1958-72.
[http://dx.doi.org/10.1016/S0140-6736(19)30041-8] [PMID: 30954305]

[10]   Micha R, Peñalvo JL, Cudhea F, Imamura F, Rehm CD, Mozaffarian D. Association between dietary factors and mortality from heart disease, stroke, and type 2 diabetes in the United States. JAMA 2017; 317(9): 912-24.
[http://dx.doi.org/10.1001/jama.2017.0947] [PMID: 28267855]

[11]   Moore KJ, Sheedy FJ, Fisher EA. Macrophages in atherosclerosis: A dynamic balance. Nat Rev Immunol 2013; 13(10): 709-21.
[http://dx.doi.org/10.1038/nri3520] [PMID: 23995626]

[12]   Davignon J, Ganz P. Role of endothelial dysfunction in atherosclerosis. Circulation 2004. 109(23); Suppl 1:III-27-32.
[http://dx.doi.org/10.1161/01.CIR.0000131515.03336.f8] [PMID: 15198963]

[13]   Gustafsson M, Borén J. Mechanism of lipoprotein retention by the extracellular matrix. Curr Opin Lipidol 2004; 15(5): 505-14.
[http://dx.doi.org/10.1097/00041433-200410000-00003] [PMID: 15361785]

[14]   Granger DN, Kubes P. The microcirculation and inflammation: Modulation of leukocyte-endothelial cell adhesion. J Leukoc Biol 1994; 55(5): 662-75.
[http://dx.doi.org/10.1002/jlb.55.5.662] [PMID: 8182345]

[15]   Remmerie A, Scott CL. Macrophages and lipid metabolism. Cell Immunol 2018; 330: 27-42.
[http://dx.doi.org/10.1016/j.cellimm.2018.01.020] [PMID: 29429624]

[16]   Pahwa R, Goyal A, Jialal I. Chronic inflammation. StatPearls . 2021.

[17]   Song P, Fang Z, Wang H, *et al.* Global and regional prevalence, burden, and risk factors for carotid atherosclerosis: a systematic review, meta-analysis, and modelling study. Lancet Glob Health 2020;

8(5): e721-9.
[http://dx.doi.org/10.1016/S2214-109X(20)30117-0] [PMID: 32353319]

[18] Pirillo A, Casula M, Olmastroni E, Norata GD, Catapano AL. Global epidemiology of dyslipidaemias. Nat Rev Cardiol 2021; 18(10): 689-700.
[http://dx.doi.org/10.1038/s41569-021-00541-4] [PMID: 33833450]

[19] Virani SS, Polsani VR, Nambi V. Novel markers of inflammation in atherosclerosis. Curr Atheroscler Rep 2008; 10(2): 164-70.
[http://dx.doi.org/10.1007/s11883-008-0024-0] [PMID: 18417072]

[20] Ridker PM. C-reactive protein and the prediction of cardiovascular events among those at intermediate risk: moving an inflammatory hypothesis toward consensus. J Am Coll Cardiol 2007; 49(21): 2129-38.
[http://dx.doi.org/10.1016/j.jacc.2007.02.052] [PMID: 17531663]

[21] Sabatine MS, Morrow DA, Jablonski KA, *et al.* Prognostic significance of the centers for disease control/american heart association high-sensitivity C-reactive protein cut points for cardiovascular and other outcomes in patients with stable coronary artery disease. Circulation 2007; 115(12): 1528-36.
[http://dx.doi.org/10.1161/CIRCULATIONAHA.106.649939] [PMID: 17372173]

[22] Pearson TA, Mensah GA, Alexander RW, *et al.* Markers of inflammation and cardiovascular disease: application to clinical and public health practice: A statement for healthcare professionals from the centers for disease control and prevention and the american heart association. Circulation 2003; 107(3): 499-511.
[http://dx.doi.org/10.1161/01.CIR.0000052939.59093.45] [PMID: 12551878]

[23] Vidula H, Tian L, Liu K, *et al.* Biomarkers of inflammation and thrombosis as predictors of near-term mortality in patients with peripheral arterial disease: A cohort study. Ann Intern Med 2008; 148(2): 85-93.
[http://dx.doi.org/10.7326/0003-4819-148-2-200801150-00003] [PMID: 18195333]

[24] Cook NR, Buring JE, Ridker PM. The effect of including C-reactive protein in cardiovascular risk prediction models for women. Ann Intern Med 2006; 145(1): 21-9.
[http://dx.doi.org/10.7326/0003-4819-145-1-200607040-00128] [PMID: 16818925]

[25] Ridker PM, Buring JE, Rifai N, Cook NR. Development and validation of improved algorithms for the assessment of global cardiovascular risk in women: The reynolds risk score. JAMA 2007; 297(6): 611-9.
[http://dx.doi.org/10.1001/jama.297.6.611] [PMID: 17299196]

[26] Rattazzi M, Puato M, Faggin E, Bertipaglia B, Zambon A, Pauletto P. C-reactive protein and interleukin-6 in vascular disease. J Hypertens 2003; 21(10): 1787-803.
[http://dx.doi.org/10.1097/00004872-200310000-00002] [PMID: 14508181]

[27] Kerr R, Stirling D, Ludlam CA. Interleukin 6 and Haemostasis. Br J Haematol 2001; 115(1): 3-12.
[http://dx.doi.org/10.1046/j.1365-2141.2001.03061.x] [PMID: 11722403]

[28] Huber SA, Sakkinen P, Conze D, Hardin N, Tracy R. Interleukin-6 exacerbates early atherosclerosis in mice. Arterioscler Thromb Vasc Biol 1999; 19(10): 2364-7.
[http://dx.doi.org/10.1161/01.ATV.19.10.2364] [PMID: 10521365]

[29] Seino Y, Ikeda U, Ikeda M, *et al.* Interleukin 6 gene transcripts are expressed in human atherosclerotic lesions. Cytokine 1994; 6(1): 87-91.
[http://dx.doi.org/10.1016/1043-4666(94)90013-2] [PMID: 8003639]

[30] Rus HG, Vlaicu R, Niculescu F. Interleukin-6 and interleukin-8 protein and gene expression in human arterial atherosclerotic wall. Atherosclerosis 1996; 127(2): 263-71.
[http://dx.doi.org/10.1016/S0021-9150(96)05968-0] [PMID: 9125317]

[31] Schieffer B, Schieffer E, Hilfiker-Kleiner D, *et al.* Expression of angiotensin II and interleukin 6 in human coronary atherosclerotic plaques: Potential implications for inflammation and plaque instability. Circulation 2000; 101(12): 1372-8.

[http://dx.doi.org/10.1161/01.CIR.101.12.1372] [PMID: 10736279]

[32]   Schieffer B, Selle T, Hilfiker A, *et al.* Impact of interleukin-6 on plaque development and morphology in experimental atherosclerosis. Circulation 2004; 110(22): 3493-500.
[http://dx.doi.org/10.1161/01.CIR.0000148135.08582.97] [PMID: 15557373]

[33]   Maier W, Altwegg LA, Corti R, *et al.* Inflammatory markers at the site of ruptured plaque in acute myocardial infarction: locally increased interleukin-6 and serum amyloid A but decreased C-reactive protein. Circulation 2005; 111(11): 1355-61.
[http://dx.doi.org/10.1161/01.CIR.0000158479.58589.0A] [PMID: 15753219]

[34]   Biasucci LM, Liuzzo G, Fantuzzi G, *et al.* Increasing levels of interleukin (IL)-1Ra and IL-6 during the first 2 days of hospitalization in unstable angina are associated with increased risk of in-hospital coronary events. Circulation 1999; 99(16): 2079-84.
[http://dx.doi.org/10.1161/01.CIR.99.16.2079] [PMID: 10217645]

[35]   Lindmark E, Diderholm E, Wallentin L, Siegbahn A. Relationship between interleukin 6 and mortality in patients with unstable coronary artery disease: Effects of an early invasive or noninvasive strategy. JAMA 2001; 286(17): 2107-13.
[http://dx.doi.org/10.1001/jama.286.17.2107] [PMID: 11694151]

[36]   Ridker PM, Rifai N, Stampfer MJ, Hennekens CH. Plasma concentration of interleukin-6 and the risk of future myocardial infarction among apparently healthy men. Circulation 2000; 101(15): 1767-72.
[http://dx.doi.org/10.1161/01.CIR.101.15.1767] [PMID: 10769275]

[37]   Pradhan AD, Manson JE, Rossouw JE, *et al.* Inflammatory biomarkers, hormone replacement therapy, and incident coronary heart disease: Prospective analysis from the Women's Health Initiative observational study. JAMA 2002; 288(8): 980-7.
[http://dx.doi.org/10.1001/jama.288.8.980] [PMID: 12190368]

[38]   Harris TB, Ferrucci L, Tracy RP, *et al.* Associations of elevated interleukin-6 and C-reactive protein levels with mortality in the elderly. Am J Med 1999; 106(5): 506-12.
[http://dx.doi.org/10.1016/S0002-9343(99)00066-2] [PMID: 10335721]

[39]   Volpato S, Guralnik JM, Ferrucci L, *et al.* Cardiovascular disease, interleukin-6, and risk of mortality in older women: The women's health and aging study. Circulation 2001; 103(7): 947-53.
[http://dx.doi.org/10.1161/01.CIR.103.7.947] [PMID: 11181468]

[40]   Gracie JA, Robertson SE, McInnes IB. Interleukin-18. J Leukoc Biol 2003; 73(2): 213-24.
[http://dx.doi.org/10.1189/jlb.0602313] [PMID: 12554798]

[41]   Gerdes N, Sukhova GK, Libby P, Reynolds RS, Young JL, Schönbeck U. Expression of interleukin (IL)-18 and functional IL-18 receptor on human vascular endothelial cells, smooth muscle cells, and macrophages: Implications for atherogenesis. J Exp Med 2002; 195(2): 245-57.
[http://dx.doi.org/10.1084/jem.20011022] [PMID: 11805151]

[42]   Nold M, Goede A, Eberhardt W, Pfeilschifter J, Mühl H. IL-18 initiates release of matrix metalloproteinase-9 from peripheral blood mononuclear cells without affecting tissue inhibitor of matrix metalloproteinases-1: Suppression by TNFα blockage and modulation by IL-10. Naunyn Schmiedebergs Arch Pharmacol 2003; 367(1): 68-75.
[http://dx.doi.org/10.1007/s00210-002-0648-5] [PMID: 12616343]

[43]   Ishida Y, Migita K, Izumi Y, *et al.* The role of IL-18 in the modulation of matrix metalloproteinases and migration of human natural killer (NK) cells. FEBS Lett 2004; 569(1-3): 156-60.
[http://dx.doi.org/10.1016/j.febslet.2004.05.039] [PMID: 15225625]

[44]   Mallat Z, Corbaz A, Scoazec A, *et al.* Expression of interleukin-18 in human atherosclerotic plaques and relation to plaque instability. Circulation 2001; 104(14): 1598-603.
[http://dx.doi.org/10.1161/hc3901.096721] [PMID: 11581135]

[45]   Mallat Z, Corbaz A, Scoazec A, *et al.* Interleukin-18/interleukin-18 binding protein signaling modulates atherosclerotic lesion development and stability. Circ Res 2001; 89(7): E41-5.

[http://dx.doi.org/10.1161/hh1901.098735] [PMID: 11577031]

[46]   Elhage R, Jawien J, Rudling M, *et al.* Reduced atherosclerosis in interleukin-18 deficient apolipoprotein E-knockout mice. Cardiovasc Res 2003; 59(1): 234-40.
[http://dx.doi.org/10.1016/S0008-6363(03)00343-2] [PMID: 12829194]

[47]   Whitman SC, Ravisankar P, Daugherty A. Interleukin-18 enhances atherosclerosis in apolipoprotein E(-/-) mice through release of interferon-γ. Circ Res 2002; 90(2): E34-8.
[http://dx.doi.org/10.1161/hh0202.105292] [PMID: 11834721]

[48]   Tenger C, Sundborger A, Jawien J, Zhou X. IL-18 accelerates atherosclerosis accompanied by elevation of IFN-γ and CXCL16 expression independently of T cells. Arterioscler Thromb Vasc Biol 2005; 25(4): 791-6.
[http://dx.doi.org/10.1161/01.ATV.0000153516.02782.65] [PMID: 15604417]

[49]   De Nooijer R, Von der Thüsen JH, Verkleij CJN, *et al.* Overexpression of IL-18 decreases intimal collagen content and promotes a vulnerable plaque phenotype in apolipoprotein-E-deficient mice. Arterioscler Thromb Vasc Biol 2004; 24(12): 2313-9.
[http://dx.doi.org/10.1161/01.ATV.0000147126.99529.0a] [PMID: 15472128]

[50]   Mallat Z, Henry P, Fressonnet R, *et al.* Increased plasma concentrations of interleukin-18 in acute coronary syndromes. Br Heart J 2002; 88(5): 467-9.
[http://dx.doi.org/10.1136/heart.88.5.467] [PMID: 12381634]

[51]   Kawasaki D, Tsujino T, Morimoto S, *et al.* Usefulness of circulating interleukin-18 concentration in acute myocardial infarction as a risk factor for late restenosis after emergency coronary angioplasty. Am J Cardiol 2003; 91(10): 1258-61.
[http://dx.doi.org/10.1016/S0002-9149(03)00279-0] [PMID: 12745116]

[52]   Narins CR, Lin DA, Burton PB, Jin ZG, Berk BC. Interleukin-18 and interleukin-18 binding protein levels before and after percutaneous coronary intervention in patients with and without recent myocardial infarction. Am J Cardiol 2004; 94(10): 1285-7.
[http://dx.doi.org/10.1016/j.amjcard.2004.07.114] [PMID: 15541247]

[53]   Blankenberg S, Tiret L, Bickel C, *et al.* Interleukin-18 is a strong predictor of cardiovascular death in stable and unstable angina. Circulation 2002; 106(1): 24-30.
[http://dx.doi.org/10.1161/01.CIR.0000020546.30940.92] [PMID: 12093765]

[54]   Tiret L, Godefroy T, Lubos E, *et al.* Genetic analysis of the interleukin-18 system highlights the role of the interleukin-18 gene in cardiovascular disease. Circulation 2005; 112(5): 643-50.
[http://dx.doi.org/10.1161/CIRCULATIONAHA.104.519702] [PMID: 16043644]

[55]   Blankenberg S, Luc G, Ducimetière P, *et al.* Interleukin-18 and the risk of coronary heart disease in european men: The prospective epidemiological study of myocardial infarction (PRIME). Circulation 2003; 108(20): 2453-9.
[http://dx.doi.org/10.1161/01.CIR.0000099509.76044.A2] [PMID: 14581397]

[56]   Koenig W, Khuseyinova N, Baumert J, Thorand B, Loewel H, Chambless L, *et al.* Increased concentrations of C-reactive protein and interleukin-6 but not interleukin-18 are independently associated with incident coronary events in middle-aged men and women. Results from the Monica/KORA Augsburg case-cohort study, 1984. Arterioscler Thromb Vasc Biol 2002. in press

[57]   Thygesen K, Alpert JS, White HD. Universal definition of myocardial infarction. J Am Coll Cardiol 2007; 50(22): 2173-95.
[http://dx.doi.org/10.1016/j.jacc.2007.09.011] [PMID: 18036459]

[58]   Antman EM, Anbe DT, Armstrong PW, *et al.* ACC/AHA guidelines for the management of patients with ST-elevation myocardial infarction; A report of the american college of cardiology/american heart association task force on practice guidelines (committee to revise the 1999 guidelines for the management of patients with acute myocardial infarction). J Am Coll Cardiol 2004; 44(3): E1-E211.
[http://dx.doi.org/10.1016/j.jacc.2004.07.014] [PMID: 15358047]

[59]   Anderson JL, Adams CD, Antman EM, *et al.* ACC/AHA 2007 guidelines for the management of patients with unstable Angina/Non–ST-Elevation myocardial infarction. J Am Coll Cardiol 2007; 50(7): e1-e157.
[http://dx.doi.org/10.1016/j.jacc.2007.02.013] [PMID: 17692738]

[60]   Schulz O, Paul-Walter C, Lehmann M, *et al.* Usefulness of detectable levels of troponin, below the 99th percentile of the normal range, as a clue to the presence of underlying coronary artery disease. Am J Cardiol 2007; 100(5): 764-9.
[http://dx.doi.org/10.1016/j.amjcard.2007.03.096] [PMID: 17719317]

[61]   Agewall S, Olsson T, Löwbeer C. Usefulness of troponin levels below the diagnostic cut-off level for acute myocardial infarction in predicting prognosis in unselected patients admitted to the coronary care unit. Am J Cardiol 2007; 99(10): 1357-9.
[http://dx.doi.org/10.1016/j.amjcard.2006.12.059] [PMID: 17493459]

[62]   Zethelius B, Johnston N, Venge P. Troponin I as a predictor of coronary heart disease and mortality in 70-year-old men: A community-based cohort study. Circulation 2006; 113(8): 1071-8.
[http://dx.doi.org/10.1161/CIRCULATIONAHA.105.570762] [PMID: 16490824]

[63]   De Lemos JA, McGuire DK, Drazner MH. B-type natriuretic peptide in cardiovascular disease. Lancet 2003; 362(9380): 316-22.
[http://dx.doi.org/10.1016/S0140-6736(03)13976-1] [PMID: 12892964]

[64]   Omland T, De Lemos JA. Amino-terminal pro-B-type natriuretic peptides in stable and unstable ischemic heart disease. Am J Cardiol 2008; 101(3) (Suppl.): S61-6.
[http://dx.doi.org/10.1016/j.amjcard.2007.11.025] [PMID: 18243861]

[65]   Khan SQ, Quinn P, Davies JE, Ng LL. N-terminal pro-B-type natriuretic peptide is better than TIMI risk score at predicting death after acute myocardial infarction. Heart 2008; 94(1): 40-3.
[http://dx.doi.org/10.1136/hrt.2006.108985] [PMID: 17488769]

[66]   Weber M, Bazzino O, Navarro Estrada JL, *et al.* N-terminal B-type natriuretic peptide assessment provides incremental prognostic information in patients with acute coronary syndromes and normal troponin T values upon admission. J Am Coll Cardiol 2008; 51(12): 1188-95.
[http://dx.doi.org/10.1016/j.jacc.2007.11.054] [PMID: 18355657]

[67]   Windhausen F, Hirsch A, Sanders GT, *et al.* N-terminal pro–brain natriuretic peptide for additional risk stratification in patients with non–ST-elevation acute coronary syndrome and an elevated troponin T: An invasive versus conservative treatment in unstable coronary syndromes (ICTUS) substudy. Am Heart J 2007; 153(4): 485-92.
[http://dx.doi.org/10.1016/j.ahj.2006.12.012] [PMID: 17383283]

[68]   Bibbins-Domingo K, Gupta R, Na B, Wu AHB, Schiller NB, Whooley MA. N-terminal fragment of the prohormone brain-type natriuretic peptide (NT-proBNP), cardiovascular events, and mortality in patients with stable coronary heart disease. JAMA 2007; 297(2): 169-76.
[http://dx.doi.org/10.1001/jama.297.2.169] [PMID: 17213400]

[69]   Omland T, Sabatine MS, Jablonski KA, *et al.* Prognostic value of B-Type natriuretic peptides in patients with stable coronary artery disease: The PEACE Trial. J Am Coll Cardiol 2007; 50(3): 205-14.
[http://dx.doi.org/10.1016/j.jacc.2007.03.038] [PMID: 17631211]

[70]   Emberson JR, Ng LL, Armitage J, Bowman L, Parish S, Collins R. N-terminal Pro-B-type natriuretic peptide, vascular disease risk, and cholesterol reduction among 20,536 patients in the MRC/BHF heart protection study. J Am Coll Cardiol 2007; 49(3): 311-9.
[http://dx.doi.org/10.1016/j.jacc.2006.08.052] [PMID: 17239712]

[71]   Olsen MH, Hansen TW, Christensen MK, *et al.* N-terminal pro-brain natriuretic peptide, but not high sensitivity C-reactive protein, improves cardiovascular risk prediction in the general population. Eur Heart J 2007; 28(11): 1374-81.
[http://dx.doi.org/10.1093/eurheartj/ehl448] [PMID: 17242007]

[72] Ix JH, Shlipak MG, Chertow GM, Whooley MA. Association of cystatin C with mortality, cardiovascular events, and incident heart failure among persons with coronary heart disease: Data from the heart and soul study. Circulation 2007; 115(2): 173-9.
[http://dx.doi.org/10.1161/CIRCULATIONAHA.106.644286] [PMID: 17190862]

[73] Maahs DM, Ogden LG, Kretowski A, *et al.* Serum cystatin C predicts progression of subclinical coronary atherosclerosis in individuals with type 1 diabetes. Diabetes 2007; 56(11): 2774-9.
[http://dx.doi.org/10.2337/db07-0539] [PMID: 17660266]

[74] Zalewski A, Macphee C. Role of lipoprotein-associated phospholipase A2 in atherosclerosis: Biology, epidemiology, and possible therapeutic target. Arterioscler Thromb Vasc Biol 2005; 25(5): 923-31.
[http://dx.doi.org/10.1161/01.ATV.0000160551.21962.a7] [PMID: 15731492]

[75] Caslake MJ, Packard CJ, Suckling KE, Holmes SD, Chamberlain P, Macphee CH. Lipoprotein-associated phospholipase A2, platelet-activating factor acetylhydrolase: A potential new risk factor for coronary artery disease. Atherosclerosis 2000; 150(2): 413-9.
[http://dx.doi.org/10.1016/S0021-9150(99)00406-2] [PMID: 10856534]

[76] MacPhee CH, Moores KE, Boyd HF, *et al.* Lipoprotein-associated phospholipase A_2, platelet-activating factor acetylhydrolase, generates two bioactive products during the oxidation of low-density lipoprotein: Use of a novel inhibitor. Biochem J 1999; 338(2): 479-87.
[http://dx.doi.org/10.1042/bj3380479] [PMID: 10024526]

[77] Packard CJ, O'Reilly DSJ, Caslake MJ, *et al.* Lipoprotein-associated phospholipase A2 as an independent predictor of coronary heart disease. N Engl J Med 2000; 343(16): 1148-55.
[http://dx.doi.org/10.1056/NEJM200010193431603] [PMID: 11036120]

[78] Ballantyne CM, Hoogeveen RC, Bang H, *et al.* Lipoprotein-associated phospholipase A_2, high-sensitivity C-reactive protein, and risk for incident coronary heart disease in middle-aged men and women in the atherosclerosis risk in communities (ARIC) study. Circulation 2004; 109(7): 837-42.
[http://dx.doi.org/10.1161/01.CIR.0000116763.91992.F1] [PMID: 14757686]

[79] Koenig W, Khuseyinova N, Löwel H, Trischler G, Meisinger C. Lipoprotein-associated phospholipase A_2 adds to risk prediction of incident coronary events by C-reactive protein in apparently healthy middle-aged men from the general population: results from the 14-year follow-up of a large cohort from southern Germany. Circulation 2004; 110(14): 1903-8.
[http://dx.doi.org/10.1161/01.CIR.0000143377.53389.C8] [PMID: 15451783]

[80] Oei HHS, van der Meer IM, Hofman A, *et al.* Lipoprotein-associated phospholipase A_2 activity is associated with risk of coronary heart disease and ischemic stroke: The Rotterdam Study. Circulation 2005; 111(5): 570-5.
[http://dx.doi.org/10.1161/01.CIR.0000154553.12214.CD] [PMID: 15699277]

[81] O'Donoghue M, Morrow DA, Sabatine MS, *et al.* Lipoprotein-associated phospholipase A_2 and its association with cardiovascular outcomes in patients with acute coronary syndromes in the PROVE IT-TIMI 22 (pravastatin or atorvastatin evaluation and infection therapy-thrombolysis in myocardial infarction) trial. Circulation 2006; 113(14): 1745-52.
[http://dx.doi.org/10.1161/CIRCULATIONAHA.105.612630] [PMID: 16537575]

[82] Oldgren J, James SK, Siegbahn A, Wallentin L. Lp-PLA_2 Does not predict mortality or new ischemic events in acute coronary syndrome patients. Circulation 2005; 112: II-387.

[83] James SK, Oldgren J, Siegbahn A, Wallentin L. No Relation between levels of Lp-PLA_2 and other inflammatory markers or outcome in non St-elevation acute coronary syndromes. Circulation 2005; 112: II-387.

[84] Çakmak HA, Demir M. MicroRNA and cardiovascular diseases. Balkan Med J 2020; 37(2): 60-71.
[http://dx.doi.org/10.4274/balkanmedj.galenos.2020.2020.1.94] [PMID: 32018347]

[85] Hosen MR, Goody PR, Zietzer A, Nickenig G, Jansen F. MicroRNAs as master regulators of atherosclerosis: From pathogenesis to novel therapeutic options. Antioxid Redox Signal 2020; 33(9):

621-44.
[http://dx.doi.org/10.1089/ars.2020.8107] [PMID: 32408755]

[86] Lu Y, Thavarajah T, Gu W, Cai J, Xu Q. Impact of miRNA in atherosclerosis. Arterioscler Thromb Vasc Biol 2018; 38(9): e159-70.
[http://dx.doi.org/10.1161/ATVBAHA.118.310227] [PMID: 30354259]

[87] Chalikiopoulou C, Bizjan BJ, Leventopoulos G, *et al.* Multiomics analysis coupled with text mining identify novel biomarker candidates for recurrent cardiovascular events. OMICS 2020; 24(4): 205-15.
[http://dx.doi.org/10.1089/omi.2019.0216] [PMID: 32176569]

[88] Urbich C, Kuehbacher A, Dimmeler S. Role of microRNAs in vascular diseases, inflammation, and angiogenesis. Cardiovasc Res 2008; 79(4): 581-8.
[http://dx.doi.org/10.1093/cvr/cvn156] [PMID: 18550634]

[89] Wang D, Deuse T, Stubbendorff M, *et al.* Local microRNA modulation using a novel anti-miR-21–eluting stent effectively prevents experimental in-stent restenosis. Arterioscler Thromb Vasc Biol 2015; 35(9): 1945-53.
[http://dx.doi.org/10.1161/ATVBAHA.115.305597] [PMID: 26183619]

[90] Berkan Ö, Arslan S, Lalem T, *et al.* Regulation of microRNAs in coronary atherosclerotic plaque. Epigenomics 2019; 11(12): 1387-97.
[http://dx.doi.org/10.2217/epi-2019-0036] [PMID: 31596136]

[91] Quan X, Ji Y, Zhang C, *et al.* Circulating MiR-146a may be a potential biomarker of coronary heart disease in patients with subclinical hypothyroidism. Cell Physiol Biochem 2018; 45(1): 226-36.
[http://dx.doi.org/10.1159/000486769] [PMID: 29357324]

[92] Tian L, Zhang L, Liu J, Guo T, Gao C, Ni J. Effects of TSH on the function of human umbilical vein endothelial cells. J Mol Endocrinol 2014; 52(2): 215-22.
[http://dx.doi.org/10.1530/JME-13-0119] [PMID: 24444496]

[93] Li K, Chen Z, Qin Y, Wei Y. MiR-664a-3p expression in patients with obstructive sleep apnea. Medicine 2018; 97(6): e9813.
[http://dx.doi.org/10.1097/MD.0000000000009813] [PMID: 29419680]

[94] Stojkovic S, Jurisic M, Kopp CW, *et al.* Circulating microRNAs identify patients at increased risk of in-stent restenosis after peripheral angioplasty with stent implantation. Atherosclerosis 2018; 269: 197-203.
[http://dx.doi.org/10.1016/j.atherosclerosis.2018.01.020] [PMID: 29366993]

[95] Jeon SB, Kang DW, Kim JS, Kwon SU. Homocysteine, small-vessel disease, and atherosclerosis: An MRI study of 825 stroke patients. Neurology 2014; 83(8): 695-701.
[http://dx.doi.org/10.1212/WNL.0000000000000720] [PMID: 25031284]

[96] Liu K, Xuekelati S, Zhou K, *et al.* Expression profiles of six atherosclerosis-associated microRNAs that cluster in patients with hyperhomocysteinemia: A clinical study. DNA Cell Biol 2018; 37(3): 189-98.
[http://dx.doi.org/10.1089/dna.2017.3845] [PMID: 29461880]

[97] Menghini R, Casagrande V, Cardellini M, *et al.* MicroRNA 217 modulates endothelial cell senescence *via* silent information regulator 1. Circulation 2009; 120(15): 1524-32.
[http://dx.doi.org/10.1161/CIRCULATIONAHA.109.864629] [PMID: 19786632]

[98] Cordes KR, Sheehy NT, White MP, *et al.* miR-145 and miR-143 regulate smooth muscle cell fate and plasticity. Nature 2009; 460(7256): 705-10.
[http://dx.doi.org/10.1038/nature08195] [PMID: 19578358]

[99] Gao J, Yang S, Wang K, Zhong Q, Ma A, Pan X. Plasma miR-126 and miR-143 as potential novel biomarkers for cerebral atherosclerosis. J Stroke Cerebrovasc Dis 2019; 28(1): 38-43.
[http://dx.doi.org/10.1016/j.jstrokecerebrovasdis.2018.09.008] [PMID: 30309729]

[100] Teruel R, Pérez-Sánchez C, Corral J, *et al.* Identification of miRNAs as potential modulators of tissue

factor expression in patients with systemic lupus erythematosus and antiphospholipid syndrome. J Thromb Haemost 2011; 9(10): 1985-92.
[http://dx.doi.org/10.1111/j.1538-7836.2011.04451.x] [PMID: 21794077]

[101] Pérez-Sánchez C, Arias-de la Rosa I, Aguirre MÁ, *et al.* Circulating microRNAs as biomarkers of disease and typification of the atherothrombotic status in antiphospholipid syndrome. Haematologica 2018; 103(5): 908-18.
[http://dx.doi.org/10.3324/haematol.2017.184416] [PMID: 29545345]

[102] Boon RA, Seeger T, Heydt S, *et al.* MicroRNA-29 in aortic dilation: Implications for aneurysm formation. Circ Res 2011; 109(10): 1115-9.
[http://dx.doi.org/10.1161/CIRCRESAHA.111.255737] [PMID: 21903938]

[103] Xiong X, Cho M, Cai X, *et al.* A common variant in pre-miR-146 is associated with coronary artery disease risk and its mature miRNA expression. Mutat Res 2014; 761: 15-20.
[http://dx.doi.org/10.1016/j.mrfmmm.2014.01.001] [PMID: 24447667]

[104] Parahuleva MS, Lipps C, Parviz B, *et al.* MicroRNA expression profile of human advanced coronary atherosclerotic plaques. Sci Rep 2018; 8(1): 7823.
[http://dx.doi.org/10.1038/s41598-018-25690-4] [PMID: 29777114]

[105] Liu X, You L, Zhou R, Zhang J. Significant association between functional microRNA polymorphisms and coronary heart disease susceptibility: A comprehensive meta-analysis involving 16484 subjects. Oncotarget 2017; 8(4): 5692-702.
[http://dx.doi.org/10.18632/oncotarget.14249] [PMID: 28035059]

[106] Condrat CE, Thompson DC, Barbu MG, *et al.* miRNAs as biomarkers in disease: Latest findings regarding their role in diagnosis and prognosis. Cells 2020; 9(2): 276.
[http://dx.doi.org/10.3390/cells9020276] [PMID: 31979244]

[107] Xiao Y, Zhao J, Tuazon JP, Borlongan CV, Yu G. MicroRNA-133a and myocardial infarction. Cell Transplant 2019; 28(7): 831-8.
[http://dx.doi.org/10.1177/0963689719843806] [PMID: 30983393]

[108] Wang GK, Zhu JQ, Zhang JT, *et al.* Circulating microRNA: A novel potential biomarker for early diagnosis of acute myocardial infarction in humans. Eur Heart J 2010; 31(6): 659-66.
[http://dx.doi.org/10.1093/eurheartj/ehq013] [PMID: 20159880]

[109] Liu X, Fan Z, Zhao T, *et al.* Plasma miR-1, miR-208, miR-499 as potential predictive biomarkers for acute myocardial infarction: An independent study of Han population. Exp Gerontol 2015; 72: 230-8.
[http://dx.doi.org/10.1016/j.exger.2015.10.011] [PMID: 26526403]

[110] Liu H, Yang N, Fei Z, *et al.* Analysis of plasma miR-208a and miR-370 expression levels for early diagnosis of coronary artery disease. Biomed Rep 2016; 5(3): 332-6.
[http://dx.doi.org/10.3892/br.2016.726] [PMID: 27602213]

[111] Chen C, Lü J, Liang Z, Liu D, Yao Q. Overview of 8 circulating microRNAs and their functions as major biomarkers for cardiovascular diseases. Clin Pract Rev Meta-analysis 2020.
[http://dx.doi.org/10.12659/CPRM.924530]

[112] De Boer HC, van Solingen C, Prins J, *et al.* Aspirin treatment hampers the use of plasma microRNA-126 as a biomarker for the progression of vascular disease. Eur Heart J 2013; 34(44): 3451-7.
[http://dx.doi.org/10.1093/eurheartj/eht007] [PMID: 23386708]

[113] Gao H, Guddeti RR, Matsuzawa Y, *et al.* Plasma levels of microRNA-145 are associated with severity of coronary artery disease. PLoS One 2015; 10(5): e0123477.
[http://dx.doi.org/10.1371/journal.pone.0123477] [PMID: 25938589]

[114] Devaux Y, Mueller M, Haaf P, *et al.* Diagnostic and prognostic value of circulating micro RNA s in patients with acute chest pain. J Intern Med 2015; 277(2): 260-71.
[http://dx.doi.org/10.1111/joim.12183] [PMID: 24345063]

[115] Schulte C, Molz S, Appelbaum S, *et al.* miRNA-197 and miRNA-223 predict cardiovascular death in a

cohort of patients with symptomatic coronary artery disease. PLoS One 2015; 10(12): e0145930.
[http://dx.doi.org/10.1371/journal.pone.0145930] [PMID: 26720041]

[116] Zoch ML, Clemens TL, Riddle RC. New insights into the biology of osteocalcin. Bone 2016; 82: 42-9.
[http://dx.doi.org/10.1016/j.bone.2015.05.046] [PMID: 26055108]

[117] Wen L, Chen J, Duan L, Li S. Vitamin K-dependent proteins involved in bone and cardiovascular health (Review). Mol Med Rep 2018; 18(1): 3-15.
[http://dx.doi.org/10.3892/mmr.2018.8940] [PMID: 29749440]

[118] Ferron M, Wei J, Yoshizawa T, *et al.* Insulin signaling in osteoblasts integrates bone remodeling and energy metabolism. Cell 2010; 142(2): 296-308.
[http://dx.doi.org/10.1016/j.cell.2010.06.003] [PMID: 20655470]

[119] Faienza MF, Luce V, Ventura A, *et al.* Skeleton and glucose metabolism: a bone-pancreas loop. Int J Endocrinol 2015; 1-7.
[http://dx.doi.org/10.1155/2015/758148] [PMID: 25873957]

[120] Booth SL, Centi A, Smith SR, Gundberg C. The role of osteocalcin in human glucose metabolism: Marker or mediator? Nat Rev Endocrinol 2013; 9(1): 43-55.
[http://dx.doi.org/10.1038/nrendo.2012.201] [PMID: 23147574]

[121] Booth SL, Rajabi AA. Determinants of vitamin K status in humans. Vitam Horm 2008; 78: 1-22.
[http://dx.doi.org/10.1016/S0083-6729(07)00001-5] [PMID: 18374187]

[122] Reyes-Garcia R, Rozas-Moreno P, Jimenez-Moleon JJ, *et al.* Relationship between serum levels of osteocalcin and atherosclerotic disease in type 2 diabetes. Diabetes Metab 2012; 38(1): 76-81.
[http://dx.doi.org/10.1016/j.diabet.2011.07.008] [PMID: 21996253]

[123] Ogawa-Furuya N, Yamaguchi T, Yamamoto M, Kanazawa I, Sugimoto T. Serum osteocalcin levels are inversely associated with abdominal aortic calcification in men with type 2 diabetes mellitus. Osteoporos Int 2013; 24(8): 2223-30.
[http://dx.doi.org/10.1007/s00198-013-2289-6] [PMID: 23563931]

[124] Evrard S, Delanaye P, Kamel S, *et al.* Vascular calcification: From pathophysiology to biomarkers. Clin Chim Acta 2015; 438: 401-14.
[http://dx.doi.org/10.1016/j.cca.2014.08.034] [PMID: 25236333]

[125] Oury F, Khrimian L, Denny CA, *et al.* Maternal and offspring pools of osteocalcin influence brain development and functions. Cell 2013; 155(1): 228-41.
[http://dx.doi.org/10.1016/j.cell.2013.08.042] [PMID: 24074871]

[126] Lee NK, Sowa H, Hinoi E, *et al.* Endocrine regulation of energy metabolism by the skeleton. Cell 2007; 130(3): 456-69.
[http://dx.doi.org/10.1016/j.cell.2007.05.047] [PMID: 17693256]

[127] Yeap BB, Chubb SAP, Flicker L, *et al.* Reduced serum total osteocalcin is associated with metabolic syndrome in older men *via* waist circumference, hyperglycemia, and triglyceride levels. Eur J Endocrinol 2010; 163(2): 265-72.
[http://dx.doi.org/10.1530/EJE-10-0414] [PMID: 20501596]

[128] Oury F, Sumara G, Sumara O, *et al.* Endocrine regulation of male fertility by the skeleton. Cell 2011; 144(5): 796-809.
[http://dx.doi.org/10.1016/j.cell.2011.02.004] [PMID: 21333348]

[129] Kanazawa I, Tanaka K, Ogawa N, Yamauchi M, Yamaguchi T, Sugimoto T. Undercarboxylated osteocalcin is positively associated with free testosterone in male patients with type 2 diabetes mellitus. Osteoporos Int 2013; 24(3): 1115-9.
[http://dx.doi.org/10.1007/s00198-012-2017-7] [PMID: 22669468]

[130] Seidu S, Kunutsor SK, Khunti K. Association of circulating osteocalcin with cardiovascular disease and intermediate cardiovascular phenotypes: Systematic review and meta-analysis. Scand Cardiovasc J 2019; 53(6): 286-95.

[http://dx.doi.org/10.1080/14017431.2019.1655166] [PMID: 31397589]

[131] Rached MT, Kode A, Xu L, *et al.* FoxO1 is a positive regulator of bone formation by favoring protein synthesis and resistance to oxidative stress in osteoblasts. Cell Metab 2010; 11(2): 147-60.
[http://dx.doi.org/10.1016/j.cmet.2010.01.001] [PMID: 20142102]

[132] Choy JC, Granville DJ, Hunt DWC, McManus BM. Endothelial cell apoptosis: Biochemical characteristics and potential implications for atherosclerosis. J Mol Cell Cardiol 2001; 33(9): 1673-90.
[http://dx.doi.org/10.1006/jmcc.2001.1419] [PMID: 11549346]

[133] Azekoshi Y, Yasu T, Watanabe S, *et al.* Free fatty acid causes leukocyte activation and resultant endothelial dysfunction through enhanced angiotensin II production in mononuclear and polymorphonuclear cells. Hypertension 2010; 56(1): 136-42.
[http://dx.doi.org/10.1161/HYPERTENSIONAHA.110.153056] [PMID: 20530293]

[134] Jung CH, Lee WJ, Hwang JY, *et al.* The preventive effect of uncarboxylated osteocalcin against free fatty acid-induced endothelial apoptosis through the activation of phosphatidylinositol 3-kinase/Akt signaling pathway. Metabolism 2013; 62(9): 1250-7.
[http://dx.doi.org/10.1016/j.metabol.2013.03.005] [PMID: 23639572]

[135] Gössl M, Mödder UI, Atkinson EJ, Lerman A, Khosla S. Osteocalcin expression by circulating endothelial progenitor cells in patients with coronary atherosclerosis. J Am Coll Cardiol 2008; 52(16): 1314-25.
[http://dx.doi.org/10.1016/j.jacc.2008.07.019] [PMID: 18929243]

[136] Flammer AJ, Gössl M, Widmer RJ, *et al.* Osteocalcin positive CD133+/CD34-/KDR+ progenitor cells as an independent marker for unstable atherosclerosis. Eur Heart J 2012; 33(23): 2963-9.
[http://dx.doi.org/10.1093/eurheartj/ehs234] [PMID: 22855739]

[137] Fadini GP, Miorin M, Facco M, *et al.* Circulating endothelial progenitor cells are reduced in peripheral vascular complications of type 2 diabetes mellitus. J Am Coll Cardiol 2005; 45(9): 1449-57.
[http://dx.doi.org/10.1016/j.jacc.2004.11.067] [PMID: 15862417]

[138] Millar SA, Patel H, Anderson SI, England TJ, O'Sullivan SE. Osteocalcin, vascular calcification, and atherosclerosis: A systematic review and meta-analysis. Front Endocrinol 2017; 8: 183.
[http://dx.doi.org/10.3389/fendo.2017.00183] [PMID: 28824544]

[139] Urano T, Shiraki M, Kuroda T, *et al.* Low serum osteocalcin concentration is associated with incident type 2 diabetes mellitus in Japanese women. J Bone Miner Metab 2018; 36(4): 470-7.
[http://dx.doi.org/10.1007/s00774-017-0857-0] [PMID: 28766135]

[140] Kanazawa I, Yamaguchi T, Yamamoto M, *et al.* Serum osteocalcin level is associated with glucose metabolism and atherosclerosis parameters in type 2 diabetes mellitus. J Clin Endocrinol Metab 2009; 94(1): 45-9.
[http://dx.doi.org/10.1210/jc.2008-1455] [PMID: 18984661]

[141] Sheng L, Cao W, Cha B, Chen Z, Wang F, Liu J. Serum osteocalcin level and its association with carotid atherosclerosis in patients with type 2 diabetes. Cardiovasc Diabetol 2013; 12(1): 22.
[http://dx.doi.org/10.1186/1475-2840-12-22] [PMID: 23342952]

[142] Yang R, Ma X, Dou J, *et al.* Relationship between serum osteocalcin levels and carotid intima-media thickness in Chinese postmenopausal women. Menopause 2013; 20(11): 1194-9.
[http://dx.doi.org/10.1097/GME.0b013e31828aa32d] [PMID: 23571521]

[143] Pennisi P, Signorelli SS, Riccobene S, *et al.* Low bone density and abnormal bone turnover in patients with atherosclerosis of peripheral vessels. Osteoporos Int 2004; 15(5): 389-95.
[http://dx.doi.org/10.1007/s00198-003-1550-9] [PMID: 14661073]

[144] Ma H, Lin H, Hu Y, *et al.* Serum levels of osteocalcin in relation to glucose metabolism and carotid atherosclerosis in Chinese middle-aged and elderly male adults: The shanghai changfeng study. Eur J Intern Med 2014; 25(3): 259-64.
[http://dx.doi.org/10.1016/j.ejim.2014.01.017] [PMID: 24521696]

[145] Osorio A, Ortega E, Torres JM, Sanchez P, Ruiz-Requena E. Biochemical markers of vascular calcification in elderly hemodialysis patients. Mol Cell Biochem 2013; 374(1-2): 21-7.
[http://dx.doi.org/10.1007/s11010-012-1500-y] [PMID: 23124853]

[146] Schurgers LJ, Barreto DV, Barreto FC, *et al.* The circulating inactive form of matrix gla protein is a surrogate marker for vascular calcification in chronic kidney disease: A preliminary report. Clin J Am Soc Nephrol 2010; 5(4): 568-75.
[http://dx.doi.org/10.2215/CJN.07081009] [PMID: 20133489]

[147] Jia F, Wang S, Jing Y, *et al.* Osteocalcin and abdominal aortic calcification in hemodialysis patients: An observational cross-sectional study. Front Endocrinol 2021; 12: 620350.
[http://dx.doi.org/10.3389/fendo.2021.620350] [PMID: 33815281]

[148] Nagata Y, Inaba M, Imanishi Y, *et al.* Increased undercarboxylated osteocalcin/intact osteocalcin ratio in patients undergoing hemodialysis. Osteoporos Int 2015; 26(3): 1053-61.
[http://dx.doi.org/10.1007/s00198-014-2954-4] [PMID: 25403902]

[149] Lin L, Chiu LT, Lee MC, Hsu BG. Serum osteocalcin level is negatively associated with vascular reactivity index by digital thermal monitoring in kidney transplant recipients. Medicina 2020; 56(8): 400.
[http://dx.doi.org/10.3390/medicina56080400] [PMID: 32784817]

[150] London GM, Pannier B, Agharazii M, Guerin AP, Verbeke FHM, Marchais SJ. Forearm reactive hyperemia and mortality in end-stage renal disease. Kidney Int 2004; 65(2): 700-4.
[http://dx.doi.org/10.1111/j.1523-1755.2004.00434.x] [PMID: 14717944]

[151] Yeap BB, Chubb SAP, Flicker L, *et al.* Associations of total osteocalcin with all-cause and cardiovascular mortality in older men. The health in men study. Osteoporos Int 2012; 23(2): 599-606.
[http://dx.doi.org/10.1007/s00198-011-1586-1] [PMID: 21359669]

[152] Hwang YC, Kang M, Cho IJ, *et al.* Association between the circulating total osteocalcin level and the development of cardiovascular disease in middle-aged men: A mean 8.7-year longitudinal follow-up study. J Atheroscler Thromb 2015; 22(2): 136-43.
[http://dx.doi.org/10.5551/jat.25718] [PMID: 25195811]

[153] Beavan SR, Prentice A, Stirling DM, *et al.* Ethnic differences in osteocalcin γ-carboxylation, plasma phylloquinone (vitamin K1) and apolipoprotein E genotype. Eur J Clin Nutr 2005; 59(1): 72-81.
[http://dx.doi.org/10.1038/sj.ejcn.1602037] [PMID: 15340366]

[154] Gafni Y, Ptitsyn AA, Zilberman Y, Pelled G, Gimble JM, Gazit D. Circadian rhythm of osteocalcin in the maxillomandibular complex. J Dent Res 2009; 88(1): 45-50.
[http://dx.doi.org/10.1177/0022034508328012] [PMID: 19131316]

[155] Popa DS, Bigman G, Rusu ME. The role of vitamin K in humans: Implication in aging and age-associated diseases. Antioxidants 2021; 10(4): 566.
[http://dx.doi.org/10.3390/antiox10040566] [PMID: 33917442]

[156] Sheng J, Xu Z. Three decades of research on angiogenin: A review and perspective. Acta Biochim Biophys Sin 2016; 48(5): 399-410.
[http://dx.doi.org/10.1093/abbs/gmv131] [PMID: 26705141]

[157] Herrero-Fernandez B, Gomez-Bris R, Somovilla-Crespo B, Gonzalez-Granado JM. Immunobiology of atherosclerosis: A complex net of interactions. Int J Mol Sci 2019; 20(21): 5293.
[http://dx.doi.org/10.3390/ijms20215293] [PMID: 31653058]

[158] Joe Y, Uddin MJ, Park J, *et al.* Chung Hun Wha Dam Tang attenuates atherosclerosis in apolipoprotein E-deficient mice *via* the NF-κB pathway. Biomed Pharmacother 2019; 120: 109524.
[http://dx.doi.org/10.1016/j.biopha.2019.109524] [PMID: 31629255]

[159] Chen PY, Schwartz MA, Simons M. Endothelial-to-mesenchymal transition, vascular inflammation, and atherosclerosis. Front Cardiovasc Med 2020; 7: 53.
[http://dx.doi.org/10.3389/fcvm.2020.00053] [PMID: 32478094]

[160] Khurana R, Simons M, Martin JF, Zachary IC. Role of angiogenesis in cardiovascular disease: A critical appraisal. Circulation 2005; 112(12): 1813-24.
[http://dx.doi.org/10.1161/CIRCULATIONAHA.105.535294] [PMID: 16172288]

[161] Moreno PR, Purushothaman KR, Fuster V, *et al.* Plaque neovascularization is increased in ruptured atherosclerotic lesions of human aorta: Implications for plaque vulnerability. Circulation 2004; 110(14): 2032-8.
[http://dx.doi.org/10.1161/01.CIR.0000143233.87854.23] [PMID: 15451780]

[162] Tello-Montoliu A, Marín F, Patel J, *et al.* Plasma angiogenin levels in acute coronary syndromes: Implications for prognosis. Eur Heart J 2007; 28(24): 3006-11.
[http://dx.doi.org/10.1093/eurheartj/ehm488] [PMID: 17981827]

[163] Heeschen C, Dimmeler S, Hamm CW, Boersma E, Zeiher AM, Simoons ML. Prognostic significance of angiogenic growth factor serum levels in patients with acute coronary syndromes. Circulation 2003; 107(4): 524-30.
[http://dx.doi.org/10.1161/01.CIR.0000048183.37648.1A] [PMID: 12566361]

[164] Jones C, Sane DC, Herrington DM. Matrix metalloproteinases A review of their structure and role in acute coronary syndrome. Cardiovasc Res 2003; 59(4): 812-23.
[http://dx.doi.org/10.1016/S0008-6363(03)00516-9] [PMID: 14553821]

[165] Kręcki R, Krzemińska-Pakuła M, Drożdż J, *et al.* Relationship of serum angiogenin, adiponectin and resistin levels with biochemical risk factors and the angiographic severity of three-vessel coronary disease. Cardiol J 2010; 17(6): 599-606.
[PMID: 21154263]

[166] Jiang H, Zhang L, Yu Y, *et al.* A pilot study of angiogenin in heart failure with preserved ejection fraction: A novel potential biomarker for diagnosis and prognosis? J Cell Mol Med 2014; 18(11): 2189-97.
[http://dx.doi.org/10.1111/jcmm.12344] [PMID: 25124701]

[167] Patel JV, Sosin M, Gunarathne A, *et al.* Elevated angiogenin levels in chronic heart failure. Ann Med 2008; 40(6): 474-9.
[http://dx.doi.org/10.1080/07853890802001419] [PMID: 19160530]

[168] Lyons SM, Fay MM, Akiyama Y, Anderson PJ, Ivanov P. RNA biology of angiogenin: Current state and perspectives. RNA Biol 2017; 14(2): 171-8.
[http://dx.doi.org/10.1080/15476286.2016.1272746] [PMID: 28010172]

[169] Sarangdhar MA, Allam R. Angiogenin (ANG)—Ribonuclease inhibitor (RNH1) system in protein synthesis and disease. Int J Mol Sci 2021; 22(3): 1287.
[http://dx.doi.org/10.3390/ijms22031287] [PMID: 33525475]

[170] Mach F. The role of chemokines in atherosclerosis. Curr Atheroscler Rep 2001; 3(3): 243-51.
[http://dx.doi.org/10.1007/s11883-001-0067-y] [PMID: 11286646]

[171] Ylä-Herttuala S, Lipton BA, Rosenfeld ME, *et al.* Expression of monocyte chemoattractant protein 1 in macrophage-rich areas of human and rabbit atherosclerotic lesions. Proc Natl Acad Sci USA 1991; 88(12): 5252-6.
[http://dx.doi.org/10.1073/pnas.88.12.5252] [PMID: 2052604]

[172] Egashira K. Molecular mechanisms mediating inflammation in vascular disease: Special reference to monocyte chemoattractant protein-1. Hypertension 2003; 41(3): 834-41.
[http://dx.doi.org/10.1161/01.HYP.0000051642.65283.36] [PMID: 12624005]

[173] Yamamoto T, Eckes B, Mauch C, Hartmann K, Krieg T. Monocyte chemoattractant protein-1 enhances gene expression and synthesis of matrix metalloproteinase-1 in human fibroblasts by an autocrine IL-1 α loop. J Immunol 2000; 164(12): 6174-9.
[http://dx.doi.org/10.4049/jimmunol.164.12.6174] [PMID: 10843667]

[174] Namiki M, Kawashima S, Yamashita T, *et al.* Local overexpression of monocyte chemoattractant

protein-1 at vessel wall induces infiltration of macrophages and formation of atherosclerotic lesion: synergism with hypercholesterolemia. Arterioscler Thromb Vasc Biol 2002; 22(1): 115-20.
[http://dx.doi.org/10.1161/hq0102.102278] [PMID: 11788470]

[175]   Inoue S, Egashira K, Ni W, *et al.* Anti-monocyte chemoattractant protein-1 gene therapy limits progression and destabilization of established atherosclerosis in apolipoprotein E-knockout mice. Circulation 2002; 106(21): 2700-6.
[http://dx.doi.org/10.1161/01.CIR.0000038140.80105.AD] [PMID: 12438296]

[176]   De Lemos JA, Morrow DA, Sabatine MS, *et al.* Association between plasma levels of monocyte chemoattractant protein-1 and long-term clinical outcomes in patients with acute coronary syndromes. Circulation 2003; 107(5): 690-5.
[http://dx.doi.org/10.1161/01.CIR.0000049742.68848.99] [PMID: 12578870]

[177]   Herder C, Baumert J, Thorand B, *et al.* Chemokines and incident coronary heart disease: Results from the MONICA/KORA Augsburg case-cohort study, 1984-2002. Arterioscler Thromb Vasc Biol 2006; 26(9): 2147-52.
[http://dx.doi.org/10.1161/01.ATV.0000235691.84430.86] [PMID: 16825597]

[178]   Iyer S, Acharya KR. Role of placenta growth factor in cardiovascular health. Trends Cardiovasc Med 2002; 12(3): 128-34.
[http://dx.doi.org/10.1016/S1050-1738(01)00164-5] [PMID: 12007738]

[179]   Luttun A, Tjwa M, Moons L, *et al.* Revascularization of ischemic tissues by PlGF treatment, and inhibition of tumor angiogenesis, arthritis and atherosclerosis by anti-Flt1. Nat Med 2002; 8(8): 831-40.
[http://dx.doi.org/10.1038/nm731] [PMID: 12091877]

[180]   Autiero M, Luttun A, Tjwa M, Carmeliet P. Placental growth factor and its receptor, vascular endothelial growth factor receptor-1: novel targets for stimulation of ischemic tissue revascularization and inhibition of angiogenic and inflammatory disorders. J Thromb Haemost 2003; 1(7): 1356-70.
[http://dx.doi.org/10.1046/j.1538-7836.2003.00263.x] [PMID: 12871269]

[181]   Khurana R, Moons L, Shafi S, *et al.* Placental growth factor promotes atherosclerotic intimal thickening and macrophage accumulation. Circulation 2005; 111(21): 2828-36.
[http://dx.doi.org/10.1161/CIRCULATIONAHA.104.495887] [PMID: 15911697]

[182]   Heeschen C, Dimmeler S, Fichtlscherer S, *et al.* Prognostic value of placental growth factor in patients with acute chest pain. JAMA 2004; 291(4): 435-41.
[http://dx.doi.org/10.1001/jama.291.4.435] [PMID: 14747500]

[183]   Lenderink T, Heeschen C, Fichtlscherer S, *et al.* Elevated placental growth factor levels are associated with adverse outcomes at four-year follow-up in patients with acute coronary syndromes. J Am Coll Cardiol 2006; 47(2): 307-11.
[http://dx.doi.org/10.1016/j.jacc.2005.08.063] [PMID: 16412852]

[184]   Bayes-Genis A, Conover CA, Overgaard MT, *et al.* Pregnancy-associated plasma protein A as a marker of acute coronary syndromes. N Engl J Med 2001; 345(14): 1022-9.
[http://dx.doi.org/10.1056/NEJMoa003147] [PMID: 11586954]

[185]   Sangiorgi G, Mauriello A, Bonanno E, *et al.* Pregnancy-associated plasma protein-a is markedly expressed by monocyte-macrophage cells in vulnerable and ruptured carotid atherosclerotic plaques: A link between inflammation and cerebrovascular events. J Am Coll Cardiol 2006; 47(11): 2201-11.
[http://dx.doi.org/10.1016/j.jacc.2005.11.086] [PMID: 16750685]

[186]   Clay Bunn R, Fowlkes JL. Insulin-like growth factor binding protein proteolysis. Trends Endocrinol Metab 2003; 14(4): 176-81.
[http://dx.doi.org/10.1016/S1043-2760(03)00049-3] [PMID: 12714278]

[187]   Lund J, Qin QP, Ilva T, *et al.* Circulating pregnancy-associated plasma protein a predicts outcome in patients with acute coronary syndrome but no troponin I elevation. Circulation 2003; 108(16): 1924-6.
[http://dx.doi.org/10.1161/01.CIR.0000096054.18485.07] [PMID: 14530192]

[188] Heeschen C, Dimmeler S, Hamm CW, Fichtlscherer S, Simoons ML, Zeiher AM. Pregnancy-associated plasma protein-A levels in patients with acute coronary syndromes. J Am Coll Cardiol 2005; 45(2): 229-37.
[http://dx.doi.org/10.1016/j.jacc.2004.09.060] [PMID: 15653020]

[189] Lund J, Qin QP, Ilva T, *et al.* Pregnancy-associated plasma protein A: A biomarker in acute ST-elevation myocardial infarction (STEMI). Ann Med 2006; 38(3): 221-8.
[http://dx.doi.org/10.1080/07853890500525883] [PMID: 16720436]

[190] Cosin-Sales J, Christiansen M, Kaminski P, *et al.* Pregnancy-associated plasma protein A and its endogenous inhibitor, the proform of eosinophil major basic protein (proMBP), are related to complex stenosis morphology in patients with stable angina pectoris. Circulation 2004; 109(14): 1724-8.
[http://dx.doi.org/10.1161/01.CIR.0000124716.67921.D2] [PMID: 15023879]

[191] Elesber AA, Conover CA, Denktas AE, *et al.* Prognostic value of circulating pregnancy-associated plasma protein levels in patients with chronic stable angina. Eur Heart J 2006; 27(14): 1678-84.
[http://dx.doi.org/10.1093/eurheartj/ehl042] [PMID: 16717071]

[192] Conti E, Andreotti F, Zuppi C. Pregnancy-associated plasma protein a as predictor of outcome in patients with suspected acute coronary syndromes. Circulation 2004; 109(18): e211-2.
[http://dx.doi.org/10.1161/01.CIR.0000127614.27267.8F] [PMID: 15136514]

[193] Qin QP, Kokkala S, Lund J, *et al.* Immunoassays developed for pregnancy-associated plasma protein-A (PAPP-A) in pregnancy may not recognize PAPP-A in acute coronary syndromes. Clin Chem 2006; 52(3): 398-404.
[http://dx.doi.org/10.1373/clinchem.2005.058396] [PMID: 16423908]

[194] Schönbeck U, Libby P. CD40 signaling and plaque instability. Circ Res 2001; 89(12): 1092-103.
[http://dx.doi.org/10.1161/hh2401.101272] [PMID: 11739273]

[195] Schönbeck U, Gerdes N, Varo N, *et al.* Oxidized low-density lipoprotein augments and 3-hydroxy-3-methylglutaryl coenzyme A reductase inhibitors limit CD40 and CD40L expression in human vascular cells. Circulation 2002; 106(23): 2888-93.
[http://dx.doi.org/10.1161/01.CIR.0000043029.52803.7B] [PMID: 12460867]

[196] Mach F, Schönbeck U, Sukhova GK, Atkinson E, Libby P. Reduction of atherosclerosis in mice by inhibition of CD40 signalling. Nature 1998; 394(6689): 200-3.
[http://dx.doi.org/10.1038/28204] [PMID: 9671306]

[197] Schönbeck U, Sukhova GK, Shimizu K, Mach F, Libby P. Inhibition of CD40 signaling limits evolution of established atherosclerosis in mice. Proc Natl Acad Sci USA 2000; 97(13): 7458-63.
[http://dx.doi.org/10.1073/pnas.97.13.7458] [PMID: 10861012]

[198] Lutgens E, Cleutjens KBJM, Heeneman S, Koteliansky VE, Burkly LC, Daemen MJAP. Both early and delayed anti-CD40L antibody treatment induces a stable plaque phenotype. Proc Natl Acad Sci USA 2000; 97(13): 7464-9.
[http://dx.doi.org/10.1073/pnas.97.13.7464] [PMID: 10861013]

[199] Blake GJ, Ostfeld RJ, Yucel EK, *et al.* Soluble CD40 ligand levels indicate lipid accumulation in carotid atheroma: An *in vivo* study with high-resolution MRI. Arterioscler Thromb Vasc Biol 2003; 23(1): e11-4.
[http://dx.doi.org/10.1161/01.ATV.0000050143.22910.62] [PMID: 12524242]

[200] Huang H, Chen G, Liao D, Zhu Y, Xue X. Effects of berries consumption on cardiovascular risk factors: A meta-analysis with trial sequential analysis of randomized controlled trials. Sci Rep 2016; 6(1): 23625.
[http://dx.doi.org/10.1038/srep23625] [PMID: 27006201]

[201] Basu A, Du M, Leyva MJ, *et al.* Blueberries decrease cardiovascular risk factors in obese men and women with metabolic syndrome. J Nutr 2010; 140(9): 1582-7.
[http://dx.doi.org/10.3945/jn.110.124701] [PMID: 20660279]

[202] Soliman GA. Dietary fiber, atherosclerosis, and cardiovascular disease. Nutrients 2019; 11(5): 1155.
        [http://dx.doi.org/10.3390/nu11051155] [PMID: 31126110]

[203] Ha V, Sievenpiper JL, De Souza RJ, *et al.* Effect of dietary pulse intake on established therapeutic
        lipid targets for cardiovascular risk reduction: A systematic review and meta-analysis of randomized
        controlled trials. CMAJ 2014; 186(8): E252-62.
        [http://dx.doi.org/10.1503/cmaj.131727] [PMID: 24710915]

[204] Zhang Z, Lanza E, Kris-Etherton PM, *et al.* A high legume low glycemic index diet improves serum
        lipid profiles in men. Lipids 2010; 45(9): 765-75.
        [http://dx.doi.org/10.1007/s11745-010-3463-7] [PMID: 20734238]

[205] Bazzano LA, He J, Ogden LG, *et al.* Legume consumption and risk of coronary heart disease in US
        men and women: NHANES I epidemiologic follow-up study. Arch Intern Med 2001; 161(21): 2573-8.
        [http://dx.doi.org/10.1001/archinte.161.21.2573] [PMID: 11718588]

[206] Rubio-Guerra AF, Cabrera-Miranda LJ, Vargas-Robles H, Maceda-Serrano A, Lozano-Nuevo JJ,
        Escalante-Acosta BA. Correlation between levels of circulating adipokines and adiponectin/resistin
        index with carotid intima-media thickness in hypertensive type 2 diabetic patients. Cardiology 2013;
        125(3): 150-3.
        [http://dx.doi.org/10.1159/000348651] [PMID: 23736118]

[207] Paulo MC, Andrade AM, Andrade ML, *et al.* Influence of n-3 polyunsaturated fatty acids on soluble
        cellular adhesion molecules as biomarkers of cardiovascular risk in young healthy subjects. Nutr
        Metab Cardiovasc Dis 2008; 18(10): 664-70.
        [http://dx.doi.org/10.1016/j.numecd.2007.11.007] [PMID: 18420395]

[208] Chi Z, Melendez AJ. Role of cell adhesion molecules and immune-cell migration in the initiation,
        onset and development of atherosclerosis. Cell Adhes Migr 2007; 1(4): 171-5.
        [http://dx.doi.org/10.4161/cam.1.4.5321] [PMID: 19262139]

[209] Buscemi S, Nicolucci A, Lucisano G, *et al.* Habitual fish intake and clinically silent carotid
        atherosclerosis. Nutr J 2014; 13(1): 2.
        [http://dx.doi.org/10.1186/1475-2891-13-2] [PMID: 24405571]

[210] Kinsella JE, Lokesh B, Stone RA. Dietary n-3 polyunsaturated fatty acids and amelioration of
        cardiovascular disease: possible mechanisms. Am J Clin Nutr 1990; 52(1): 1-28.
        [http://dx.doi.org/10.1093/ajcn/52.1.1] [PMID: 2193500]

[211] Cuevas-Ramos D, Almeda-Valdés P, Chávez-Manzanera E, *et al.* Effect of tomato consumption on
        high-density lipoprotein cholesterol level: A randomized, single-blinded, controlled clinical trial.
        Diabetes Metab Syndr Obes 2013; 6: 263-73.
        [http://dx.doi.org/10.2147/DMSO.S48858] [PMID: 23935376]

[212] Jacques PF, Lyass A, Massaro JM, Vasan RS, D'Agostino RB Sr. Relationship of lycopene intake and
        consumption of tomato products to incident CVD. Br J Nutr 2013; 110(3): 545-51.
        [http://dx.doi.org/10.1017/S0007114512005417] [PMID: 23317928]

[213] Valderas-Martinez P, Chiva-Blanch G, Casas R, *et al.* Tomato sauce enriched with olive oil exerts
        greater effects on cardiovascular disease risk factors than raw tomato and tomato sauce: A randomized
        trial. Nutrients 2016; 8(3): 170.
        [http://dx.doi.org/10.3390/nu8030170] [PMID: 26999197]

[214] Palozza P, Parrone N, Simone RE, Catalano A. Lycopene in atherosclerosis prevention: An integrated
        scheme of the potential mechanisms of action from cell culture studies. Arch Biochem Biophys 2010;
        504(1): 26-33.
        [http://dx.doi.org/10.1016/j.abb.2010.06.031] [PMID: 20599665]

[215] Olas B. Anti-aggregatory potential of selected vegetables-promising dietary components for the
        prevention and treatment of cardiovascular disease. Adv Nutr 2019; 10(2): 280-90.
        [http://dx.doi.org/10.1093/advances/nmy085] [PMID: 30759176]

[216] Blekkenhorst LC, Bondonno CP, Lewis JR, *et al.* Cruciferous and allium vegetable intakes are inversely associated with 15-year atherosclerotic vascular disease deaths in older adult women. J Am Heart Assoc 2017; 6(10): e006558.
[http://dx.doi.org/10.1161/JAHA.117.006558] [PMID: 29066442]

[217] Mahmoud AM, Hernández Bautista RJ, Sandhu MA, Hussein OE. Beneficial effects of citrus flavonoids on cardiovascular and metabolic health. Oxid Med Cell Longev 2019; 1-19.
[http://dx.doi.org/10.1155/2019/5484138] [PMID: 30962863]

[218] Gorinstein S, Caspi A, Libman I, *et al.* Red grapefruit positively influences serum triglyceride level in patients suffering from coronary atherosclerosis: Studies *in vitro* and in humans. J Agric Food Chem 2006; 54(5): 1887-92.
[http://dx.doi.org/10.1021/jf058171g] [PMID: 16506849]

[219] Miwa Y, Yamada M, Sunayama T, *et al.* Effects of glucosyl hesperidin on serum lipids in hyperlipidemic subjects: Preferential reduction in elevated serum triglyceride level. J Nutr Sci Vitaminol 2004; 50(3): 211-8.
[http://dx.doi.org/10.3177/jnsv.50.211] [PMID: 15386934]

[220] Tsui PF, Lin CS, Ho LJ, Lai JH. Spices and atherosclerosis. Nutrients 2018; 10(11): 1724.
[http://dx.doi.org/10.3390/nu10111724] [PMID: 30423840]

[221] Son D, Akiba S, Hong J, *et al.* Piperine inhibits the activities of platelet cytosolic phospholipase A2 and thromboxane A2 synthase without affecting cyclooxygenase-1 activity: different mechanisms of action are involved in the inhibition of platelet aggregation and macrophage inflammatory response. Nutrients 2014; 6(8): 3336-52.
[http://dx.doi.org/10.3390/nu6083336] [PMID: 25153972]

[222] Zeng HH, Tu PF, Zhou K, Wang H, Wang BH, Lu JF. Antioxidant properties of phenolic diterpenes from Rosmarinus officinalis. Acta Pharmacol Sin 2001; 22(12): 1094-8.
[PMID: 11749806]

[223] Mohammadi A, Sahebkar A, Iranshahi M, *et al.* Effects of supplementation with curcuminoids on dyslipidemia in obese patients: A randomized crossover trial. Phytother Res 2013; 27(3): 374-9.
[http://dx.doi.org/10.1002/ptr.4715] [PMID: 22610853]

[224] DiSilvestro RA, Joseph E, Zhao S, Bomser J. Diverse effects of a low dose supplement of lipidated curcumin in healthy middle aged people. Nutr J 2012; 11(1): 79.
[http://dx.doi.org/10.1186/1475-2891-11-79] [PMID: 23013352]

[225] Francis AA, Deniset JF, Austria JA, *et al.* Effects of dietary flaxseed on atherosclerotic plaque regression. Am J Physiol Heart Circ Physiol 2013; 304(12): H1743-51.
[http://dx.doi.org/10.1152/ajpheart.00606.2012] [PMID: 23585134]

[226] Prasad K, Jadhav A. Prevention and treatment of atherosclerosis with flaxseed -derived compound secoisolariciresinol diglucoside. Curr Pharm Des 2015; 22(2): 214-20.
[http://dx.doi.org/10.2174/1381612822666151112151130] [PMID: 26561066]

[227] Lidder S, Webb AJ. Vascular effects of dietary nitrate (as found in green leafy vegetables and beetroot) *via* the nitrate-nitrite-nitric oxide pathway. Br J Clin Pharmacol 2013; 75(3): 677-96.
[http://dx.doi.org/10.1111/j.1365-2125.2012.04420.x] [PMID: 22882425]

[228] Raubenheimer K, Hickey D, Leveritt M, *et al.* Acute effects of nitrate-rich beetroot juice on blood pressure, hemostasis and vascular inflammation markers in healthy older adults: A randomized, placebo-controlled crossover study. Nutrients 2017; 9(11): 1270.
[http://dx.doi.org/10.3390/nu9111270] [PMID: 29165355]

[229] Jacobs DR Jr, Gallaher DD. Whole grain intake and cardiovascular disease: A review. Curr Atheroscler Rep 2004; 6(6): 415-23.
[http://dx.doi.org/10.1007/s11883-004-0081-y] [PMID: 15485586]

[230] Anderson JW, Hanna TJ, Peng X, Kryscio RJ. Whole grain foods and heart disease risk. J Am Coll

Nutr 2000; 19(3); Suppl: 291S-9S.
[http://dx.doi.org/10.1080/07315724.2000.10718963] [PMID: 10875600]

[231] Andersson KE, Svedberg KA, Lindholm MW, Öste R, Hellstrand P. Oats (*Avena sativa*) reduce atherogenesis in LDL-receptor-deficient mice. Atherosclerosis 2010; 212(1): 93-9.
[http://dx.doi.org/10.1016/j.atherosclerosis.2010.05.001] [PMID: 20553794]

[232] Thongoun P, Pavadhgul P, Bumrungpert A, Satitvipawee P, Harjani Y, Kurilich A. Effect of oat consumption on lipid profiles in hypercholesterolemic adults. J Med Assoc Thai 2013; 96; Suppl 5: S25-32.
[PMID: 24851570]

[233] Thomas M, Kim S, Guo W, Collins FW, Wise ML, Meydani M. High levels of avenanthramides in oat-based diet further suppress high fat diet-induced atherosclerosis in Ldlr-/- Mice. J Agric Food Chem 2018; 66(2): 498-504.
[http://dx.doi.org/10.1021/acs.jafc.7b04860] [PMID: 29298067]

[234] Sang S, Chu Y. Whole grain oats, more than just a fiber: Role of unique phytochemicals. Mol Nutr Food Res 2017; 61(7): 1600715.
[http://dx.doi.org/10.1002/mnfr.201600715] [PMID: 28067025]

[235] Wu JR, Leu HB, Yin WH, *et al.* The benefit of secondary prevention with oat fiber in reducing future cardiovascular event among CAD patients after coronary intervention. Sci Rep 2019; 9(1): 3091.
[http://dx.doi.org/10.1038/s41598-019-39310-2] [PMID: 30816213]

[236] Djoussé L, Hopkins PN, Arnett DK, *et al.* Chocolate consumption is inversely associated with calcified atherosclerotic plaque in the coronary arteries: The NHLBI family heart study. Clin Nutr 2011; 30(1): 38-43.
[http://dx.doi.org/10.1016/j.clnu.2010.06.011] [PMID: 20655129]

[237] Loffredo L, Perri L, Catasca E, *et al.* Dark chocolate acutely improves walking autonomy in patients with peripheral artery disease. J Am Heart Assoc 2014; 3(4): e001072.
[http://dx.doi.org/10.1161/JAHA.114.001072] [PMID: 24990275]

[238] Widmer RJ, Freund MA, Flammer AJ, *et al.* Beneficial effects of polyphenol-rich olive oil in patients with early atherosclerosis. Eur J Nutr 2013; 52(3): 1223-31.
[http://dx.doi.org/10.1007/s00394-012-0433-2] [PMID: 22872323]

[239] Gorzynik-Debicka M, Przychodzen P, Cappello F, *et al.* Potential health benefits of olive oil and plant polyphenols. Int J Mol Sci 2018; 19(3): 686.
[http://dx.doi.org/10.3390/ijms19030686] [PMID: 29495598]

[240] Kelly JH Jr, Sabaté J. Nuts and coronary heart disease: An epidemiological perspective. Br J Nutr 2006; 96(S2) (Suppl. 2): S61-7.
[http://dx.doi.org/10.1017/BJN20061865] [PMID: 17125535]

[241] Kris-Etherton PM. Walnuts decrease risk of cardiovascular disease: A summary of efficacy and biologic mechanisms. J Nutr 2014; 144(4) (Suppl.): 547S-54S.
[http://dx.doi.org/10.3945/jn.113.182907] [PMID: 24500935]

[242] De Oliveira Otto MC, Wu JHY, Baylin A, *et al.* Circulating and dietary omega-3 and omega-6 polyunsaturated fatty acids and incidence of CVD in the multi-ethnic study of atherosclerosis. J Am Heart Assoc 2013; 2(6): e000506.
[http://dx.doi.org/10.1161/JAHA.113.000506] [PMID: 24351702]

[243] Bertoia ML, Triche EW, Michaud DS, *et al.* Mediterranean and dietary approaches to stop hypertension dietary patterns and risk of sudden cardiac death in postmenopausal women. Am J Clin Nutr 2014; 99(2): 344-51.
[http://dx.doi.org/10.3945/ajcn.112.056135] [PMID: 24351877]

[244] Saulle R, La Torre G. The mediterranean diet, recognized by UNESCO as a cultural heritage of humanity. Ital J Public Health 2012; 7(4)

[245] Gardener H, Wright CB, Cabral D, *et al.* Mediterranean diet and carotid atherosclerosis in the Northern Manhattan Study. Atherosclerosis 2014; 234(2): 303-10.
[http://dx.doi.org/10.1016/j.atherosclerosis.2014.03.011] [PMID: 24721190]

[246] Esposito K, Marfella R, Ciotola M, *et al.* Effect of a mediterranean-style diet on endothelial dysfunction and markers of vascular inflammation in the metabolic syndrome: a randomized trial. JAMA 2004; 292(12): 1440-6.
[http://dx.doi.org/10.1001/jama.292.12.1440] [PMID: 15383514]

[247] Keys A, Mienotti A, Karvonen MJ, *et al.* The diet and 15-year death rate in the seven countries study. Am J Epidemiol 1986; 124(6): 903-15.
[http://dx.doi.org/10.1093/oxfordjournals.aje.a114480] [PMID: 3776973]

[248] Estruch R, Ros E, Salas-Salvadó J, *et al.* Primary prevention of cardiovascular disease with a Mediterranean diet supplemented with extra-virgin olive oil or nuts. N Engl J Med 2018; 378(25): e34.
[http://dx.doi.org/10.1056/NEJMoa1800389] [PMID: 29897866]

[249] Yan SH, Zhao NW, Geng ZR, *et al.* Modulations of Keap1-Nrf2 signaling axis by TIIA ameliorated the oxidative stress-induced myocardial apoptosis. Free Radic Biol Med 2018; 115: 191-201.
[http://dx.doi.org/10.1016/j.freeradbiomed.2017.12.001] [PMID: 29221988]

[250] Saita E, Kondo K, Momiyama Y. Anti-inflammatory diet for atherosclerosis and coronary artery disease: Antioxidant foods. Clin Med Insights Cardiol 2015; 8 (Suppl. 3): 61-5.
[http://dx.doi.org/10.4137/CMC.S17071] [PMID: 26279633]

[251] Harris WS. The prevention of atherosclerosis with antioxidants. Clin Cardiol 1992; 15(9): 636-40.
[http://dx.doi.org/10.1002/clc.4960150904] [PMID: 1395197]

[252] Wattanapitayakul S, Bauer JA. Oxidative pathways in cardiovascular disease: roles, mechanisms, and therapeutic implications. Pharmacol Ther 2001; 89(2): 187-206.
[http://dx.doi.org/10.1016/S0163-7258(00)00114-5] [PMID: 11316520]

[253] Moser M, Chun O. Vitamin C and heart health: A review based on findings from epidemiologic studies. Int J Mol Sci 2016; 17(8): 1328.
[http://dx.doi.org/10.3390/ijms17081328] [PMID: 27529239]

[254] Meydani M, Kwan P, Band M, *et al.* Long-term vitamin E supplementation reduces atherosclerosis and mortality in Ldlr−/− mice, but not when fed Western style diet. Atherosclerosis 2014; 233(1): 196-205.
[http://dx.doi.org/10.1016/j.atherosclerosis.2013.12.006] [PMID: 24529144]

[255] Chan AC. Vitamin E and atherosclerosis. J Nutr 1998; 128(10): 1593-6.
[http://dx.doi.org/10.1093/jn/128.10.1593] [PMID: 9772122]

[256] Azzi A, Boscoboinik D, Marilley D, Ozer NK, Stäuble B, Tasinato A. Vitamin E: A sensor and an information transducer of the cell oxidation state. Am J Clin Nutr 1995; 62(6) (Suppl.): 1337S-46S.
[http://dx.doi.org/10.1093/ajcn/62.6.1337S] [PMID: 7495229]

[257] Bendich A, D'Apolito P, Gabriel E, Machlin LJ. Interaction of dietary vitamin C and vitamin E on guinea pig immune responses to mitogens. J Nutr 1984; 114(9): 1588-93.
[http://dx.doi.org/10.1093/jn/114.9.1588] [PMID: 6332184]

[258] Boscoboinik D, Szewczyk A, Hensey C, Azzi A. Inhibition of cell proliferation by alpha-tocopherol. Role of protein kinase C. J Biol Chem 1991; 266(10): 6188-94.
[http://dx.doi.org/10.1016/S0021-9258(18)38102-X] [PMID: 2007576]

[259] Buettner GR. The pecking order of free radicals and antioxidants: Lipid peroxidation, α-tocopherol, and ascorbate. Arch Biochem Biophys 1993; 300(2): 535-43.
[http://dx.doi.org/10.1006/abbi.1993.1074] [PMID: 8434935]

[260] Chan AC. Partners in defense, vitamin E and vitamin C. Can J Physiol Pharmacol 1993; 71(9): 725-31.
[http://dx.doi.org/10.1139/y93-109] [PMID: 8313238]

[261] Chan AC, Leith MK. Decreased prostacyclin synthesis in vitamin E-deficient rabbit aorta. Am J Clin Nutr 1981; 34(11): 2341-7.
[http://dx.doi.org/10.1093/ajcn/34.11.2341] [PMID: 7030047]

[262] Chan AC, Tran K, Pyke DD, Powell WS. Effects of dietary vitamin E on the biosynthesis of 5-lipoxygenase products by rat polymorphonuclear leukocytes (PMNL). Biochim Biophys Acta Lipids Lipid Metab 1989; 1005(3): 265-9.
[http://dx.doi.org/10.1016/0005-2760(89)90047-7] [PMID: 2508746]

[263] Chan AC, Tran K, Raynor T, Ganz PR, Chow CK. Regeneration of vitamin E in human platelets. J Biol Chem 1991; 266(26): 17290-5.
[http://dx.doi.org/10.1016/S0021-9258(19)47372-9] [PMID: 1910041]

[264] Chan AC, Wagner M, Kennedy C, Mroske C, Proulx P, Laneuville O, *et al.* Vitamin E up-regulates phospholipase A~ 2, arachidonic acid release and cyclooxygenase in endothelial cells. Aktuel Ernahrungsmed 1998; 23: 152-9.

[265] Chatelain E, Boscoboinik DO, Bartoli GM, *et al.* Inhibition of smooth muscle cell proliferation and protein kinase C activity by tocopherols and tocotrienols. Biochim Biophys Acta Mol Cell Res 1993; 1176(1-2): 83-9.
[http://dx.doi.org/10.1016/0167-4889(93)90181-N] [PMID: 7680904]

[266] Cominacini L, Garbin U, Pasini AF, *et al.* Antioxidants inhibit the expression of intercellular cell adhesion molecule-1 and vascular cell adhesion molecule-1 induced by oxidized LDL on human umbilical vein endothelial cells. Free Radic Biol Med 1997; 22(1-2): 117-27.
[http://dx.doi.org/10.1016/S0891-5849(96)00271-7] [PMID: 8958136]

[267] Ramji DP. Polyunsaturated fatty acids and atherosclerosis: Insights from pre-clinical studies. Eur J Lipid Sci Technol 2019; 121(1): 1800029.
[http://dx.doi.org/10.1002/ejlt.201800029]

[268] Moss JWE, Williams JO, Ramji DP. Nutraceuticals as therapeutic agents for atherosclerosis. Bio chem Biophys Acta Mol Basis Dis 2018; 1864(5) (5 Pt A): 1562-72.
[http://dx.doi.org/10.1016/j.bbadis.2018.02.006] [PMID: 29454074]

[269] Moss JWE, Ramji DP. Nutraceutical therapies for atherosclerosis. Nat Rev Cardiol 2016; 13(9): 513-32.
[http://dx.doi.org/10.1038/nrcardio.2016.103] [PMID: 27383080]

[270] Buckley ML, Ramji DP. The influence of dysfunctional signaling and lipid homeostasis in mediating the inflammatory responses during atherosclerosis. Biochim Biophys Acta Mol Basis Dis 2015; 1852(7): 1498-510.
[http://dx.doi.org/10.1016/j.bbadis.2015.04.011] [PMID: 25887161]

[271] Ramji DP, Davies TS. Cytokines in atherosclerosis: Key players in all stages of disease and promising therapeutic targets. Cytokine Growth Factor Rev 2015; 26(6): 673-85.
[http://dx.doi.org/10.1016/j.cytogfr.2015.04.003] [PMID: 26005197]

[272] Calder PC. The role of marine omega-3 (*n*-3) fatty acids in inflammatory processes, atherosclerosis and plaque stability. Mol Nutr Food Res 2012; 56(7): 1073-80.
[http://dx.doi.org/10.1002/mnfr.201100710] [PMID: 22760980]

[273] Campbell AP. DASH eating plan: An eating pattern for diabetes management. Diabetes Spectr 2017; 30(2): 76-81.
[http://dx.doi.org/10.2337/ds16-0084] [PMID: 28588372]

[274] Fuentes MC, Lajo T, Carrión JM, Cuñé J. Cholesterol-lowering efficacy of *Lactobacillus plantarum* CECT 7527, 7528 and 7529 in hypercholesterolaemic adults. Br J Nutr 2013; 109(10): 1866-72.
[http://dx.doi.org/10.1017/S000711451200373X] [PMID: 23017585]

[275] Jones ML, Martoni CJ, Prakash S. Cholesterol lowering and inhibition of sterol absorption by *Lactobacillus reuteri* NCIMB 30242: A randomized controlled trial. Eur J Clin Nutr 2012; 66(11):

1234-41.
[http://dx.doi.org/10.1038/ejcn.2012.126] [PMID: 22990854]

[276] Costabile A, Buttarazzi I, Kolida S, *et al.* An *in vivo* assessment of the cholesterol-lowering efficacy of *Lactobacillus plantarum* ECGC 13110402 in normal to mildly hypercholesterolaemic adults. PLoS One 2017; 12(12): e0187964.
[http://dx.doi.org/10.1371/journal.pone.0187964] [PMID: 29228000]

[277] Zhu L, Zhang D, Zhu H, *et al.* Berberine treatment increases Akkermansia in the gut and improves high-fat diet-induced atherosclerosis in Apoe$^{-/-}$ mice. Atherosclerosis 2018; 268: 117-26.
[http://dx.doi.org/10.1016/j.atherosclerosis.2017.11.023] [PMID: 29202334]

[278] Bird JK, Raederstorff D, Weber P, Steinert RE. Cardiovascular and antiobesity effects of resveratrol mediated through the gut microbiota. Adv Nutr 2017; 8(6): 839-49.
[http://dx.doi.org/10.3945/an.117.016568] [PMID: 29141969]

[279] Chen M, Yi L, Zhang Y, *et al.* Resveratrol attenuates trimethylamine-N-oxide (TMAO)-induced atherosclerosis by regulating TMAO synthesis and bile acid metabolism *via* remodeling of the gut microbiota. MBio 2016; 7(2): e02210-15.
[http://dx.doi.org/10.1128/mBio.02210-15] [PMID: 27048804]

[280] Ahmadi Khatir S, Bayatian A, Barzegari A, *et al.* Saffron (*Crocus sativus* L.) supplements modulate circulating MicroRNA (miR-21) in atherosclerosis patients: A randomized, double-blind, placebo-controlled trial. Iran Red Crescent Med J 2018; In Press.
[http://dx.doi.org/10.5812/ircmj.80260]

CHAPTER 8

Immunomodulating Botanicals: An Overview of the Bioactive Phytochemicals for the Management of Autoimmune Disorders

Ami P. Thakkar[1], **Amisha Vora**[1], **Harpal S. Buttar**[2] and **Ginpreet Kaur**[1,*]

[1] *Shobhaben Pratapbhai Patel School of Pharmacy and Technology Management, Shri Vile Parle Kelavani Mandal's Narsee Monjee Institute of Management Studies, Mumbai, Maharashtra, India*

[2] *Department of Pathology & Laboratory Medicine, Faculty of Medicine, University of Ottawa, Ottawa, Ontario, Canada*

Abstract: Immunomodulation refers to the mechanism by which the response of the immune system is modified by the regulation of antibody synthesis, leading to either an increase or a decrease in its levels in the circulation and body organs. Owing to their immunomodulation and remedial benefits, a broad range of herbal remedies have been shown to be effective in the treatment of autoimmune diseases such as multiple sclerosis, rheumatoid arthritis, myasthenia gravis, and systemic lupus erythematosus. The ancient Indian system of Ayurveda and different other alternative therapeutic methods have acknowledged the potential benefits of herbal-based remedies to upregulate or suppress the immune response in the human body. The conventional pharmacotherapies used for the management of autoimmune ailments are documented to cause serious drug-induced adverse reactions (ADRs). Whereas, some phytotherapies have proven safe, reliable, and efficient alternatives for the existing drug regimens with lesser ADRs. For instance, *Withania somnifera, Andrographis paniculate, Tinospora cordifolia, Glycyrrhiza glabra,* and *Berberis arista* are a few herbs whose bioactive phytoconstituents have been reported to possess powerful immunomodulation properties. Based on their purported immunomodulatory mechanisms, they can be used for the management of autoimmune conditions. The focus of this review is to highlight the key inflammatory biomarkers such as TNF-α and interleukin 1, 6 involved in the distortion of the immune system in humans. Also, we will discuss the usefulness of animal models for understanding the underlying mechanisms of autoimmune disorders. In addition, we will describe the patents of phytomedicine formulations filed by different manufacturers for the management of autoimmune disorders, as well as futuristic opportunities that should be explored for discovering the therapeutic functions of alternate remedies for treating autoimmune diseases.

* **Corresponding author Ginpreet Kaur:** Shobhaben Pratapbhai Patel School of Pharmacy and Technology Management, Shri Vile Parle Kelavani Mandal's Narsee Monjee Institute of Management Studies, Mumbai, Maharashtra, India; E-mail: Ginpreet.Kaur@nmims.edu

Pardeep Kaur, Tewin Tencomnao, Robin and Rajendra G. Mehta (Eds.)

Keywords: *Andrographis paniculate*, Autoimmune disorders, Animal models of autoimmune diseases, *Berberis arista*, Formulation patents, *Glycyrrhiza glabra*, Immunomodulators, *Tinospora cordifolia*, *Withania somnifera*.

INTRODUCTION

Antimicrobial resistance can be tackled by improving the host immune system [1]. The immune system is highly precised and developed, and prevents the host from the spectrum of foreign substances and infections [2]. The host immune system developed largely to protect the host against pathogenic germs, providing a survival benefit. The hosts try to resist the diseases, while the pathogens try to avoid the host's developing defenses [3]. Activated immune system causes coordinated release of various cells like natural killer cells, T cells, polymorphonuclear leukocytes, dendritic cells, macrophages, and B cells. These cells elimate the pathogens and maintain host immunity. The immune cells are produced by the primary lymphoid organs, like bone marrow, thymus, and secondary lymphatic tissues, like the spleen and lymph node [4]. Development of T cell and B cell occurs in thymus and bone marrow respectively [5]. Various immune cells are stored in the spleen and are circulated through the blood throughout the body when required. The lymphatic nodules contain plenty of white blood cells and the nodules present near the throat prevent the host from foreign particle invasion [6]. Natural killer cells can detect and eliminate tumor cells without any prior antigenic activation and secrete cytokines such as tumor necrosis factor-alpha (TNF-α) and interferon-gamma (IFN-γ) to improve immune responses [7].

The immune system consists of cells and chemical mediators that protect the organism's integrity against foreign microorganisms, and its perfect operation and stability are required to avoid a variety of immunomodulatory diseases [8]. Rheumatoid arthritis (RA) is an immunomodulatory condition that affects synovial joints. RA begins as painful inflammation of the joints and worsens, leading to joint deterioration and irreversible damage to joints [9]. The predominant factors involved in acute and chronic inflammation are cytokines, such as IL-17, IL-7, IL-1β, IL-6, IL-35 and TNF-α. They stimulate and activate dendritic cells, B cells and T cells, thereby leading to the activation of receptor complexes through Janus kinase (JAK). Furthermore, monocyte recruitment and macrophage differentiation lead to the inflammation of synoviocytes in RA [10]. Multiple sclerosis (MS) is a neurodegenerative disorder of the central nervous system leading to chronic inflammation and demyelination of neurons that is affected by both genetic and environmental factors [11]. In systemic lupus erythematosus (SLE), the cells are attacked by the host's own immune system, resulting in widespread inflammation and tissue damage in the affected organs.

Body parts most likely to be affected include the brain, kidneys, lungs, skin, joints, and blood vessels [12]. The pathogenesis is mediated by cytokine IFN-α, which upon induction by the immune complexes upregulates several inflammatory proteins. T cell-derived cytokines like IFN-γ, IL-2, IL-6, IL-17, and IL-21 are dysregulated in SLE. A T cell phenotype is induced by the T cell-derived cytokines, characterized by the enhanced secretion of B cells and proinflammatory cytokines, and reduced expression of suppressive T cells, as well as a decrease in activation-induced cell death [13]. The neuromuscular disorder, myasthenia gravis (MS), weakens skeletal muscles due to impairment in the signalling between muscles and nerve cells [14]. In addition to cytokines, *anti-acetylcholine receptor* antibodies and complement proteins significantly contribute the progression of inflammation at the neuromuscular junction. The pathogenesis of MS can be attributed to the increased proportion of Th1 (type 1 helper T cell) and Th17 cells, whereas its development is ameliorated by Th2 and Treg (regulatory T cell) cells. Downregulation of IL-4 levels and upregulation of IL-17 are reported in patients with MS [15]. Fig. (**1**) shows the various immune cells that lead to immunomodulation in various diseases.

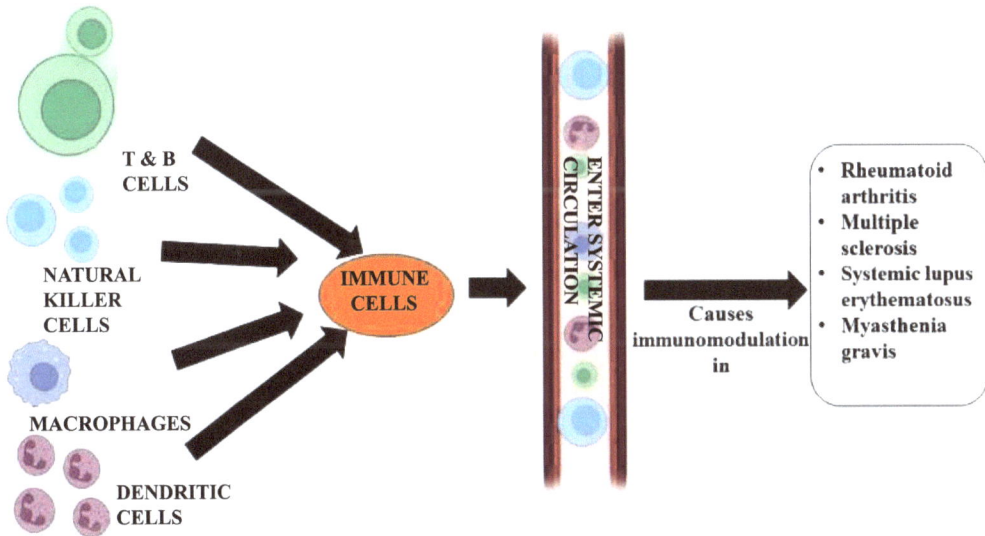

Fig. (1). Illustrates various immune cells that enter into the systemic circulation leading to immunomodulation [16, 17].

Research on these autoimmune illnesses has been conducted using a variety of animal models, each of which has a specific objective, rationale, and approach. Animal models have been utilized not just for fundamental scientific study but also for the development and evaluation of new vaccines and medicines, which has led to a number of important scientific breakthroughs [18]. Animal experimental models of autoimmune disorders may be broken down into two distinct categories: spontaneous models, in which the animals acquire the disease on their own, with or without any genetic changes; and induced models, in which the disease is purposefully produced [19]. Table **1** shows the various models explored for the various above-mentioned immunomodulatory diseases. It also illustrates the characteristics of each animal model concerning the inducers used for them.

Table 1. Clinical features of autoimmune diseases and the role of animal models in understanding the underlying mechanisms of autoimmune disorders.

Disease	Models for Autoimmune Diseases	Clinical Features of the Disease Model	References
Rheumatoid arthritis	Collagen-induced arthritis	• Stimulates a response from T cells as well as antibody. • Inoculation with mimicking collagen causes recurrent and intermittent episodes of arthritis.	[20,21]
	Antigen-induced arthritis	• The administration of antigens calls for a high level of technical understanding. • Stimulates both the humoral and cell-mediated immune responses.	[22,23]
	Collagen-antibody-induced arthritis	• Commencement in less than 48 hours. • Stimulates macrophages as well as polymorphonuclear cells. • No participation of the T cell or the B cell.	[24,25]
	Spontaneous occurrence in transgenic animals	• Comprises KBxN, DNaseII−/−IFN-IR−/−, and human TNF-α transgenic mice. • The sudden and severe development of arthritis, with a prevalence of one hundred percent.	[26,27]
	Zymosan-induced autoimmune disorder	• Progression of monoarthritis afterward 3 days of inoculation that recedes within day 7. • Need a TLR2 receptor. • Could be induced in a number of different mouse strains.	[28,29]

(Table 1) cont.....

Disease	Models for Autoimmune Diseases	Clinical Features of the Disease Model	References
Multiple sclerosis (MS)	Experimental autoimmune encephalomyelitis (EAE)	• Immunization of rodents with a complete Freund's adjuvant and an antigen linked with the central nervous system. • The progression of the illness is determined by the peptide antigen and the mice strain. • Actively inducing autoreactive T cells *via* peripheral immunization.	[30,31]
	Lysolecithin-induced MS	• Both demyelination and remyelination can be studied. • Therapeutical trials can be designed to suppress demyelination or accelerate remyelination.	[32,33]
	Cuprizone-induced MS	• Animal models have shown the occurrence of oligodendrocyte death and the progressive process of demyelination. • High level of reproducibility and can be readily adopted. • Produce demyelinating lesions consistently.	[34,35]
	Theiler's murine encephalomyelitis virus	• In vulnerable mouse strains, it may cause both neurological and gastrointestinal disorders. • Investigations can be done on damage to axons as well as inflammation-induced demyelination.	[36,37]
	EAE in transgenic mice	• Investigation can be done on activation of the immune system and neurological inflammation. • SJL/J mice immunization with PLP. • C57BL/6J mice immunization with MOG • Stimulation of relapsing/remitting MS. • The study of relapse rates can be undertaken. • Evaluation of potential therapeutic agents.	[32,33]

(Table 1) cont.....

Disease	Models for Autoimmune Diseases	Clinical Features of the Disease Model	References
Systemic lupus erythematosus	Pristane-induced lupus model	• Preference for rodent species of the female gender. • Mediated by Type I interferon. • Produces autoantibodies, arthritis, serositis, glomerulonephritis, anemia. • Suitable for the investigation of the associations between dysregulated type I interferon generation and the development of systemic lupus erythematosus (SLE) in humans.	[38,39]
	Induced Chronic Graft-versu--Host Disease	• Produces autoantibodies, T cell activation, glomerulonephritis, and proteinuria (donor CD4$^+$ T cell-dependent) polyclonal B cell activation. • B cells and T cells may also play a role in the progression of illness *via* other methods.	[40,41]
	Spontaneous autoimmune disease models	• F1 hybrid following cross between New Zealand blank mouse (NZB) and New Zealand white mouse (NZW) strains *lpr* mutation in Fas gene on MRL background. • Backcross of NZW and NZB/W F1 followed by siblings breeding. • Backcross between B6 X SB/Le F1 and SB/Le.	-
Myasthenia gravis	Acetylcholine receptor-experimental autoimmune myasthenia gravis	• Injection of complete Freuds' adjuvant + Acetylcholine receptor antibody (AChR) generates antibodies to counter AChR. • AChR introduction to antibody facilitates antibody binding.	[42,43]
	Experimental humanized mouse model	• The introduction of a thymic fragment to a mouse model results in the generation of antibodies and the accumulation of lymphocytes.	[44]
	Muscle-specific kinase myasthenia (MuSK) active immunization models	• Injection of MuSK+CFA results in the generation of antibodies targeting MuSK. • Injection of antibody to MuSK leads to binding of the antibody.	[44,45]

Immunomodulation is the process that brings about modification in the response of immune system by increasing or decreasing the production of serum antibodies. In clinical practice, immunomodulators are generally classified as immunostimulants, immunoadjuvants, and immunosuppressants, which effectively regulate immune response [46]. Fig. (**2**) illustrates the herb or its parts affecting innate and adaptive immunity. The Indian medical literature has shed light on a large number of medicinal plants that possess immunomodulatory activities and can be used in Rasayanas.

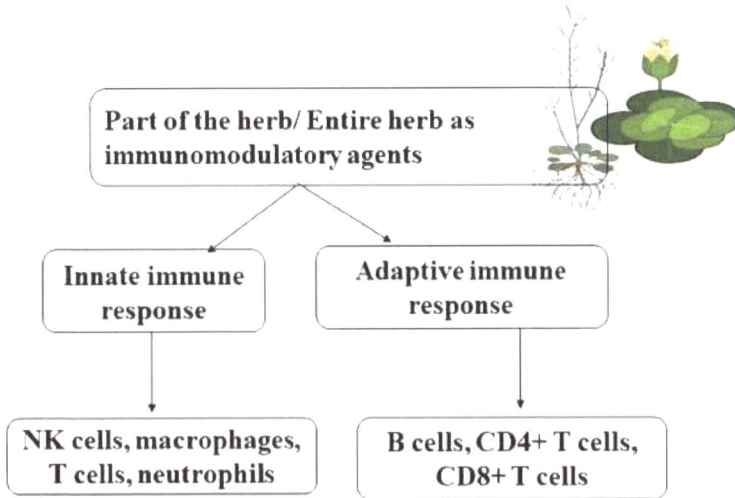

Fig. (2). Diagrammatic illustration of the entire herb or its parts affecting the innate and adaptive immunity.

Because of their immunomodulatory capabilities, medicinal plants can be used instead of conventional chemotherapy to treat disorders that threaten the host defense mechanism [47]. Although the development of modern therapeutics has reduced the use of traditional medicine, the potential of herbal therapy for both humans and animals remains undeniable [46]. As the World Health Organization (WHO) estimates, 80% of people worldwide, mostly in developing countries, prefer herbal medication for treating different diseases, including immune-related diseases. Moreover, approximately 30% of all drugs approved by the Food and Drug Administration (FDA) are derived from botanical sources [48]. The development of modern multi-herb prescriptions requires accurate investigations at the molecular level and standardized clinical trials. The discovery and utilization of the medicinal properties of plants have been made easier by emerging technologies like genomics and synthetic biology [49].

There has been an increasing surge in the use of herbals across the globe and India has been a leading exporter in supplying herbal medicines across the globe [50]. Fig. (**3**) illustrates the export trade value in million United States Dollars (USD) of India from the financial year 2010 to 2021.

**Export trade value in million USD
vs Financial year**

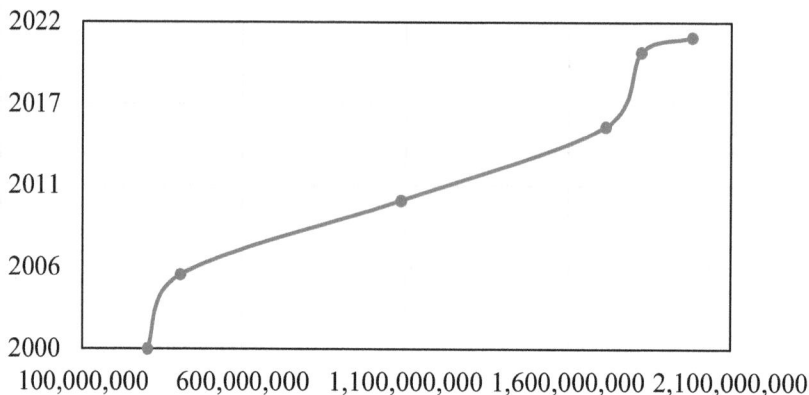

Fig. (3). Export trade value in million USD from India during the financial year 2010 to 2021 on COMTRADE statistics accessed *via* ITC 'Trade Map'.

HERBAL AND ALTERNATIVE REMEDIES USED FOR THE MANAGEMENT OF AUTOIMMUNE DISORDERS

Most traditional medications for the treatment of autoimmune illnesses are known to have serious side responses, and they are also expensive. Natural plant products are utilized in complementary and alternative medicine (CAM) to treat inflammatory and immunological problems [51]. The medicinal plant *Withania somnifera* can weaken or enhance the host's capacity to non-specifically resist infection and tumors or react specifically to a foreign substance [46]. *Tinospora cordifolia* shows lymphoproliferative and macrophage-activating properties, thus, proposing its use as an immunomodulator. Specific dosages of plant extracts and herbal-fed additions boost the effectiveness of cell-mediated immune responses. Because of their great effectiveness, low toxicity, and low cost, botanical compounds with potential therapeutic uses are in high demand [52]. A few examples of such therapeutic molecules include the cardiac stimulant digoxin which is obtained from *Digitalis purpurea;* antimalarials like quinine obtained from *Cinchona* bark; reserpine, an antipsychotic and antihypertensive drug from *Rauwolfia spp.*; salicylic acid, a precursor of aspirin, derived from *Salix spp* [53]. Immunostimulants like antigens stimulate the intracellular signaling pathway, leading to the expression of proinflammatory genes and cytokines, such as interleukin (IL)-2, IL-6, TNF-α, and IFN-α [54]. *Curcuma longa* (turmeric) has been of much interest for its action as an immunomodulatory agent that induces immune cells, such as B cells, T cells, dendritic cells, and macrophages. Similarly, the effect of *Echinacea* on immune cells has been studied extensively

[52]. The cytokine signature of each immunosuppressant is distinct, which can be used to determine the level of immunosuppression (under or over-immunosuppression) in transplant recipients. Modification of immunosuppressants could improve the cytokine profiles, maximizing the immunosuppressive effects and minimizing infection risk. Furthermore, immunosuppressants may inhibit the production of various cytokines, such as IL-1β, IL-10, IFN-γ, IL-13, TNF-α, IL-2, IL-4, IL-5, IL-6, IL-8, and granulocyte colony-stimulating factor [55]. In mouse splenocytes, the use of herbs like Ashwagandha and *Berberis arista* showed significant downregulation in the expressions of TNF-α, IL-1β, and MIP-1α, whereas IFN-γ levels were significantly upregulated. The regulation of the proinflammatory cytokines was hypothesized to occur *via* the NF-κB pathway [56, 57]. *Withania somnifera,* also called "Indian Ginseng or Ashwagandha", is a medicinal plant belonging to the Indian subcontinent. Its spectrum of phytochemicals is diverse and has a broad range of biological implications. The active constituents of *Withania somnifera* include withanoside IV, withanone, withaferin A, withanoside VII, withanoside V, withanolide A, withanolide B, viscosalactone B, 12-deoxywithastramonolide, 27-hydroxywithanone, and dihydrowithaferin A [58]. Furthermore, *Tinospora cordifolia* is another ayurvedic medicinal plant that is easily found in the Indian subcontinent and China.

The use of this plant, both alone and in combination, has been described in folk medicine as well as in the Ayurvedic system of medicine. The active constituents of *Tinospora cordifolia* include alkaloids; steroids; terpenoids; sesquiterpenoids; lignans; amritosides A, B, C, and D; and aliphatic compounds [59, 60]. One of the most popular medicinal plants, *Andrographis paniculate,* has been used traditionally for the treatment of an array of diseases. Its phytochemical constituents are unique, possessing interesting biological properties [61]. The active constituents of *Andrographis paniculata* are a new diterpene 21-nor-3,-9-isopropylidine-14-deoxy-ent-labda-8(17),13-dien-16,15-olide (1); five known labdane type diterpenes, such as andrographolide 3, 14- deoxyandrographolide 4, 14-deoxy-12-hydroxyandrographolide5, 14-deoxy-11,12-dihydroandrographolide 6, neoandrographolide 7; and two acids, like cinnamic acid 8, and ferulic acid 9 [62, 63]. *Curcuma longa* L. (turmeric), cultivated in southeast Asian countries, is one of the oldest cultivated spice plants belonging to the ginger family. In recent years, detailed *in-vitro* and *in-vivo* tests along with clinical trials have revealed its anti-inflammatory, antioxidant, and anti-cancer properties [64, 65]. Similarly, *Punica granatum,* a plant possessing remarkable medicinal properties along with a prominent medical history, has been the subject of current attraction due to its wide variety of therapeutic indications [66]. The active constituents are ellagic acid, punicalagin, punicalagin A&B, corilagin, gallic acid, punicalin, punicalin A&B, ascorbic acid, isovitexin, catechin, arjunic acid, and chebulaginic acid [67, 68]. The extract of another popular herb, *Camellia sinensis,* has been widely utilized in the traditional Chinese medicinal system and has currently gained special attention and popularity due to its beneficial effects in this modern era of changing lifestyles [69]. Its active constituents include (+)-catechin, (-)-epicatechin, (+)-gallocatechin, (-)-epigallocatechin, (-)-gallocatechin-3-O-gallate, (-)-epigallocatechin-3-O-gallate, and (-)-epicatechin-3-O-gallate [70]. The immunomodulatory and immunity booster herbal preparations have been used for various autoimmune diseases like RA, MS, and SLE [71]. The article covers the description of the established plants that act as immunomodulators, including plant parts and their active phytoconstituents, immunomodulatory mechanisms, and indications, as shown in Table **2**. Besides, patents registered for the plant herbs have also been illustrated.

Table 2. List of patents showing plant-based formulations with promising therapeutic potential for the management of autoimmune disorders.

Botanical Name	Family Name	Part of the Plant Used	Active Constituents	Immunomodulatory Mechanism	Indications	Patent No.	References
T. wilfordii Hook	Celastraceae	Roots	Diterpenes triptolide, tripdiolide, triptonide, 16-hydroxytriptolide, (5R)-5-hydroxytriptolide, tripchloride and celastrol	Activation of B cells and plasma cells leads to activation of macrophages /macrophages, astrocytes, and monocytes. These cells produce matrix metalloproteinases, autoantibodies against neurons/oligodendrocytes, chemokines, and inflammatory cytokines.	RA, MS	US5846742A US5580562A EP2414542B1	[72–76]
Withania somnifera	Solanaceae	Roots, leaves	Withanolides, withanosides withaferins, sitoindoside VII and VIII, isopellertierine, and anferine (1).	Downregulates the expression of proinflammatory cytokines, such as IFN-γ, IL-1β, TNF-α, and MIP-1α.	RA, MS, SLE	US9987323B2 US10646532B2 AU2020201462B2 EP1740196B1	[56,77–82]
Tinospora cordifolia	Menispermaceae	Stems	Cordifolioside A, 20-hydroxy ecdysone, tinosporaside, 8-hydroxy tinosporide, tinosporide, alkaloids like columbin, berberine, and tinosporic acid.	Macrophage activation. *Tinospora cordifolia* and lipopolysaccharide enhance lysozyme secretion in the J774A macrophage cell line.	RA, Diabetes, SLE, MS	WO2018/042229A1 US9675582B2	[83–86]
Andrographis paniculata	Acanthaceae	Entire herb	Diterpenoid lactones (andrographolides), panniculitis, farnesols, and flavonoids.	Inhibits inflammatory responses of neutrophils. Prevents the production of reactive oxygen species.	RA, MS	US7749547 US10786522B2 AU2011343634 B2	[56, 81, 87 - 89]
Berberis arista	Berberidaceae	Root, stem, leaf, fruit.	Isoquinoline, and alkaloids (the majority being berberine).	Inhibits T-cell response against allogenic or antigenic stimuli, which in turn inhibits or blocks the activation of T cells and suppresses TNF-induced reactions.	RA	US8163312B2 US9167842B2 US9623108B2 US9233133B2	[90 - 95]
Glycyrrhiza glabra	Fabaceae	Root, bark	Glycyrrhizin, glycyrrhetinic acid, and liquiritigenin	Interferes with IgE production by decreasing IgE-stimulating cytokine and subsequently inhibits the recruitment of neutrophils, macrophages, and lymphocytes.	RA	US20100221363A1 US20180200320A1 US10111912B2 US10111925B2	[96 - 101]
Zingiber Officinalis	Zingiberaceae	Rhizome	Zingerone, shogaols, gingerols, volatile oils, gingediol, and galanolactone.	Attenuates COX-1/Tx synthase enzymatic activity. Inhibits macrophage activation.	RA	US10016478B2 US20170136076A1 US9283259B2 CA2597900C US10751282B2	[99, 102 - 107]

(Table 2) cont.....

Botanical Name	Family Name	Part of the Plant Used	Active Constituents	Immunomodulatory Mechanism	Indications	Patent No.	References
Ocimum tenuiflorum	Lamiaceae	Leaves, stem	Oleanolic acid, ursolic acid, rosmarinic acid, eugenol, carvacrol, linalool, and β-caryophyllene.	Blocks cyclooxygenase and lipoxygenase pathways of arachidonate metabolism.	Immunity booster	US20150297652A1 US2015/0190446A1 WO2015000064A1 US2015/0374624A1 US9795647B2	[108 - 115]
Cinnamomum zelynicum	Lauraceae	Bark, inner bark	Cinnamaldehyde, eugenol, trans-cinnamic acid, phenolic compounds, catechins, terpenoids gum, mucilage, resin, starch, and sugar.	Reduces the expression of IL-6, IL-1β, TNF, and Cyclooxygenase (COX) enzymes.	RA	-	[116, 117]
Curcuma longa	Zingiberaceae	Rhizomes	Curcumin, tumerone, atlantone, zingiberene, demethoxycurcumin, and bisdemethoxycurcumin.	Inhibits COX-2, TNF-α, and activation factor NF-κB.	MS, RA	US9833491B2 PH22018001155Y1 716A1 US9585822B2	[118 - 123]
Punica granatum	Punicaceae	Fruits, seeds, peels	Punicalagins, gallo tannins, ellagitannins, flavonoids like delphinidin, cyanidin, pelargonidin, anthocyanins, gallic acid, caffeic acid, catechin, quercetin, rutin, and minerals.	Inhibits invasion/motility, cell cycle, apoptosis, and enzymes, such as COX, lipoxygenases, CYP450, PLA2	RA, Diabetes	FR2968214A1 US9795645B2 CN101983722B	[119 - 128]
Camellia sinensis	Theaceae	Leaves	Theobromine, theophylline, epicatechin, gallocatechin, and theasinensin.	Reduces ROS production, lowers protein oxidation and decreases IL-6 secretion.	RA	US2013010160A1	[121, 129, 130]
Boswellia serrata	Burseraceae	Resins from the tree trunk	β-boswellic acid, acetyl--boswellic acid, 11-keto-β-boswellic acid, and acetyl-11-keto-β-boswellic acid	Inhibits pro-inflammatory enzymes. Inhibits the synthesis of the proinflammatory enzyme 5-LO, including 5-hydroxyeicosatetraenoic acid and LTB-4.	RA, OA	EP2444081B1 US2011/0165136A1 CN102218075A US10029082B2	[129, 131 - 133]
Harpagophytum procumbens	Pedaliaceae	Roots	Harpagoside, glycosides of harpagoside, and acteoside	Inhibits 5-LO and COX2 activity and leukotriene biosynthesis.	OA, RA	ES2385683B1 US2011/0212193A1	[132 - 137]
Rosa canina	Rosaceae	Fruits, leaves, petals	Vitispiran, α-E-acaridial, hexadecanoic acid, and heptanal	Decreases the expression of matrix MMP-9 and inhibits NF-κB signaling pathway. Decreases the expression of crucial proinflammatory cytokines, like IFN-γ, TNF-α, IL-1β, IL-6, and IL-12 as well of chemokines like chemokine receptor 5	OA, RA	US8877239B2	[138 - 140]
Uncaria tomentosa	Rubiaceae	Root, bark	Ajmalicine, campesterol, carboxyl alkyl esters, akuammigine, sitosterols, rutin, chlorogenic acid, speciophylline, catechin, and cinchonain	Enhances lymphocyte production and inhibits NF-κB and TNF-α secretion.	OA, RA	-	[141, 142]
Urtica dioica	Urticaceae	Stem, leaves, flowers	Methanoic acid, histamine, flavonoids, tannins, volatile compounds, fatty acids, and polysaccharides	Stimulates the proliferation of human lymphocytes and interferon secretion.	OA, RA, IBD	-	[143, 144]
Argemone Mexicana	Papaveraceae	Entire herb	Dehydrocorydalmine, jatrorrhizine, columbamine, N-demethyloxysanguimarine, and oxyberberine	Inhibits lipid peroxidation and protects from free radicals damage.	Psoriasis	CN105250748A CN104127804A	[145 - 148]
Humulus lupus	Cannabaceae	Leaves, flower	Xanthohumol, humulone, cohumulone, and adhumulone.	Induces proliferation of T cells, production of Th1 cytokines (IL-2, IFN-γ, and TNF-α), and development of LAK (IL--activated) cells.	Immunity booster	-	[149 - 151]
Artemisia annua	Asteraceae	Leaves, fruits, seeds	Artemisinin, artesunate sesquiterpenoids, triterpenoids, monoterpenoids, steroids, and flavonoids.	Decreases TLR4 and TLR9 mRNA expression. Blocks the inactivation of NF-κB and the production of proinflammatory cytokines.	SLE, RA	US2016/0317653A1 CN104686867A	[152 - 156]

(Table 2) cont.....

Botanical Name	Family Name	Part of the Plant Used	Active Constituents	Immunomodulatory Mechanism	Indications	Patent No.	References
Smilax spp.	Smilacaceae	Root, rhizome	Saponins, such as sarasapogenin, smilagenin, β-sitosterol, and stigmasterol.	Inhibits TNF-α-induced NF-κB activation.	RA	US10226499B2 US20180036402A1 US2015/014.0068A1	[157 - 161]
Hemidesmus indicus	Asclepiadaceae	Entire herb	Benzaldehyde, lupanone, hemidesmin 1, hemidesmin 2, and α-amyrin.	Regulates IgG secretion and adenosine deaminase activity.	RA	-	[162, 163]
Ganoderma spp.	Ganodermataceae	Stem, butt, and root rot.	β-D-glucans, peptidoglycans, arabinose, galactose, glucose, xylose, and mannose.	Protects macrophage mitochondrial membrane and alleviates free radicals-induced membrane injury. Potential antioxidant and ROS effects.	SLE, RA	US20150216918A1	[157, 163 - 165]
Rehmannia glutinosa	Scrophulariaceae	Root, rhizome	Catalpol,dihydrocatalpol, danmellittoside, acetylcatalpol, leonuride, aucubin, melittoside, and rehmaglutin A, B, C, D.	Inhibits TNF-α and IL-1 secretion.	RA	TW201832774A US9974822B2 CN110693893A	[160, 166 - 169]
Chelidonium majus	Papaveraceae	Root, shoot, leaves	Sanguinarine, chelidonine, chelerythrine, berberine, and coptisisine.	Generation of activated killer cells, the proliferation of splenocytes, and activation of macrophages and granulocyte macrophage-colony forming cells.	Immunity booster	EP2787958B1 US20190022162A1 CN104892789A	[170 - 174]
Allium sativum	Alliaceae	Bulb	Alliinase, allicin, scordinin A and B, and alliin.	Downregulates PKB1/TGF--activated kinase-1, MAPK, and NF-κB pathways.	Immunity booster	-	[175, 176]
Citrus sps	Rutaceae	Peel, leaf, flower	d-Limonene, linalool, linalyl acetate, β-pinene, γ-terpinene.	Adjusts oxidation/antioxidation imbalance, down-regulates connective tissue growth factor and mRNA expression in lung tissues, and reduces collagen deposition and fibrosis.	Immunity booster	-	[177, 178]
Zingiber officinale	Zingiberaceae	Root	6-Gingerol, 8-gingerol, and 10-gingerol, quercetin, zingerone, gingerenone-A, and 6-dehydrogingerdione.	Stimulates the expression of several antioxidant enzymes and reduces the generation of ROS and lipid peroxidation.	Immunity booster	US20120244086A1 US20160317599A1 US9381221B2 US9283259B2	[104, 179 - 184]
Emblica officinalis	Euphorbiaceae	Fruits, seeds, leaves, root bark, flowers.	Emblicanin A, emblicanin B, punigluconin and pedunculagin, gallic acid, ellagic acid, chebulinic acid, quercetin, chebulagic acid, corilagin, isostrictiniin, methyl gallate, and luteolin.	Protects against the devastating effects of free radicals, non-radicals, and transition metal-induced oxidative stress.	Immunity booster	-	[185 - 187]
Moringa oleifera	Moringaceae	Leaves, fruit, flower pods.	Moringine, moringinine, vanillin, β-sitosterol, β-sitostenone, 4-hydroxymellin, and octacosanoic acid.	Exhibits strong *in-vitro* antioxidant and radical scavenging activity and reduces oxidative stress.	Immunity booster	CN105265955A	[188 - 191]

DISCUSSION

Indian-origin medicinal plants form an integral part of healthcare products such as traditional medicines, nutraceuticals, functional foods, and dietary supplements. These plants have been used all over the world for well-being. In many countries, these plant formulations have been used in the indigenous system of medicine and modern nutraceuticals. Approximately 80% of the global population is largely dependent on traditional plant-derived drugs for their primary healthcare. In contrast, the modern pharmaceutical industry is based on discrete active compounds, used only after determining their precise modes of action. The increasing popularity and widespread clinical use of these natural plant products and their analogs have led to the development of highly effective drugs. Despite this development, an effective cure for complex human diseases, such as autoimmune disorders, cancer, degenerative diseases, and diabetes has remained elusive. However, we are now in an interesting era where the amalgamation of ancient wisdom and traditional herbal medicines with modern science is being used for the development of cosmetics, health supplements, herbal tea, nutraceuticals, and various other products. Consequently, natural plant products have garnered global recognition and paved the way for research in medicinal plants, with India being one of the forerunners. The updated knowledge about the mechanism of action of various herbs would help the readers to have a clear knowledge of herbal drugs. We believe this article would help the readers explore and gain knowledge about the already patented herbal products.

CONCLUSION

There is an unmet need for the treatment of immunological disorders or diseases. Although herbal products are popular at present, it needs a more focused approach. The herbs discussed in the present work need further consideration in immunomodulation research. Many herbs whose immunological benefits have been proven are also part of the diet. In other words, herbs having neutraceutical value need further preference in immunological research, as their safety would not be a major concern if found immunologically beneficial. Besides, it would be cost-effective as well. Specifically, the herbs mentioned in the article may contribute significantly to the treatment of autoimmune disorders. Overall, there is a greater need for exploring the therapeutic role of neutraceutical herbs as pharmacotherapeutic agents. These would promote a safe and effective replacement of the current drug regimen with reduced side effects. This article will provide better insight to promote future research on immunomodulatory concepts with proper correlation to animal models, indications, and patents. Furthermore, the immunomodulatory function of the herbals would help in better control and management of autoimmune diseases.

ABBREVIATIONS

ADRs	Drug-induced Adverse Reactions
TNF-α	Tumor Necoris Factor-alpha
IFN-γ	Interferon-gamma
RA	Rheumatoid Arthritis
JAK	Janus Kinase
MS	Multiple Sclerosis

SLE	Systemic Lupus Erythematosus
Th1	Type 1 helper T cell
Treg	Regulatory T cell
EAE	Experimental Autoimmune Encephalomyelitis
NZB	New Zealand Blank Mouse
NZW	New Zealand White Mouse
AChR	Acetylcholine Receptor Antibody
MuSK	Muscle-specific Kinase Myasthenia
WHO	World Health Organization
FDA	Food and Drug Administration
USD	United States Dollars
CAM	Complementary and Alternative Medicine
IL	Interleukin
COX	Cyclooxygenase
MOG	Myelin Oligodendrocyte Glycoprotein
TLR	Toll-like Receptors

CONFLICT OF INTEREST

The authors declare that the study was conducted in the absence of any commercial or financial relationships that could be construed as a potential conflict of interest.

REFERENCES

[1] Mahima RA, Rahal A, Deb R, *et al.* Immunomodulatory and therapeutic potentials of herbal, traditional/indigenous and ethnoveterinary medicines. Pak J Biol Sci 2012; 15(16): 754-74.
[http://dx.doi.org/10.3923/pjbs.2012.754.774] [PMID: 24175417]

[2] Sharma P, Kumar P, Sharma R, Gupta G, Chaudhary A. Immunomodulators: Role of medicinal plants in immune system. National Journal of Physiology, Pharmacy and Pharmacology. Mr Bhawani Singh 2017; 7: pp. 552-6.

[3] Woolhouse MEJ, Webster JP, Domingo E, Charlesworth B, Levin BR. Biological and biomedical implications of the co-evolution of pathogens and their hosts. Nat Genet 2002; 32(4): 569-77.
[http://dx.doi.org/10.1038/ng1202-569] [PMID: 12457190]

[4] Review on immunomodulation and immunomodulatory activity of some herbal plants. Available from: https://www.researchgate.net/publication/285964504_Review_on_immunomodulation_and_immunom odulatory_activity_of_some_herbal_plants

[5] Ruiz-Argüelles A. T lymphocytes in autoimmunity. 2013.

[6] What are the organs of the immune system? : InformedHealth.org ; NCBI Bookshelf. Available from: https://www.ncbi.nlm.nih.gov/books/NBK279395/

[7] Total and specific IgG4 antibody levels in atopic eczema : PubMed. Available from: https://pubmed.ncbi.nlm.nih.gov/6744664/

[8]   Chamani S, Moossavi M, Naghizadeh A, *et al.* Immunomodulatory effects of curcumin in systemic autoimmune diseases. Phytother Res 2022; 36(4): 1616-32. https://onlinelibrary.wiley.com/doi/full/10.1002/ptr.7417
[http://dx.doi.org/10.1002/ptr.7417] [PMID: 35302258]

[9]   Doshi G, Thakkar A. Deciphering role of cytokines for therapeutic strategies against rheumatoid arthritis. Curr Drug Targets 2021; 22(7): 803-15.https://pubmed.ncbi.nlm.nih.gov/33109042/
[http://dx.doi.org/10.2174/1389450121666201027124625] [PMID: 33109042]

[10]   Doshi G, Thakkar A. Deciphering role of cytokines for therapeutic strategies against rheumatoid arthritis. Curr Drug Targets 2020; 21.
[PMID: 33109042]

[11]   Filippi M, Bar-Or A, Piehl F, Preziosa P, Solari A, Vukusic S, *et al.* Multiple sclerosis. Nature Reviews Disease Primers 2018; 4(1): 1-27. Available from: https://www.nature.com/articles/s41572-018-0041-4 [cited 2022 Dec 29].

[12]   Jolly M, Pickard SA, Mikolaitis RA, Rodby RA, Sequeira W, Block JA. LupusQoL-US benchmarks for US patients with systemic lupus erythematosus. J Rheumatol 2010; 37(9): 1828-33.
[http://dx.doi.org/10.3899/jrheum.091443] [PMID: 20716659]

[13]   Ohl K, Tenbrock K. Inflammatory cytokines in systemic lupus erythematosus. 2011. J Biomed Biotechnol 2011; 2011: 1-14.
[http://dx.doi.org/10.1155/2011/432595]

[14]   Ha JC, Richman DP. Myasthenia gravis and related disorders: Pathology and molecular pathogenesis. Biochimica et Biophysica Acta : Molecular Basis of Disease. Elsevier B.V. 2015; 1852: pp. 651-7.

[15]   Uzawa A, Kanai T, Kawaguchi N, Oda F, Himuro K, Kuwabara S. Changes in inflammatory cytokine networks in myasthenia gravis. Sci Rep 2016; 6(1): 25886.
[http://dx.doi.org/10.1038/srep25886] [PMID: 27172995]

[16]   Muire PJ, Mangum LH, Wenke JC. Time course of immune response and immunomodulation during normal and delayed healing of musculoskeletal wounds. Front Immunol 2020; 11: 1056.
[http://dx.doi.org/10.3389/fimmu.2020.01056] [PMID: 32582170]

[17]   Almeida CR, Bottazzi B, De Nardo D, Lawlor KE. Editorial: Immunomodulation of innate immune cells. Front Immunol 2020; 11: 101.
[http://dx.doi.org/10.3389/fimmu.2020.00101] [PMID: 32117255]

[18]   Barré-Sinoussi F, Montagutelli X. Animal models are essential to biological research: Issues and perspectives. Future Science OA. Future Medicine Ltd 2015; 1.

[19]   Yu X, Petersen F. A methodological review of induced animal models of autoimmune diseases. Autoimmunity Reviews. Elsevier B.V. 2018; 17: pp. 473-9.

[20]   Asquith DL, Miller AM, McInnes IB, Liew FY. Animal models of rheumatoid arthritis. Eur J Immunol 2009; 39(8): 2040-4.
[http://dx.doi.org/10.1002/eji.200939578] [PMID: 19672892]

[21]   Grötsch B, Bozec A, Schett G. *In vivo* models of rheumatoid arthritis. Methods in Molecular Biology. Humana Press Inc. 2019; pp. 269-80.

[22]   van den Berg WB, Joosten LAB, van Lent PLEM. Murine antigen-induced arthritis. Methods Mol Med 2007; 136: 243-53.
[http://dx.doi.org/10.1007/978-1-59745-402-5_18] [PMID: 17983153]

[23]   Bendele AM. Animal models of rheumatoid arthritis. 1. J Musculoskelet Neuronal Interact 2001.

[24]   Nandakumar KS, Holmdahl R. Collagen antibody induced arthritis. Methods Mol Med 2007; 136: 215-23.
[http://dx.doi.org/10.1007/978-1-59745-402-5_16] [PMID: 17983151]

[25]   Khachigian LM. Collagen antibody-induced arthritis. Nat Protoc 2006; 1(5): 2512-6.
[http://dx.doi.org/10.1038/nprot.2006.393] [PMID: 17406499]

[26]   Cuzzocrea S. Characterization of a novel and spontaneous mouse model of inflammatory arthritis. Arthritis Research and Therapy. BioMed Central 2011; 13: p. 126.

[27]   Schinnerling K, Rosas C, Soto L, Thomas R, Aguillón JC. Humanized mouse models of rheumatoid arthritis for studies on immunopathogenesis and preclinical testing of cell-based therapies. Frontiers in Immunology. Frontiers Media S.A. 2019; 10: p. 203.

[28]   Guazelli CFS, Staurengo-Ferrari L, Zarpelon AC, *et al.* Quercetin attenuates zymosan-induced arthritis in mice. Biomed Pharmacother 2018; 102: 175-84.
[http://dx.doi.org/10.1016/j.biopha.2018.03.057] [PMID: 29554596]

[29]   Chaves HV, Ribeiro RDA, De Souza AMB, Silva AARE, Gomes AS, Vale ML, *et al.* Experimental model of zymosan-induced arthritis in the rat temporomandibular joint: Role of nitric oxide and neutrophils. J Biomed Biotechnol 2011.

[30]   Kipp M, Nyamoya S, Hochstrasser T, Amor S. Multiple sclerosis animal models: a clinical and histopathological perspective. 2017.

[31]   Constantinescu CS, Farooqi N, O'Brien K, Gran B. Experimental autoimmune encephalomyelitis (EAE) as a model for multiple sclerosis (MS). British J Pharmacol. Wiley-Blackwell 2011; 164: pp. 1079-6.

[32]   Keough MB, Jensen SK, Yong VW. Experimental demyelination and remyelination of murine spinal cord by focal injection of lysolecithin. J Vis Exp 2015; (97): 52679.
[PMID: 25867716]

[33]   Dousset V, Brochet B, Vital A, *et al.* Lysolecithin-induced demyelination in primates: preliminary *in vivo* study with MR and magnetization transfer. AJNR Am J Neuroradiol 1995; 16(2): 225-31.
[PMID: 7726066]

[34]   Vega-Riquer JM, Mendez-Victoriano G, Morales-Luckie RA, Gonzalez-Perez O. Five Decades of Cuprizone, an Updated Model to Replicate Demyelinating Diseases. Curr Neuropharmacol 2019; 17(2): 129-41.
[http://dx.doi.org/10.2174/1570159X15666170717120343] [PMID: 28714395]

[35]   Mohamed A, Al-Kafaji G, Almahroos A, *et al.* Effects of enhanced environment and induced depression on cuprizone mouse model of demyelination. Exp Ther Med 2019; 18(1): 566-72.
[http://dx.doi.org/10.3892/etm.2019.7654] [PMID: 31281443]

[36]   Dal Canto MC, Kim BS, Miller SD, Melvold RW. Theiler's murine encephalomyelitis virus (TMEV)-induced demyelination: A model for human multiple sclerosis. Methods: A Companion to Methods in Enzymology 1996; 10(3): 453-61.

[37]   Oleszak EL, Chang JR, Friedman H, Katsetos CD, Platsoucas CD. Theiler's Virus Infection: A Model for Multiple Sclerosis. 2004.

[38]   Reeves WH, Lee PY, Weinstein JS, Satoh M, Lu L. Induction of autoimmunity by pristane and other naturally occurring hydrocarbons. Trends in Immunology. NIH Public Access 2009; 30: pp. 455-64.

[39]   Freitas EC, De Oliveira MS, Monticielo OA. Pristane-induced lupus: Considerations on this experimental model. Clin Rheumatol 2017; 36(11): 2403-14.
[http://dx.doi.org/10.1007/s10067-017-3811-6] [PMID: 28879482]

[40]   Martin PJ. Biology of chronic graft-versus-host disease: Implications for a future therapeutic approach. Keio Journal of Medicine. NIH Public Access 2008; 57: pp. 177-83.

[41]   Hamilton BL, Parkman R. Acute and chronic graft-versus-host disease induced by minor histocompatibility antigens in mice. Transplantation 1983; 36(2): 150-4.
[http://dx.doi.org/10.1097/00007890-198308000-00008] [PMID: 6349039]

[42]   Graus YMF, van BREDA VRIESMAN PJC, De BAETS MH. Characterization of anti-acetylcholine receptor (AChR) antibodies from mice differing in susceptibility for experimental autoimmune myasthenia gravis (EAMG). Clin Exp Immunol 2008; 92(3): 506-13.
[http://dx.doi.org/10.1111/j.1365-2249.1993.tb03429.x] [PMID: 8513583]

[43]   Mantegazza R, Cordiglieri C, Consonni A, Baggi F. Animal models of myasthenia gravis: Utility and limitations. International Journal of General Medicine. Dove Medical Press Ltd 2016; 9: pp. 53-64.

[44]   Kusner LL, Le Panse R, Losen M, Phillips WD. Animal models of myasthenia gravis for preclinical evaluation. Current Clinical Neurology. Humana Press Inc. 2018; pp. 61-70.

[45]   Richman DP, Nishi K, Ferns MJ, *et al.* Animal models of antimuscle-specific kinase myasthenia. Ann N Y Acad Sci 2012; 1274(1): 140-7.
[http://dx.doi.org/10.1111/j.1749-6632.2012.06782.x] [PMID: 23252909]

[46]   Kumar D, Arya V, Kaur R, Bhat ZA, Gupta VK, Kumar V. A review of immunomodulators in the Indian traditional health care system. J Microbiol Immunol Infect 2012; 45(3): 165-84.
[http://dx.doi.org/10.1016/j.jmii.2011.09.030] [PMID: 22154993]

[47]   Virendra Kumar S, Pramod Kumar S, Rupesh D, Nitin K. Immunomodulatory effects of some traditional medicinal plants. J Chem Pharm Res 2011; 3(1): 675-84.

[48]   Wen CC, Chen HM, Yang NS. Developing Phytocompounds from Medicinal Plants as Immunomodulators. Advances in Botanical Research. Academic Press Inc. 2012; pp. 197-272.

[49]   Li FS, Weng JK. Demystifying traditional herbal medicine with modern approaches. Nature Plants. Palgrave Macmillan Ltd. 2017; 3..

[50]   Polshettiwar SA, Sawant DH, Abhale NB, *et al.* Review on regulation of herbal products used as a medicine across the globe: A case study on turmeric : Golden Medicine. Biomed Pharmacol J 2022; 15(3): 1227-37.
[http://dx.doi.org/10.13005/bpj/2458]

[51]   Moudgil KD, Venkatesha SH, Rajaiah R, Berman BM. Immunomodulation of autoimmune arthritis by herbal CAM. Evidence-based Complementary and Alternative Medicine. Evid Based Complement Alternat Med 2011..

[52]   A review on herbal plants as immunomodulators | international journal of pharmaceutical sciences and research. Available from: https://ijpsr.com/bft-article/a-review-on-herbal-plants-as-immunomo-dulators/

[53]   Wells TNC. Natural products as starting points for future anti-malarial therapies: going back to our roots? Vol. 10, Malaria Journal. 2011.
[http://dx.doi.org/10.1186/1475-2875-10-S1-S3] [PMID: 21411014]

[54]   Felippe MJB. Immunotherapy. Equine Infectious Diseases. 2nd. Elsevier Inc. 2013; pp. 584-597.e5.

[55]   Liu Z, Yuan X, Luo Y, *et al.* Evaluating the effects of immunosuppressants on human immunity using cytokine profiles of whole blood. Cytokine 2009; 45(2): 141-7.
[http://dx.doi.org/10.1016/j.cyto.2008.12.003] [PMID: 19138532]

[56]   Jana S, Trivedi MK, Mondal SC, Gangwar M. Effect of a novel ashwagandha-based herbomineral formulation on pro-inflammatory cytokines expression in mouse splenocyte cells: A potential immunomodulator. Pharmacogn Mag 2017; 13(49) (Suppl. 1): 90.
[http://dx.doi.org/10.4103/0973-1296.197709] [PMID: 28479732]

[57]   Kumar R, Gupta YK, Singh S. Anti-inflammatory and anti-granuloma activity of *Berberis aristata* DC. in experimental models of inflammation. Indian J Pharmacol 2016; 48(2): 155-61.
[http://dx.doi.org/10.4103/0253-7613.108299] [PMID: 27114638]

[58]   Girme A, Saste G, Pawar S, *et al.* Investigating 11 withanosides and withanolides by UHPLC-PDA and mass fragmentation studies from ashwagandha (*Withania somnifera*). ACS Omega 2020; 5(43): 27933-43.

[http://dx.doi.org/10.1021/acsomega.0c03266] [PMID: 33163776]

[59]   Sharma P, Dwivedee BP, Bisht D, Dash AK, Kumar D. The chemical constituents and diverse pharmacological importance of *Tinospora cordifolia*. Heliyon. Elsevier Ltd 2019; 5.
[http://dx.doi.org/10.1016/j.heliyon.2019.e02437]

[60]   Upadhyay A, Kumar K, Kumar A, Mishra H. *Tinospora cordifolia* (Willd.) Hook. f. and Thoms. (Guduchi) : Validation of the Ayurvedic pharmacology through experimental and clinical studies. Int J Ayurveda Res 2010; 1(2): 112-21.
[http://dx.doi.org/10.4103/0974-7788.64405] [PMID: 20814526]

[61]   Okhuarobo A, Ehizogie Falodun J, Erharuyi O, Imieje V, Falodun A, Langer P. Harnessing the medicinal properties of *Andrographis paniculata* for diseases and beyond: a review of its phytochemistry and pharmacology. Asian Pac J Trop Dis 2014; 4(3): 213-22.
[http://dx.doi.org/10.1016/S2222-1808(14)60509-0]

[62]   Xu C. Chemical constituents from roots of *Andrographis paniculata*. Acta pharmaceutica Sinica 2011. Available from: https://pubmed.ncbi.nlm.nih.gov/21626787/.

[63]   Xu C, Chou GX, Wang ZT. A new diterpene from the leaves of *Andrographis paniculata* Nees. Fitoterapia 2010; 81(6): 610-3.
[http://dx.doi.org/10.1016/j.fitote.2010.03.003] [PMID: 20230876]

[64]   Girme A, Saste G, Balasubramaniam AK, Pawar S, Ghule C, Hingorani L. Assessment of *Curcuma longa* extract for adulteration with synthetic curcumin by analytical investigations. J Pharm Biomed Anal 2020; 191: 113603.
[http://dx.doi.org/10.1016/j.jpba.2020.113603] [PMID: 32957065]

[65]   Karłowicz-Bodalska KA, Han ST, Freier J, Smoleński MBA. 2017. Available from: https://pubmed.ncbi.nlm.nih.gov/29624265/

[66]   Bassiri-Jahromi S. *Punica granaturn* (Pomegranate) activity in health promotion and cancer prevention. Oncology Reviews Page Press Publications 2018; 12: 1-7.

[67]   Mayasankaravalli C, Deepika K, Esther Lydia D, *et al.* Profiling the phyto-constituents of *Punica granatum* fruits peel extract and accessing its *in-vitro* antioxidant, anti-diabetic, anti-obesity, and angiotensin-converting enzyme inhibitory properties. Saudi J Biol Sci 2020; 27(12): 3228-34.
[http://dx.doi.org/10.1016/j.sjbs.2020.09.046] [PMID: 33304128]

[68]   Rena K, Palida AZX. 2009. Available from: https://pubmed.ncbi.nlm.nih.gov/19565710/

[69]   Saeed M, Naveed M, Arif M, Kakar MU, Manzoor R, Abd El-Hack ME, *et al.* Green tea (*Camellia sinensis*) and L-theanine: Medicinal values and beneficial applications in humans—A comprehensive review. Biomedicine and Pharmacotherapy Elsevier Masson SAS 2017; 95: 1260-75.

[70]   Xu J, Wang M, Zhao J, Wang YH, Tang Q, Khan IA. Yellow tea (*Camellia sinensis* L.), a promising Chinese tea: Processing, chemical constituents and health benefits. Food Research International. Elsevier Ltd 2018; 107: pp. 567-77.

[71]   Jantan I, Ahmad W, Bukhari SNA. Plant-derived immunomodulators: An insight on their preclinical evaluation and clinical trials. Frontiers in Plant Science. Frontiers Research Foundation 2015; 6..

[72]   De Oliveira DP, Braga FC, Teixeira MM. Medicinal plants and their potential use in the treatment of rheumatic diseases. Inflammation and Natural Products. Elsevier 2021; pp. 205-34.
[http://dx.doi.org/10.1016/B978-0-12-819218-4.00014-6]

[73]   Wang Q, Meng J, Dong A, Yu JZ, Zhang GX, Ma CG. The pharmacological effects and mechanism of *Tripterygium wilfordii* Hook F in central nervous system autoimmunity. J Alternat Complement Med. Mary Ann Liebert Inc. 2016; 22: pp. 496-502.

[74]   Lipsky PE, Tao XL, Cai J, Kovacs WJON. Selecting substances for treating glucocorticoid-mediated inflammation or immune diseases using *Tripterygium wilfordii* Hook F extracts. US5846742, 1998.

[75]   Lipsky PE, Tao XLCJ. Preparations and uses thereof for immunosuppression. 1996.

[76]   Achiron AGM. Methods of predicting clinical course and treating multiple sclerosis. 2012.

[77]   Uddin Q, Samiulla L, Singh Vk, Jamil Ss, Rao S, *et al.* Propagation of *Withania Somnifera* and estimation of Withanolides for Neurological disorders. 71. J Appl Pharm Sci 2010.

[78]   Wadhwa Renu. Water Extract of Ashwagandha Leaves Has Anticancer Activity : Identification of an Active Component and Its Mechanism of Action. Chemical and Pharmaceutical Bulletin. PCT Pub 2007; 55..

[79]   Antony BI. Process to enhance the bioactivity of Ashwagandha extracts. 2018.

[80]   Nelson SK, Bose SK, Grunwald GK, Myhill P, McCord JM. The induction of human superoxide dismutase and catalase *in vivo* : A fundamentally new approach to antioxidant therapy. Free Radic Biol Med 2006; 40(2): 341-7.
[http://dx.doi.org/10.1016/j.freeradbiomed.2005.08.043] [PMID: 16413416]

[81]   Bharti VK, Malik JK, Gupta RC. Ashwagandha: Multiple health benefits. Nutraceuticals: Efficacy, Safety and Toxicity. Elsevier Inc. 2016; pp. 717-33.
[http://dx.doi.org/10.1016/B978-0-12-802147-7.00052-8]

[82]   Classification | USDA PLANTS Available from: https://plants.usda.gov/java/ClassificationServlet?source=profile&symbol=WISO&display=31

[83]   Dayanath DIAS. Pharmaceutical or medicinal preparation comprising a combination of two herbs *Emblica officinalis* (nelli) and *Tinospora cordifolia* (rasakinda) to be administered together for targeted stimulation of immue system for prophylaxis and treatment of oral cancer - Google Patents WO2018042229A1. 2018.

[84]   Rosen BD. Alternative ACT with natural botanical active GRAS ingredients for treatment and prevention of the Zika virus. United States patent US 9,675,582 2017.

[85]   Ghosh S, Saha S. *Tinospora cordifolia*: One plant, many roles. Anc Sci Life 2012; 31(4): 151-9.
[http://dx.doi.org/10.4103/0257-7941.107344] [PMID: 23661861]

[86]   Aranha I, Clement F, Venkatesh YP. Immunostimulatory properties of the major protein from the stem of the Ayurvedic medicinal herb, guduchi (*Tinospora cordifolia*). J Ethnopharmacol 2012; 139(2): 366-72.
[http://dx.doi.org/10.1016/j.jep.2011.11.013] [PMID: 22119223]

[87]   Heuer MA, Clement K, Chaudhuri S, Ramsbottom JDTM. Nutritional composition and method for increasing creatine uptake and retention in skeletal muscle, increasing muscle mass and strength, increasing exercise capacity and for aiding recovery following exercise. United States patent US 7,749,547 2016.

[88]   Burgos R, Hancke J, Jara EHM. Compositions that include anthocyanidins and methods of use. United States patent US 10,786,522 2020.

[89]   Alonso RM, Schmeichel KL, Lafosse-Marin I, *et al.* Blister cards promoting intuitive dosing. United States patent US 8,752,704 2014.

[90]   Krishnan GG. Herbal formulation for prevention and treatment of diabetes and associated complications. United States patent US 8,163,312 2012.

[91]   Buonamici G. Functional food preparation and use thereof United States patent US 9,167,842 2015.

[92]   Senin P, Setnikar IRLA. Formulation for oral administration with beneficial effects on the cardiovascular system. United States patent US 9,623,108 2016.

[93]   Chaudhary M. Detoxifier herbal formulation United States patent US 9,233,133 2016.

[94]   Rathi B, Sahu J, Koul S, Kosha RL. Detailed pharmacognostical studies on *Berberis aristata* DC plant. Anc Sci Life 2013; 32(4): 234-40.
[http://dx.doi.org/10.4103/0257-7941.131981] [PMID: 24991073]

[95] Potdar D, Hirwani RR, Dhulap S. Phyto-chemical and pharmacological applications of *Berberis aristata*. Fitoterapia 2012; 83(5): 817-30.
[http://dx.doi.org/10.1016/j.fitote.2012.04.012] [PMID: 22808523]

[96] Konstantinidou-Doltsinis S, Schmitt A, Cergel S, Kleeberg HRJ. Process for the production of a storage stable fungicidal extract of Glycyrrhiza glabra for the control of phytopathogenic fungi and other plant diseases. United States patent application US 12/668,802 2010.

[97] Langland J, Denzler K, Jacobs BWR. Method and compositions for the use of botanical extracts in the treatment of viral infections, cancer, pain, itch, and inflammation. United States patent application US 14/443,767 2018.

[98] *Glycyrrhiza glabra*: A phytopharmacological review International Journal of pharmaceutical sciences and research 2013; 4(7): 2470-7. Available from: https://www.researchgate.net/publication/ 260082960_Glycyrrhiza_glabra_A_phytopharmacological_review'_International_Journal_of_pharma ceutical_sciences_and_research'_R_Kaur_and_HPKaur_2013_47_2470-2477

[99] Gulati K, Rai N, Chaudhary S, Ray A. Nutraceuticals in respiratory disorders. Nutraceuticals: Efficacy, Safety and Toxicity. Elsevier Inc. 2016; pp. 75-86.
[http://dx.doi.org/10.1016/B978-0-12-802147-7.00006-1]

[100] Cifter Ü, Arabacioglu NTÖ. Herbal formulations. United States patent US 10,111,912 2018.

[101] Cifter Ü, Arabacioglu NTÖ. Formulations comprising plant extracts United States patent US 10,111,925 2018.

[102] Bombardelli E, Morazzoni P. Combinations of extracts of *Serenoa repens* and lipophilic extracts of *Zingiber officinalis* and *Echinacea angustifolia*, the use thereof, and formulations containing them. United States patent US 10,016,478 2018.

[103] Soman GSPS. Therapeutic compositions comprising herbal extracts and essential oils for smoking and vaporization United States patent application US 15/343,022 2017.

[104] Bombardelli EMP. Formulations containing extracts of *Echinacea angustifolia* and *Zingiber officinale* which are useful in reducing inflammation and peripheral pain United States patent US 9,283,259 2016.

[105] Shew FL. Arthritis gone CA2597900C 2007.

[106] Ragot P, Pons E, Mompon BRC. Edible product comprising reconstituted plant material United States patent US 10,751,282 2020.

[107] Mbaveng AT, Kuete V. *Zingiber officinale*. Medicinal Spices and Vegetables from Africa: Therapeutic Potential Against Metabolic, Inflammatory, Infectious and Systemic Diseases. Elsevier Inc. 2017; pp. 627-39.
[http://dx.doi.org/10.1016/B978-0-12-809286-6.00030-3]

[108] Balaraman B. Compositions and methods for their dermatological use. United States patent application US 14/646,049 2015.

[109] D.F. . Herbal compositions for the treatment of diabetes and/or conditions associated therewith. United States patent application US20150190446A1 2010.

[110] Evans D ES. Composition for treating pain and/or inflammation comprising eugenol and betacaryophyllene WO2015000064A1 2013.

[111] Ragot P, Mompon B, Rousseau C, Pons EPC. Composition for Making a Tea Beverage or Herbal and Vegetable Broths United States patent application US 14/193,910 2014.

[112] Mehta, Han; Effect of n-3 Polysaturated Fatty Acids on Barrett's Epithelium in the Human Lower Esophagus. All Office Actions issued in U S Appl No Hardman 2014; 320.

[113] Cohen MM. Tulsi - Ocimum sanctum: A herb for all reasons. J Ayurveda Integr Med 2014; 5: 251-9.

[114] Suppakul P, Miltz J, Sonneveld K, Bigger SW. Antimicrobial properties of basil and its possible application in food packaging. J Agric Food Chem 2003; 51(11): 3197-207.
[http://dx.doi.org/10.1021/jf021038t] [PMID: 12744643]

[115] Panchal P, Parvez N. Phytochemical analysis of medicinal herb (*Ocimum sanctum*). Int J Nanomater Nanotechnol Nanomed 2019; 5(2): 8-11.

[116] SEEMA JAIN, SPARSH GUPTA. Effects of *Cinnamomum zeylanicum* bark extract on nociception and anxiety like behavior in mice. Asian J Pharm Clin Res 2019; 236-41.
[http://dx.doi.org/10.22159/ajpcr.2019.v12i9.31287]

[117] Ranasinghe P, Pigera S, Premakumara GAS, Galappaththy P, Constantine GR, Katulanda P. Medicinal properties of 'true' cinnamon (*Cinnamomum zeylanicum*): A systematic review. BMC Complement Altern Med 2013; 13(1): 275.
[http://dx.doi.org/10.1186/1472-6882-13-275] [PMID: 24148965]

[118] TC S. *Curcuma longa* (turmeric) based herbal compound formulations as dietary supplements United States patent US 9,833,491 2017.

[119] Ida T, Suico YTG. Turmeric (*Curcuma longa*) and ginger (*Zingiber officinale*) tea PH22018001155Y1 2018.

[120] Lewis IJDJ. Methods of preparing and using botanical antioxidant compositions United States patent US 9,585,822 2017.

[121] Bui Thanh T, Đồng N, Dang Kim T. *Curcuma longa*, the polyphenolic curcumin compound and pharmacological effects on liver.

[122] Nair A, Chattopadhyay D, Saha B. Plant-derived immunomodulators. New Look to Phytomedicine: Advancements in Herbal Products as Novel Drug Leads. Elsevier 2018; pp. 435-99.

[123] Dasgupta A. Antiinflammatory herbal supplements. Translational Inflammation. Elsevier 2018; pp. 69-91.

[124] Duranton A. Use of combination of extract of lotus, extract of pomegranate (*Punica granatum*) and methylxanthine comprising e.g. caffeine and theophylline, or plant extract rich in methylxanthines, as agent to prevent signs of aging of skin or hair FR2968214A1 2010.

[125] Mastaloudis A, Wood S, Weindruch R, *et al.* Oral formulations for counteracting effects of aging United States patent US 9,795,645 2017.

[126] Bai Houzeng Jiao Ying, Yang Zeyi, Zhu Lianjun SG. Composition for preventing and treating joint soft tissue injury and complications thereof. CN101983722B 2010.

[127] Viuda-Martos M, Fernández-López J, Pérez-Álvarez JA. Pomegranate and its many functional components as related to human health: A review. Compr Rev Food Sci Food Saf 2010; 9(6): 635-54.
[http://dx.doi.org/10.1111/j.1541-4337.2010.00131.x] [PMID: 33467822]

[128] Rahimi HR, Arastoo M, Ostad SN. A comprehensive review of *Punica granatum* (Pomegranate) properties in toxicological, pharmacological, cellular and molecular biology researches Iran J Pharm Res 2012; 385-400.

[129] Supplements and methods of supplementation. United States patent application, US 2013 01 01690A1 2013.

[130] Pivari F, Mingione A, Brasacchio C, Soldati L. Curcumin and type 2 diabetes mellitus: Prevention and treatment. Nutrients 2019; 11(8): 1837.
[http://dx.doi.org/10.3390/nu11081837] [PMID: 31398884]

[131] Bertocchi M, Isani G, Medici F, Andreani G, Usca IT, Roncada P, *et al.* Anti-inflammatory activity of *Boswellia serrata* extracts: An *in vitro* study on porcine aortic endothelial cells Oxid Med Cell Longev 2018.

[132] Siddiqui MZ. *Boswellia serrata*, a potential antiinflammatory agent: An overview. Indian J Pharm Sci

2011; 73(3): 255-61.
[PMID: 22457547]

[133] Ross RF. Device for delivery of rheumatoid arthritis medication United States patent US 10029082B2 2018.

[134] Compositions for the treatment of pain and / or inflammation ES2385683B1 2010.

[135] Urschel MJ, Urschel TLMK. Herbal ointment for musculoskeletal and joint-related conditions. United States patent US 20140348960A1 2014.

[136] Williams CA. Specialized dietary supplements. Equine Applied and Clinical Nutrition: Health, Welfare and Performance. Elsevier Ltd. 2013; pp. 351-66.
[http://dx.doi.org/10.1016/B978-0-7020-3422-0.00019-5]

[137] McGregor GP. Harpagophytum procumbens – Traditional anti-inflammatory herbal drug with broad therapeutic potential. Herbal Drugs. Ethnomedicine to Modern Medicine. Springer Berlin Heidelberg 2008; pp. 81-95.

[138] Settineri RPJ. Lipid supplements for maintaining health and treatment of acute and chronic disorders. United States patent US 8,877,239 2014.

[139] Essential Oils in Food Preservation, Flavor and Safety 2016.

[140] Mármol I, Sánchez-De-Diego C, Jiménez-Moreno N, Ancín-Azpilicueta C, Rodríguez-Yoldi M. Therapeutic applications of rose hips from different Rosa species. International Journal of Molecular Sciences. MDPI AG 2017; 18..

[141] Batiha GES, Beshbishy AM, Wasef L, Elewa YHA, El-Hack MEA, Taha AE, et al. Applied Sciences. *Uncaria tomentosa* (Willd. ex Schult.) DC.: A review on chemical constituents and biological activities.Switzerland: MDPI AG 2020; 10: p. 2668.

[142] Romm A, Clare B, Alschuler L, Hobbs C, Upton R. Vaginal infections and sexually transmitted diseases. Botanical Medicine for Women's Health. Elsevier Inc. 2010; pp. 256-89.
[http://dx.doi.org/10.1016/B978-0-443-07277-2.00010-6]

[143] De Vico G, Guida V, Carella F. *Urtica dioica* (stinging nettle): A neglected plant with emerging growth promoter/immunostimulant properties for farmed fish. Frontiers in Physiology Frontiers Media SA 2018; 9.

[144] Phytochemical and pharmacological importance of genus urtica – a review. Int J Pharm Sci Res Available from: https://ijpsr.com/bft-article/phytochemical-and-pharmacological-importance-of-genus-urtica-a-review/

[145] Tan Zhen JY. Traditional Chinese medicine for treating cervical cancer and preparation method CN105250748A 2015.

[146] Hongping H. Traditional Chinese medicine capable of treating diabetic foot ulcer CN104127804A 2014.

[147] Sharma RA, Goswami M, Yadav A, Bhardwaj R, Joshi YC. Antioxidant properties of methanolic extracts of *Argemone mexicana*. Res J Med Plant 2014; 8(4): 167-77.
[http://dx.doi.org/10.3923/rjmp.2014.167.177]

[148] A review on *Argemone mexicana* linn. – an indian medicinal plant Int J Pharm Sci Res Available from: https://ijpsr.com/bft-article/a-review-on-argemone-mexicana-linn-an-indian-medicinal-plant/?view=fulltext

[149] McCallum JL, Nabuurs MH, Gallant ST, Kirby CW, Mills AAS. Phytochemical characterization of wild hops (*Humulus lupulus* ssp. *lupuloides*) Germplasm resources from the maritimes region of Canada. Front Plant Sci 2019; 10: 1438.
[http://dx.doi.org/10.3389/fpls.2019.01438] [PMID: 31921222]

[150] Chadwick LR, Pauli GF, Farnsworth NR. The pharmacognosy of *Humulus lupulus* L. (hops) with an

emphasis on estrogenic properties. Phytomedicine 2006; 13(1-2): 119-31.
[http://dx.doi.org/10.1016/j.phymed.2004.07.006] [PMID: 16360942]

[151] Gao X, Deeb D, Liu Y, Gautam S, Dulchavsky SA, Gautam SC. Immunomodulatory activity of xanthohumol: inhibition of T cell proliferation, cell-mediated cytotoxicity and Th1 cytokine production through suppression of NF-κB. Immunopharmacol Immunotoxicol 2009; 31(3): 477-84.
[http://dx.doi.org/10.1080/08923970902798132] [PMID: 19555200]

[152] Cook DN, Berry DA, Von Maltzahn G, Henn MR, Zhang HGB. Bacterial compositions and methods of use thereof for treatment of immune system disorders. United States patent US 20160317653A1 2014.

[153] Meng Yanqiang TX. Chicken fodder for enhancing immunity and preparation method thereof CN104686867A 2015.

[154] Septembre-Malaterre A, Rakoto ML, Marodon C, Bedoui Y, Nakab J, Simon E, *et al. Artemisia annua*, a traditional plant brought to light. International Journal of Molecular Sciences MDPI AG 2020; 21: 1-34.

[155] Bora KS, Sharma A. The genus Artemisia: A comprehensive review. Pharm Biol 2011; 49(1): 101-9.
[http://dx.doi.org/10.3109/13880209.2010.497815] [PMID: 20681755]

[156] Alesaeidi S, Miraj S. A systematic review of anti-malarial properties, immunosuppressive properties, anti-inflammatory properties, and anti-cancer properties of *Artemisia annua*. Electron Physician 2016; 8(10): 3150-5.
[http://dx.doi.org/10.19082/3150] [PMID: 27957318]

[157] Rozenblat S, Jung D, Moh S, Kim SLJ. Plant extracts for the treatment and prevention of infections. United States patent US 10,226,499 2019.

[158] Berti F, Contorni M, Costantino P, Finco O, Grandi G, Maione DTJ. Immunogenic compositions. United States patent application US 20180036402A1 2011.

[159] Barnett S, Bannerjee K. Immunogenc compositions and uses thereof United States Patent US 20150140068A1 2015.

[160] Zampieron ER, Kamhi EJ. Natural support for autoimmune and inflammatory disease. J Restor Med 2012; 1(1): 38-47.
[http://dx.doi.org/10.14200/jrm.2012.1.1003]

[161] Smilax ornate / Smilax spp. | Materia Medica Available from: https://herbalmateriamedica. wordpress.com/2014/08/08/smilax-ornate-smilax-spp/

[162] Nandy S, Mukherjee A, Pandey DK, Ray P, Dey A. Indian Sarsaparilla (*Hemidesmus indicus*): Recent progress in research on ethnobotany, phytochemistry and pharmacology. J Ethnopharmacol 2020; 254.

[163] Kües U, Nelson DR, Liu C, *et al.* Genome analysis of medicinal *Ganoderma* spp. with plant-pathogenic and saprotrophic life-styles. Phytochemistry 2015; 114: 18-37.
[http://dx.doi.org/10.1016/j.phytochem.2014.11.019] [PMID: 25682509]

[164] Lin Z. Cellular and molecular mechanisms of immuno-modulation by *Ganoderma lucidum*. J Pharmacol Sci 2005; 99: 144-53.

[165] Suárez-Arroyo I, Loperena-Alvarez Y, Rosario-Acevedo R, Martínez-Montemayor M. *Ganoderma* spp.: A Promising adjuvant treatment for breast cancer. Medicines 2017; 4(1): 15.
[http://dx.doi.org/10.3390/medicines4010015] [PMID: 28758107]

[166] Park J, Lee SH, Song M, Aihong KIKH. Composition containing composite extract of *Rehmannia glutinosa* and *Pueraria lobata* for preventing or treating menopausal symptoms United States patent US 9,974,822 2018.

[167] Wenting SJ. Extract from *Rehmannia glutinosa* used as a therapeutic agent for multiple sclerosis CN110693893A 2019.

[168]   Zhang RX, Li MX, Jia ZP. *Rehmannia glutinosa*: Review of botany, chemistry and pharmacology. J Ethnopharmacol 2008; 117(2): 199-214.
[http://dx.doi.org/10.1016/j.jep.2008.02.018] [PMID: 18407446]

[169]   Dai X, Su S, Cai H, *et al.* Protective effects of total glycoside from *Rehmannia glutinosa* leaves on diabetic nephropathy rats *via* regulating the metabolic profiling and modulating the TGF-β1 and Wnt/β-catenin signaling pathway. Front Pharmacol 2018; 9(SEP): 1012.
[http://dx.doi.org/10.3389/fphar.2018.01012] [PMID: 30271343]

[170]   Anna Bianucci, Alice Borghini, Simone Del Corso, Imbriani Marcello PD. *Cheudonium majus* extracts and their use in the treatment of skin disorders and promotion of skin regeneration EP2787958A2 2011.

[171]   Batistoni R, Bianucci AM, Ferrari A, *et al.* Combination anticancer endowed with antitumor activity, comprising alkaloids of *Chelidonium majus*. United States patent Application US 20190022162A1 2016.

[172]   Liu Fugang, Jiong Liu, Wang Yanzhi, Yang Yun ZJ. Celandine polysaccharide extracted from *Chelidonium majus* and application of celandine polysaccharide CN104892789A 2015.

[173]   Biswas SJ, Khuda-Bukhsh AR. Effect of a homeopathic drug, Chelidonium, in amelioration of p-DAB induced hepatocarcinogenesis in mice. BMC Complement Altern Med 2002; 2(1): 4.
[http://dx.doi.org/10.1186/1472-6882-2-4] [PMID: 11943072]

[174]   Song JY, Yang HO, Pyo SN, Jung IS, Yi SY, Yun YS. Immunomodulatory activity of protein-bound polysaccharide extracted from *Chelidonium majus*. Arch Pharm Res 2002; 25(2): 158-64.
[http://dx.doi.org/10.1007/BF02976557] [PMID: 12009029]

[175]   Rybak ME, Calvey EM, Harnly JM. Quantitative determination of allicin in garlic: Supercritical fluid extraction and standard addition of alliin. J Agric Food Chem 2004; 52(4): 682-7.
[http://dx.doi.org/10.1021/jf034853x] [PMID: 14969516]

[176]   Krest I, Keusgen M. Quality of herbal remedies from *Allium sativum*: Differences between alliinase from garlic powder and fresh garlic. Planta Med 1999; 65(2): 139-43.
[http://dx.doi.org/10.1055/s-1999-13975] [PMID: 10193205]

[177]   Dosoky NS, Setzer WN. Biological activities and safety of *Citrus* spp. Essential oils. Int J Mol Sci 2018; 19.

[178]   Mabberley DJ. Citrus (Rutaceae): A review of recent advances in etymology, systematics and medical applications. Blumea: Journal of Plant Taxonomy and Plant Geography Nationaal Herbarium Nederland 2004; 49: 481-98.

[179]   Trivedi HMGE. Oral compositions containing extracts of *Zingiber officinale* and related methods United States patent Application US 20120244086A1 2010.

[180]   Dale MJDJ. Treatment of pain United States patent Application US 20160317599A1 2014.

[181]   H de JVR. Phytocomposition for the treatment of pain related to joint diseases United States patent US 9,381,221 2016.

[182]   Mao QQ, Xu XY, Cao SY, Gan RY, Corke H, Beta T, *et al.* Bioactive compounds and bioactivities of ginger (*Zingiber officinale* roscoe). Foods MDPI Multidisciplinary Digital Publishing Institute. 2019; 8..

[183]   Stoner GD. Ginger: Is it ready for prime time? Cancer Prev Res 2013; 6(4): 257-62.
[http://dx.doi.org/10.1158/1940-6207.CAPR-13-0055] [PMID: 23559451]

[184]   Han Y, Song C, Koh W, *et al.* Anti-inflammatory effects of the *Zingiber officinale* roscoe constituent 12-dehydrogingerdione in lipopolysaccharide-stimulated Raw 264.7 cells. Phytother Res 2013; 27(8): 1200-5.
[http://dx.doi.org/10.1002/ptr.4847] [PMID: 23027684]

[185] Hasan MR, Islam MN, Islam MR. Phytochemistry, pharmacological activities and traditional uses of *Emblica officinalis*: A review. Int Curr Pharm J 2016; 5(2): 14-21.
[http://dx.doi.org/10.3329/icpj.v5i2.26441]

[186] A review on medicinal importance of *Emblica officinalis*. Int J Pharm Sci Res Available from: https://ijpsr.com/bft-article/a-review-on-medicinal-importance-of-emblica-officinalis/ [cited 2021 Jun 27].

[187] Gantait S, Mahanta M, Bera S, Verma SK. Advances in biotechnology of *Emblica officinalis* Gaertn. syn. *Phyllanthus emblica* L.: A nutraceuticals-rich fruit tree with multifaceted ethnomedicinal uses. 3 Biotech 2021; 11(2): 66.

[188] Li Jianhui, Shan Lin, Xu Hezhuang YY. Solid *Moringa oleifera* leaf drink. CN105265955A 2015.

[189] Posmontier B. The medicinal qualities of *Moringa oleifera*. Holist Nurs Pract 2011; 25(2): 80-7.
[http://dx.doi.org/10.1097/HNP.0b013e31820dbb27] [PMID: 21325908]

[190] Anwar F, Latif S, Ashraf M, Gilani AH. *Moringa oleifera* : A food plant with multiple medicinal uses. Phytother Res 2007; 21(1): 17-25.
[http://dx.doi.org/10.1002/ptr.2023] [PMID: 17089328]

[191] Paikra BK, Dhongade HKJ, Gidwani B. Phytochemistry and pharmacology of *Moringa oleifera* Lam. J Pharmacopuncture 2017; 20: 194-200.

SUBJECT INDEX

A

Abnormal protein aggregation 111
Accumulation, neointimal macrophage 166
Acid(s) 26, 29, 31, 38, 39, 51, 54, 55, 56, 61,
 86, 113, 115, 117, 133, 139, 170, 173,
 179, 180, 212, 213, 214, 215, 216
 amino 29, 31, 38, 39, 54, 173, 180
 applanoxidic 56
 arachidonic 139, 170
 astraodoric 55
 bile (ba) 179
 boswellic 215
 caffeic 117, 215
 chebulagic 216
 chebulaginic 213
 chebulinic 216
 cinnamic 61, 213
 ellagic 213, 216
 ferulic 213
 gallic 61, 86, 213, 215, 216
 ganoderic 51, 61
 glycyrrhetinic 214
 glycyrrhizic 115
 hexadecanoic 215
 hydroxybenzoic 61, 113
 hydroxycinnamic 113
 nucleic 26
 octacosanoic 216
 oleanolic 215
 organic 61
 rosmarinic 215
 salicylic 212
 tinosporic 214
 zoledronic 133
Action 4, 140, 178, 179
 anti-osteoporotic 140
 cytoprotective 179
 modulatory 178
 neuronal 4
Activation 35, 36, 60, 114, 118, 119, 141, 176,
 178, 206, 209, 214, 216

 macrophage 176, 214, 216
Activator protein 35
Activities 28, 30, 38, 39, 52, 54, 57, 60, 79,
 81, 84, 86, 87, 88, 90, 113, 118, 134,
 135, 138,
 alkaline phosphatase 138
 anti-aging 38
 anti-microbial 57
 anti-parasitic 79
 anti-protozoa 84
 anti-tumor 60
 anti-viral 54
 antimalarial 90
 antioxidative 86
 antiviral 52
 autophagic 118
 enzyme-catalyzed 30
 estrogen 134
 glutathione peroxidase 87
 inhibitory 39
 leishmanicidal 81, 88
 mediated antitumor 60
 mineral binding 52
 mitochondrial 28
 mitogenic 60
 neuroprotective 113
 osteoblastic 135
 telomerase 60
Acute 71, 75, 152, 155, 157, 158, 164, 165,
 166, 167
 coronary syndrome (ACS) 152, 155, 157,
  158, 164, 165, 166, 167
 respiratory distress syndrome (ARDS) 71,
  75
Adhesion 36, 169, 176, 177, 179, 216
 deaminase activity 216
 molecules, cell membrane 169
 monocyte 177, 179
Adipocytes 162, 163
Adipogenesis 135, 138
 inhibiting 135
Adiponectin 162, 164

www.ingramcontent.com/pod-product-compliance
Lightning Source LLC
Chambersburg PA
CBHW050826220326
41598CB00006B/319